Preterm Birth: Causes, Consequences and Prevention

Preterm Birth: Causes, Consequences and Prevention

Editor: Natasha Page

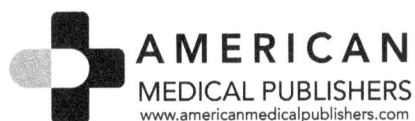

AMERICAN
MEDICAL PUBLISHERS
www.americanmedicalpublishers.com

AMERICAN
MEDICAL PUBLISHERS
www.americanmedicalpublishers.com

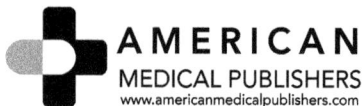

Cataloging-in-Publication Data

Preterm birth : causes, consequences and prevention / edited by Natasha Page.
   p. cm.
Includes bibliographical references and index.
ISBN 978-1-63927-166-5
1. Premature labor. 2. Premature infants. 3. Pregnancy--Duration.
4. Labor (Obstetrics)--Complications. I. Page, Natasha.
RG649 .P74 2022
618.397--dc23

American Medical Publishers,
41 Flatbush Avenue,
1st Floor, New York,
NY 11217, USA

ISBN 978-1-63927-166-5 (Hardback)

Contents

Preface...IX

Chapter 1 **Antenatal corticosteroids for management of preterm birth: a multi-country analysis of health system bottlenecks and potential solutions**...........................1
Grace Liu, Joel Segrè, A Metin Gülmezoglu, Matthews Mathai,
Jeffrey M Smith, Jorge Hermida, Aline Simen-Kapeu, Pierre Barker,
Mercy Jere, Edward Moses, Sarah G Moxon, Kim E Dickson,
Joy E Lawn and Fernando Althabe

Chapter 2 **Time trends and risk factor associated with premature birth and infants deaths due to prematurity in Hubei Province, China from 2001 to 2012**.........................17
Haiqing Xu, Qiong Dai, Yusong Xu, Zhengtao Gong, Guohong Dai,
Ming Ding, Christopher Duggan, Zubin Hu and Frank B. Hu

Chapter 3 **Neonatal and maternal outcomes following midtrimester preterm premature rupture of the membranes**...26
Laura Aoife Linehan, Jennifer Walsh, Aoife Morris, Louise Kenny,
Keelin O'Donoghue, Eugene Dempsey and Noirin Russell

Chapter 4 **Risk factors for small-for-gestational-age and preterm births among 19,269 Tanzanian newborns**..33
Alfa Muhihi, Christopher R. Sudfeld, Emily R. Smith, Ramadhani A. Noor,
Salum Mshamu, Christina Briegleb, Mohamed Bakari, Honorati Masanja,
Wafaie Fawzi and Grace Jean-Yee Chan

Chapter 5 **Is maternal trait anxiety a risk factor for late preterm and early term deliveries?** 45
Margarete Erika Vollrath, Verena Sengpiel, Markus A. Landolt,
Bo Jacobsson and Beatrice Latal

Chapter 6 **Maternal intake of seafood and supplementary long chain n-3 poly-unsaturated fatty acids and preterm delivery**...51
Anne Lise Brantsæter, Linda Englund-Ögge, Margareta Haugen,
Bryndis Eva Birgisdottir, Helle Katrine Knutsen, Verena Sengpiel,
Ronny Myhre, Jan Alexander, Roy M. Nilsen, Bo Jacobsson and
Helle Margrete Meltzer

Chapter 7 **Specialist antenatal clinics for women at high risk of preterm birth** 66
Reem Malouf and Maggie Redshaw

Chapter 8 **Morbidity and mortality among very preterm singletons following fertility treatment in Australia and New Zealand, a population cohort study**..............83
Alex Y Wang, Abrar A. Chughtai, Kei Lui and Elizabeth A. Sullivan

Chapter 9   **Congenital tuberculosis in an extremely preterm infant conceived after in vitro fertilization** 93
Veronica Samedi, Stephen K. Field, Essa Al Awad, Gregory Ratcliffe and
Kamran Yusuf

Chapter 10   **The prevalence and risk factors of preterm small-for-gestational-age infants: a population-based retrospective cohort study in rural Chinese population** 97
Shi Chen, Rong Zhu, Huijuan Zhu, Hongbo Yang, Fengying Gong,
Linjie Wang, Yu Jiang, Bill Q. Lian, Chengsheng Yan, Jianqiang Li, Qing Wang,
Shi-kun Zhang and Hui Pan

Chapter 11   **Histologic chorioamnionitis does not modulate the oxidative stress and antioxidant status in pregnancies complicated by spontaneous preterm delivery** 105
Laura Fernandes Martin, Natália Prearo Moço, Moisés Diôgo de Lima,
Jossimara Polettini, Hélio Amante Miot, Camila Renata Corrêa,
Ramkumar Menon and Márcia Guimarães da Silva

Chapter 12   **What is the safest mode of delivery for extremely preterm cephalic/non-cephalic twin pairs?** 113
Catherine Dagenais, Anne-Mary Lewis-Mikhael, Marinela Grabovac,
Amit Mukerji and Sarah D. McDonald

Chapter 13   **Influence of weight gain, according to Institute of Medicine 2009 recommendation, on spontaneous preterm delivery in twin pregnancies** 125
Paola Algeri, Francesca Pelizzoni, Davide Paolo Bernasconi, Francesca Russo,
Maddalena Incerti, Sabrina Cozzolino, Salvatore Andrea Mastrolia and
Patrizia Vergani

Chapter 14   **Prevalence and factors associated with preterm birth at kenyatta national hospital** 132
Peter Wagura, Aggrey Wasunna, Ahmed Laving, Dalton Wamalwa and
Paul Ng'ang'a

Chapter 15   **Cerclage is associated with the increased risk of preterm birth in women who had cervical conization** 140
Geum Joon Cho, Yung-Taek Ouh, Log Young Kim, Tae-Seon Lee, Geun U. Park,
Ki Hoon Ahn, Soon-Cheol Hong, Min-Jeong Oh and Hai-Joong Kim

Chapter 16   **Nausea and vomiting during pregnancy associated with lower incidence of preterm births: the Japan Environment and Children's Study (JECS)** 145
Naomi Mitsuda, Masamitsu Eitoku, Keiko Yamasaki, Masahiko Sakaguchi,
Kahoko Yasumitsu-Lovell, Nagamasa Maeda, Mikiya Fujieda and
Narufumi Suganuma

Chapter 17   **Folic acid supplementation, preconception body mass index, and preterm delivery: findings from the preconception cohort data in a Chinese rural population** 151
Yuanyuan Wang, Zongfu Cao, Zuoqi Peng, Xiaona Xin, Ya Zhang, Ying Yang,
Yuan He, Jihong Xu and Xu Ma

Chapter 18   **The association between fine particulate matter exposure during pregnancy and preterm birth**..160
Xiaoli Sun, Xiping Luo, Chunmei Zhao, Rachel Wai Chung Ng,
Chi Eung Danforn Lim, Bo Zhang and Tao Liu

Chapter 19   **Serum screening in first trimester to predict pre-eclampsia, small for gestational age and preterm delivery**..172
Yan Zhong, Fufan Zhu and Yiling Ding

Chapter 20   **How many preterm births in England are due to excision of the cervical transformation zone? Nested case control study**..182
R. Wuntakal, Alejandra Castanon, R. Landy and P. Sasieni

Chapter 21   **Maternal history of childhood sexual abuse and preterm birth**..189
Adaeze C. Wosu, Bizu Gelaye and Michelle A. Williams

Permissions

List of Contributors

Index

Preface

Preterm birth is the birth of a baby at less than 37 weeks into gestation. Certain risk factors for preterm birth are diabetes, obesity, high blood pressure, being pregnant with two or more babies, vaginal infections, psychological stress and tobacco smoking, among others. The medical reason for early delivery is preeclampsia. Premature babies are considered at risk of developing cerebral palsy, developmental delays, auditory and sight problems. It is therefore not recommended to medically induce labor before 39 weeks, unless otherwise indicated due to certain clinical scenarios. In mothers who are considered at high risk of preterm delivery, it is recommended to take the hormone progesterone and folic acid before pregnancy. In other cases, medications such as nifedipine and corticosteroids can improve outcomes. Calcium supplementation for women with low dietary calcium, smoking cessation, routine ultrasound evaluation, etc. are certain tactics for reducing the chances of preterm birth. This book provides comprehensive insights into the causes, consequences and prevention of preterm birth. It consists of contributions made by international experts in obstetrics and gynecology. The topics covered in this book offer the readers new insights in preterm birth.

The information contained in this book is the result of intensive hard work done by researchers in this field. All due efforts have been made to make this book serve as a complete guiding source for students and researchers. The topics in this book have been comprehensively explained to help readers understand the growing trends in the field.

I would like to thank the entire group of writers who made sincere efforts in this book and my family who supported me in my efforts of working on this book. I take this opportunity to thank all those who have been a guiding force throughout my life.

Editor

Antenatal corticosteroids for management of preterm birth: a multi-country analysis of health system bottlenecks and potential solutions

Grace Liu[1], Joel Segrè[2], A Metin Gülmezoglu[3], Matthews Mathai[4], Jeffrey M Smith[5], Jorge Hermida[6], Aline Simen-Kapeu[7], Pierre Barker[8,9], Mercy Jere[10], Edward Moses[10], Sarah G Moxon[11,12,13], Kim E Dickson[7], Joy E Lawn[11,12,13]*, Fernando Althabe[14], Working Group for the UN Commission of Life Saving Commodities Antenatal Corticosteroids

Abstract

Background: Preterm birth complications are the leading cause of deaths for children under five years. Antenatal corticosteroids (ACS) are effective at reducing mortality and serious morbidity amongst infants born at <34 weeks gestation. WHO guidelines strongly recommend use of ACS for women at risk of imminent preterm birth where gestational age, imminent preterm birth, and risk of maternal infection can be assessed, and appropriate maternal/newborn care provided. However, coverage remains low in high-burden countries for reasons not previously systematically investigated.

Methods: The bottleneck analysis tool was applied in 12 countries in Africa and Asia as part of the *Every Newborn* Action Plan process. Country workshops involved technical experts to complete the survey tool, which is designed to synthesise and grade health system "bottlenecks", factors that hinder the scale up, of maternal-newborn intervention packages. We used quantitative and qualitative methods to analyse the bottleneck data, combined with literature review, to present priority bottlenecks and actions relevant to different health system building blocks for ACS.

Results: Eleven out of twelve countries provided data in response to the ACS questionnaire. Health system building blocks most frequently reported as having significant or very major bottlenecks were health information systems (11 countries), essential medical products and technologies (9 out of 11 countries) and health service delivery (9 out of 11 countries). Bottlenecks included absence of coverage data, poor gestational age metrics, lack of national essential medicines listing, discrepancies between prescribing authority and provider cadres managing care, delays due to referral, and lack of supervision, mentoring and quality improvement systems.

Conclusions: Analysis centred on health system building blocks in which 9 or more countries (>75%) reported very major or significant bottlenecks. Health information systems should include improved gestational age assessment and track ACS coverage, use and outcomes. Better health service delivery requires clarified policy assigning roles by level of care and cadre of provider, dependent on capability to assess gestational age and risk of preterm birth, and the implementation of guidelines with adequate supervision, mentoring and quality improvement systems, including audit and feedback. National essential medicines lists should include dexamethasone for antenatal use, and dexamethasone should be integrated into supply logistics.

* Correspondence: joy.lawn@lshtm.ac.uk
[11]Maternal, Adolescent, Reproductive and Child Health (MARCH) Centre, London School of Hygiene and Tropical Medicine, London, WC1E 7HT, UK
Full list of author information is available at the end of the article

Background

Each year, an estimated 15 million infants are born premature, representing over one in ten live births [1]. Complications from prematurity are the leading global cause of deaths in children under five [2], with over one million annual deaths [3], particularly from pulmonary immaturity and resultant respiratory distress syndrome (RDS) [4,5]. A preventive approach, first demonstrated to be effective in 1972, is the administration of antenatal corticosteroids (ACS) to mothers at risk of imminent preterm birth in order to stimulate fetal lung maturation [6]. Subsequent trials have established the safety and efficacy of ACS for women at risk of imminent preterm birth, with a meta-analysis of 21 studies finding a roughly one-third reduction in risk of neonatal death [4]. A subgroup analysis of the four trials conducted in middle-income countries (MICs) found a further reduction of around 50% in mortality, suggesting possible greater benefit in lower-resource settings [7].

Reducing the burden of preterm birth requires effective maternal care including comprehensive obstetric care (with caesarean section, if needed [8]), and specific care for the preterm newborn [9-11]. ACS administration is a critical component of this care. A recent large, six-country study (Antenatal Corticosteroids Trial, or ACT) extending ACS to community and primary care settings with lower level workers, found adverse outcomes in neonatal mortality, stillbirth and maternal infection, underlining the importance of trained health professionals able to accurately assess gestational age and provide ACS in hospital settings with adequate supportive care [12]. Currently, organisations including the new WHO guidelines on interventions to improve preterm birth outcomes [13] recommend a single course of ACS (dexamethasone or betamethasone, 24 mg administered by intramuscular injection in divided doses) to mothers less than 34 completed weeks of gestation, with risk of imminent preterm birth (anticipated within the subsequent 7 days) [15-20]. Safe and effective use of ACS depends on the accuracy of gestational age assessment, correct diagnosis of imminent preterm birth, and adequate maternal and newborn care (Figure 1). ACS is contraindicated for women with chorioamnionitis.

There has been rapid adoption of ACS use in high-income countries (HICs) since the mid-1990s [20], with coverage rates of over 90%. Yet coverage appears to remain low in low- and middle-income countries (LMICs), where 99% of all neonatal deaths occur [21]. Available estimates suggest that coverage varies greatly in LMIC facilities but is generally low even at the highest levels of care (Table 1). Increased safe and effective use of ACS has the potential to save an estimated 214,300 newborns each year with use for those births already occurring in hospitals with the appropriate package of linked care [22].

ACS is only one part of obstetric and preterm birth management [8] and should be part of initiatives to increase institutional birth rates and improve antenatal and intrapartum care coverage, quality and equity. Effectiveness and safety also critically require adequate neonatal care including thermal care, breastfeeding, resuscitation [11], kangaroo mother care [10], and availability of inpatient care of small and sick newborns [9].

Low coverage of ACS has been variously attributed to lack of guidelines, prescribing authority, provider awareness or skills, drug availability, and patient access to appropriate facilities [23]. However, the health system barriers to increased uptake of ACS have not previously been systematically examined.

This paper presents the results of a systematic multi-country analysis of barriers to uptake of ACS for preterm birth. In this analysis, we aim to identify priority health system building blocks facing common and critical bottlenecks to scaling up this life-saving intervention. We additionally discuss policy and programmatic implications and recommend priority actions drawn from the survey responses, existing evidence, and programme experience.

Objectives of this paper are as follows:

1. Use a 12-country analysis to explore health system bottlenecks affecting the scale-up of ACS.
2. Present the solutions to overcome the most significant bottlenecks including insights from respondent countries, literature review and programme experience.
3. Discuss policy and programmatic implications and propose priority actions.

Methods

This study used quantitative and qualitative research methods to collect information, assess health system bottlenecks and identify solutions to scale-up of maternal and newborn care interventions in 12 countries: Afghanistan, Cameroon, Democratic Republic of Congo (DRC), Kenya, Malawi, Nigeria, Uganda, Bangladesh, India, Nepal, Pakistan and Vietnam. The methodology has been discussed in detail previously and in paper 1 of this supplement [24,25].

Data collection

The maternal-newborn bottleneck analysis tool was developed as part of the *Every Newborn* Action Plan (ENAP) process to assist countries in identifying context-specific bottlenecks to the scale-up and provision of maternal and newborn health interventions across seven health system building blocks [25]. The tool was utilised during a series of national consultations supported by the global *Every Newborn* Steering Group between July 1st and December 31st 2013 (see Additional file 1). The

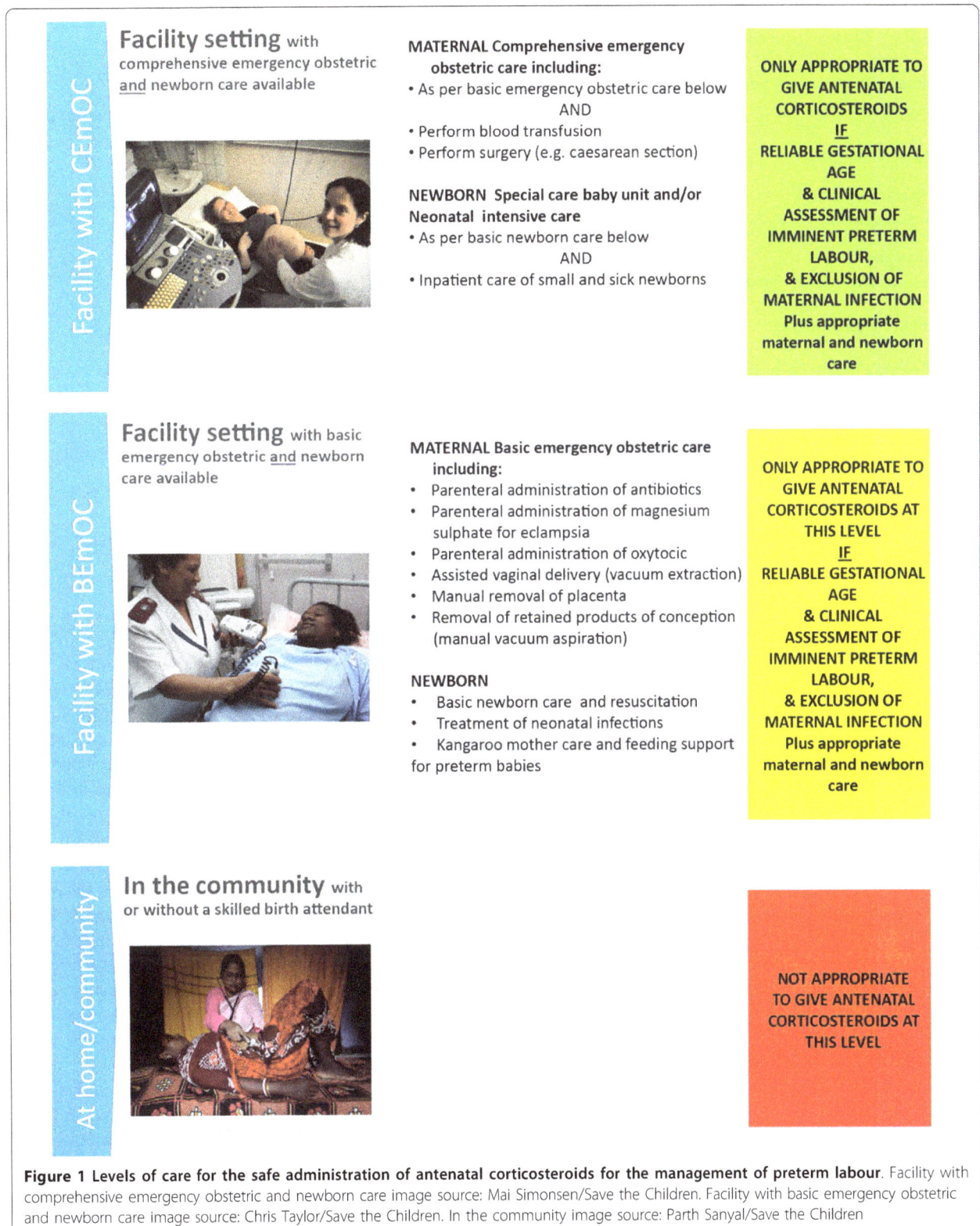

Facility setting with comprehensive emergency obstetric <u>and</u> newborn care available

MATERNAL Comprehensive emergency obstetric care including:
• As per basic emergency obstetric care below
AND
• Perform blood transfusion
• Perform surgery (e.g. caesarean section)

NEWBORN Special care baby unit and/or Neonatal intensive care
• As per basic newborn care below
AND
• Inpatient care of small and sick newborns

ONLY APPROPRIATE TO GIVE ANTENATAL CORTICOSTEROIDS
IF
RELIABLE GESTATIONAL AGE & CLINICAL ASSESSMENT OF IMMINENT PRETERM LABOUR, & EXCLUSION OF MATERNAL INFECTION
Plus appropriate maternal and newborn care

Facility setting with basic emergency obstetric <u>and</u> newborn care available

MATERNAL Basic emergency obstetric care including:
• Parenteral administration of antibiotics
• Parenteral administration of magnesium sulphate for eclampsia
• Parenteral administration of oxytocic
• Assisted vaginal delivery (vacuum extraction)
• Manual removal of placenta
• Removal of retained products of conception (manual vacuum aspiration)

NEWBORN
• Basic newborn care and resuscitation
• Treatment of neonatal infections
• Kangaroo mother care and feeding support for preterm babies

ONLY APPROPRIATE TO GIVE ANTENATAL CORTICOSTEROIDS AT THIS LEVEL
IF
RELIABLE GESTATIONAL AGE & CLINICAL ASSESSMENT OF IMMINENT PRETERM LABOUR, & EXCLUSION OF MATERNAL INFECTION
Plus appropriate maternal and newborn care

In the community with or without a skilled birth attendant

NOT APPROPRIATE TO GIVE ANTENATAL CORTICOSTEROIDS AT THIS LEVEL

Facility with CEmOC

Facility with BEmOC

At home/community

Figure 1 Levels of care for the safe administration of antenatal corticosteroids for the management of preterm labour. Facility with comprehensive emergency obstetric and newborn care image source: Mai Simonsen/Save the Children. Facility with basic emergency obstetric and newborn care image source: Chris Taylor/Save the Children. In the community image source: Parth Sanyal/Save the Children

workshops for each country included participants from national ministries of health, United Nations (UN) agencies, the private sector, non-governmental organisations, professional bodies, academia, bilateral agencies, and other stakeholders. For each workshop, a facilitator, orientated on the tool, coordinated the process and

Table 1. Existing estimates of antenatal corticosteroid coverage using World Bank income groupings

Country	Coverage estimate (%)	Indicator	Year
42 countries with 90% of child deaths	5	**All preterm births**	2000 [38]
In facility			
WHO Multi-country Survey 7 low income countries 19 middle income countries	27 58	Eligible women 26-34 weeks at facilities with >1,000 deliveries per year and capacity for caesarean section	2014 [39]
75 Countdown countries 34 low income countries + 40 middle income countries	41	Preterm births in secondary and tertiary facilities	2014 [40]
Cameroon (middle income country)	10	Facility-based RH providers using ACS	2005 [41]
Brazil (middle income country)	4	Eligible women 28-33^{+6} weeks in public maternal hospitals in Rio de Janeiro	1999 [42]
Ecuador (middle income country)	35	Eligible women 24-34^{+6} weeks in influential reference hospitals in capital cities	2010 [43]
El Salvador (middle income country)	55		
Uruguay (high income country)	71		
Indonesia (middle income country)	8	Eligible women <34 weeks in tertiary and district hospitals	2008 [44]
Malaysia (middle income country)	28		
Philippines (middle income country)	7		
Thailand (middle income country)	74		

facilitated groups to reach consensus on the specific bottlenecks for each health system building block. This paper, third in the series, is focused on antenatal corticosteroids for the management of preterm birth.

Data analysis methods

We graded bottlenecks for each health system building block using one of the following options: not a bottleneck (=1), minor bottleneck (=2), significant bottleneck (=3), or **very** major bottleneck (=4). We first present the grading in heat maps according to the very major or significant health system bottlenecks as reported by all 12 countries, then by mortality contexts (neonatal mortality rate (NMR) <30 or NMR ≥30 deaths per 1000 live births) and by region (countries in Africa and countries in Asia). We developed a second heat map showing the specific grading of bottlenecks for each health system building block by individual country. Survey responses were analysed for common specific bottlenecks, defined to be those reported by at least 3 countries. Where the same specific bottleneck was reported under more than one building block, it was categorised in accordance with the relevant survey question, or under the building block where most countries reported the specific bottleneck.

Finally, we categorised context-specific solutions for scaling up under the subcategories of corresponding bottlenecks within each health system building block.

Results

Eleven out of twelve country teams submitted their responses to the ACS questionnaire. Cameroon, Democratic Republic of the Congo (DRC), Kenya, Malawi, Nigeria, Uganda, Bangladesh, Nepal, and Vietnam returned national-level responses. Pakistan provided sub-national data from all provinces, Gilgit-Baltistan, and Azad Jammu and Kashmir, excluding two tribal territories. Sindh province, Pakistan, did not provide a grade for community ownership and partnership. India returned data from three states: Andhra Pradesh, Odisha, and Rajasthan. Rajasthan state completed the questionnaire and listed specific bottlenecks, but did not provide ratings for any building block. India responded to the earlier version of the questionnaire with fewer questions. Afghanistan, the twelfth country, returned national-level survey data without responses to the ACS portion and therefore is not included in our analysis.

An overview of grading for the health system building blocks, for all countries and by mortality setting and geography, is shown in Figure 2. More building blocks were graded as having significant or very major bottlenecks in countries with higher NMR; all four countries with NMR ≥30 (DRC, Nigeria, India, and Pakistan) reported very major or significant bottlenecks across all seven health system building blocks. Health system building blocks were graded poorly by a comparable proportion of countries in Africa and Asia, except for leadership and governance,

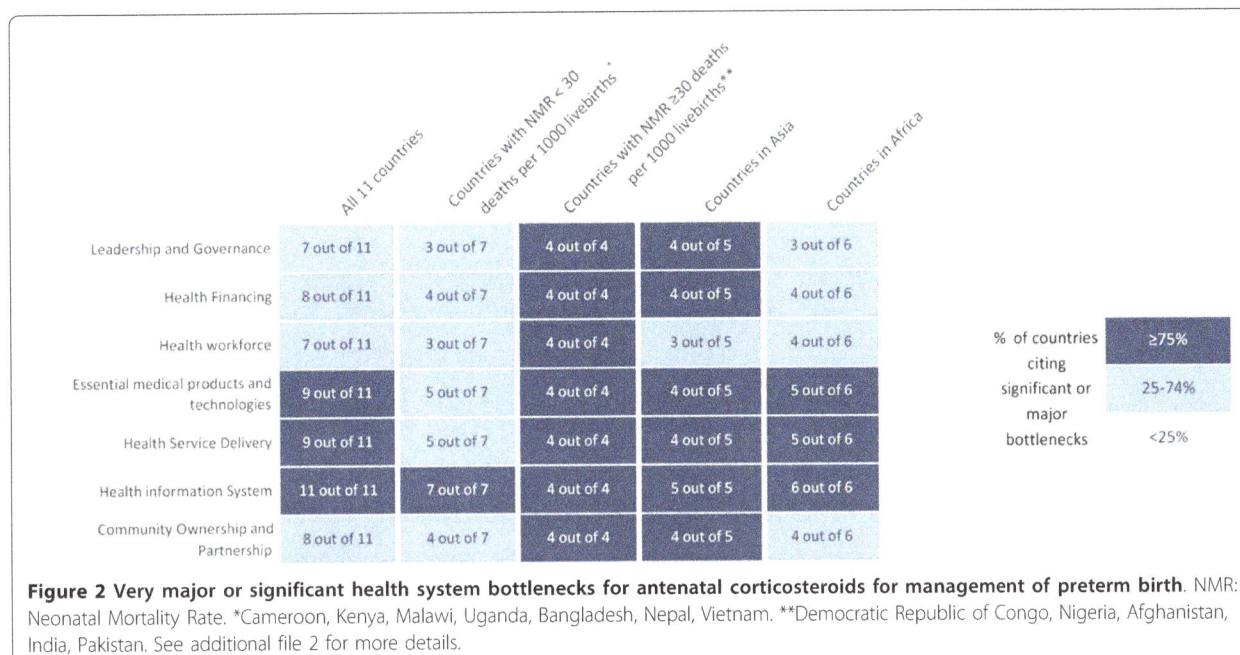

	All 11 countries	Countries with NMR < 30 deaths per 1000 livebirths *	Countries with NMR ≥30 deaths per 1000 livebirths **	Countries in Asia	Countries in Africa
Leadership and Governance	7 out of 11	3 out of 7	4 out of 4	4 out of 5	3 out of 6
Health Financing	8 out of 11	4 out of 7	4 out of 4	4 out of 5	4 out of 6
Health workforce	7 out of 11	3 out of 7	4 out of 4	3 out of 5	4 out of 6
Essential medical products and technologies	9 out of 11	5 out of 7	4 out of 4	4 out of 5	5 out of 6
Health Service Delivery	9 out of 11	5 out of 7	4 out of 4	4 out of 5	5 out of 6
Health information System	11 out of 11	7 out of 7	4 out of 4	5 out of 5	6 out of 6
Community Ownership and Partnership	8 out of 11	4 out of 7	4 out of 4	4 out of 5	4 out of 6

% of countries citing significant or major bottlenecks
≥75%
25-74%
<25%

Figure 2 Very major or significant health system bottlenecks for antenatal corticosteroids for management of preterm birth. NMR: Neonatal Mortality Rate. *Cameroon, Kenya, Malawi, Uganda, Bangladesh, Nepal, Vietnam. **Democratic Republic of Congo, Nigeria, Afghanistan, India, Pakistan. See additional file 2 for more details.

more commonly reported as a very major or significant bottleneck by African respondents.

Building block grading for each respondent country is summarised in Figure 3. Very major or significant bottlenecks were reported by at least 75% of country teams (at least 9 of 11) in three building blocks: health information systems (all countries), essential medical products and technologies (9 of 11 countries) and health service delivery (9 of 11 countries).

Table 2 summarises priority actions proposed by country teams to address specific bottlenecks to ACS scale-up. These solutions are grouped by health system building block. Common bottlenecks (reported by at least 3 countries) to scale-up of ACS are summarised in additional file 2 (table S1), along with underlying causes where reported.

Leadership and governance bottlenecks and solutions
Leadership and governance was graded as a very major or significant bottleneck by 7 of 11 country teams (Figure 2), representing a larger proportion of Asian countries (4 of 5 countries in Asia, compared to 3 of 6 countries in Africa). The most commonly cited specific bottleneck was inadequate guidelines on ACS use, cited by 9 of 11 country teams. Of these, 5 country teams (4 in Asia) reported no clear guidelines on ACS for management of preterm birth, and 4 country teams (all in Africa) reported available guidelines, which were either outdated or not disseminated.

Proposed solutions included development (or update) and dissemination of national guidelines and protocols

on prevention and management of preterm labour, including ACS. Updated WHO guidelines will be useful to inform national guidelines.

Health financing bottlenecks and solutions
Health financing was graded as a very major or significant bottleneck by 8 of 11 country teams. The most commonly cited specific bottleneck was insufficient funding, reported by 9 country teams, with 8 indicating a lack of priority or policy as the underlying cause.

Proposed solutions included increased advocacy and leadership, particularly with funding and budget allocation, for preterm birth prevention, management and care including ACS.

Health workforce bottlenecks and solutions
Health workforce was graded as a very major or significant bottleneck by 7 of 11 country teams. All country teams questioned reported a shortage of health workers especially in higher cadres, inadequate training, and inadequate supervision or mentoring. India did not provide an answer to the question on health worker shortages.

Proposed solutions included integration of ACS into pre-service and in-service training, development and dissemination of job aids, and consideration of expanded prescription authority for more cadres of health workers.

Essential medical products and technologies bottlenecks and solutions
Essential medical products and technologies was graded as a very major or significant bottleneck by 9 of 11 country teams. All 11 country teams cited as a specific

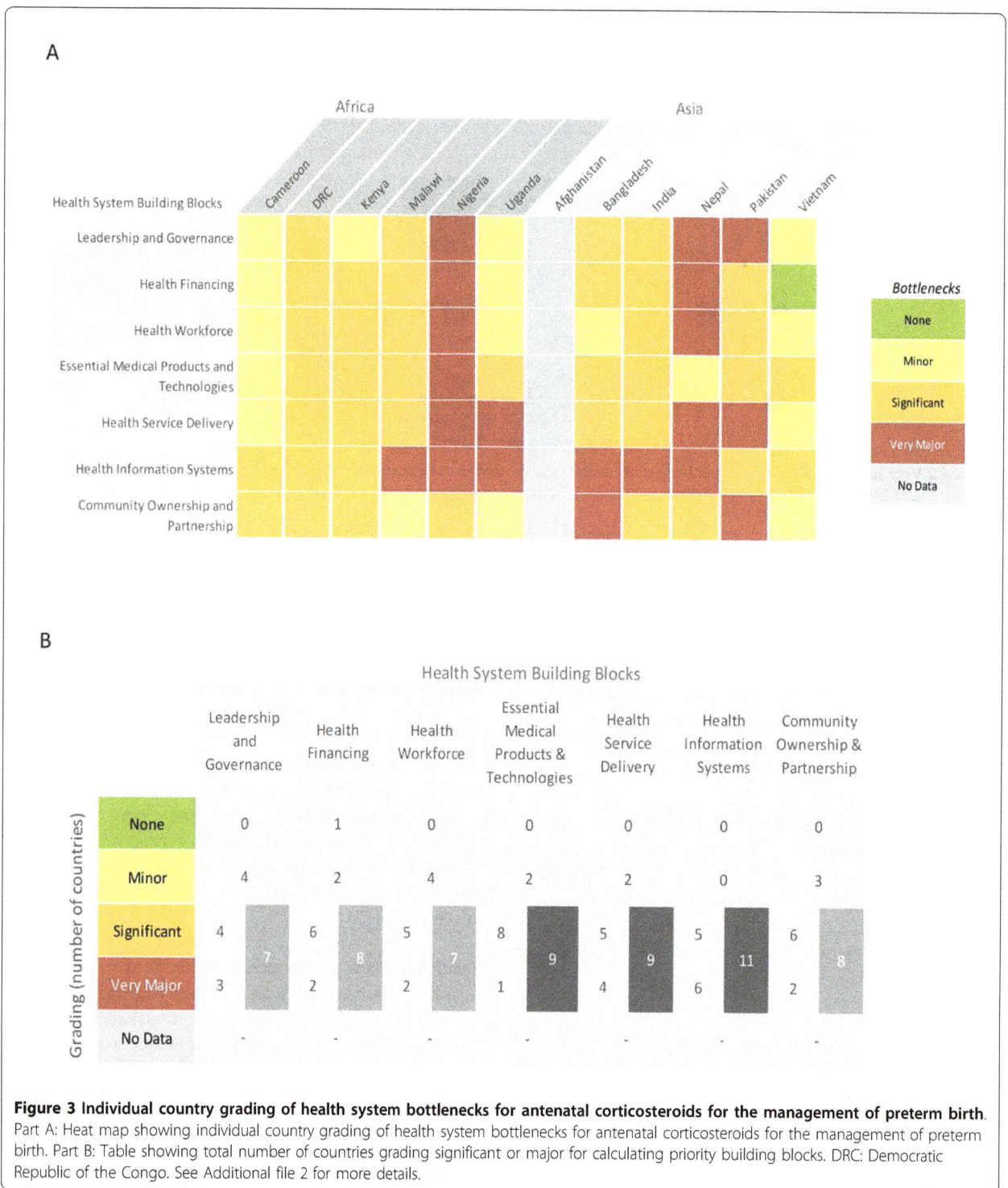

Figure 3 Individual country grading of health system bottlenecks for antenatal corticosteroids for the management of preterm birth. Part A: Heat map showing individual country grading of health system bottlenecks for antenatal corticosteroids for the management of preterm birth. Part B: Table showing total number of countries grading significant or major for calculating priority building blocks. DRC: Democratic Republic of the Congo. See Additional file 2 for more details.

bottleneck the lack of inclusion of ACS on the national essential medicines list (NEML) for fetal lung maturation, though all included dexamethasone for other indications. Of 8 country teams reporting inadequate procurement or distribution of ACS, 6 cited the lack of policy or NEML listing for fetal lung (or other lack of alignment between supply chain policy and ACS recommendations) as a direct cause of lack of integration into supply chain system. Additionally, no respondent country included ACS in quantification and forecasting, and none reported having an indicator for ACS drug availability.

Table 2. Country-recommended priority actions for addressing common bottlenecks to scaling up antenatal corticosteroids

Health system building block	Sub-category	Priority actions
Leadership and governance	*Policy and guidelines*	• Develop, update and disseminate the national policy on prevention and management of preterm labour; this should include policy on ACS use • Advocate for newborn health to be made as a priority • Develop national clinical protocols and guidelines on management of preterm labour
Health financing	*Funding/budget allocation*	• Increase funding / budget allocation for newborn care • Advocate and lobby for more funding from partners in newborn health
	Cost of antenatal corticosteroids	• Assess financial implications and develop financial policy for supplies and services to deliver this intervention to beneficiaries • Include antenatal corticosteroids as part of the free MNCH policy • Scale up obstetric kits by including relevant newborn drugs such as antenatal corticosteroids
Health workforce	*Policy restriction for prescription and administration*	• Authorise all skilled births attendants to prescribe and administer ACS
	Job descriptions/job aids	• Develop and disseminate job aids
	Shortage of qualified staff	• Recruit and train competent health providers • Develop an electronic database to track training activities and identify needs • Ensure staffing norms are in line with WHO recommendations
	Competency and training	• Strengthen competency based pre-service and in-service training, and on job training to capture use of ACS by health providers for fetal lung maturation • Include ACS training in skilled birth attendant evaluation
Health service delivery	*Service availability*	• Develop and disseminate national guidelines in health facilities • Establish follow-up visits to monitor availability and use of ACS in all health facilities
	Quality of care	• Establish a supportive supervision and mentoring mechanism with a reward system; • Regular integrated monitoring visits to ensure compliance to protocols; • Integrate ACS use in clinical audits and reviews;
	Referral systems	• Involve all stakeholders to improve infrastructure for timely referral (road network) • Build district-level capacity to monitor appropriate use of ambulances and ensure adequate maintenance
Essential medical products and technologies	*Procurement policy*	• Include ACS in national essential medicines list with appropriate indication (fetal lung maturation)
	Drug availability	• Develop and disseminate policy in health facilities to enhance procurement
	Logistics management information systems (LMIS)	• Estimate needs based on number/estimate of preterm birth load at health facilities • Build staff capacity for logistics management
Health information system	*Data collection and reporting*	• Define indicator(s) for tracking ACS use and incorporate into national system • Strengthen monitoring mechanisms such as regular monitoring and evaluation visits, documentation through use of program data. • Conduct regular review meetings on data management at all levels
Community ownership and participation	*Knowledge / awareness*	• Conduct integrated community maternal and newborn education and campaigns in local languages • Improve community awareness on newborn health by adding newborn information to maternal awareness documents, campaigns, media, etc.
	Community participation / engagement	• Strengthen community leaders and male involvement through innovative approaches; • Strengthen functioning of existing community units with nationwide community awareness initiatives on newborn health • Health facilities to come up with innovative ways of involving men e.g. set aside time for couples during antenatal visits and time for adolescents
	Demand for preterm birth care	• Scale up tribal empowerment project to address socio-cultural barriers to newborn care • Utilise community radio and mobile applications

Proposed solutions included listing of ACS drugs on NEMLs for a fetal lung maturation indication, development and dissemination of guidelines, and software to support needs-based forecasting and procurement.

Health service delivery bottlenecks and solutions

Health service delivery was graded as a very major or significant bottleneck by 9 of 11 country teams. All country teams reported having inadequate or non-existent quality monitoring and improvement systems, and 9 country teams noted a lack of alignment between ACS prescribing authority and health worker cadres providing care for women at risk of preterm birth. Additionally, 7 countries cited delays due to referrals as a specific bottleneck. Table S3 and S4 of the Additional file 2 summarises levels of care where ACS is allowed and health worker cadres permitted to prescribe and/or administer ACS, as reported by country teams.

Proposed solutions included development and dissemination of guidelines across facilities, creation of supervision and mentoring systems, integration into clinical audits and reviews, and strengthened referral systems.

Health information system bottlenecks and solutions

Health information system was identified as the most problematic building block, with all 11 country teams reporting very major or significant bottlenecks. Responses to health information systems questions revealed an almost complete absence of defined and standardised indicators for ACS use, with the exception of Nepal and one province in Pakistan, where country teams reported that ACS use was tracked on partographs. No countries reported having an indicator for ACS drug availability. Moreover, no countries included ACS use in clinical audits or perinatal reviews.

Proposed solutions included creation of indicator(s) for ACS use and integration of ACS data into record-keeping systems and regular reviews.

Community ownership and partnership bottlenecks and solutions

Community engagement was graded as a very major or significant bottleneck by 8 of 11 country teams. The most commonly cited specific bottlenecks were lack of awareness and initiatives targeted at raising awareness of preterm birth risks and management (9 countries), and the absence of an accessible facility or transportation to reach a facility where ACS could be administered (9 countries).

Proposed solutions included leveraging existing community outreach infrastructure, such as community groups, opinion leaders, and media.

Discussion

This systematic analysis of ACS use in 11 high-burden countries, which together account for over half of maternal and newborn deaths, has identified commonly experienced health system bottlenecks to scaling up ACS for management of preterm birth. A comprehensive approach to preterm birth should include strategies for prevention as well as management; however, the menu for high-impact, evidence-based preterm birth prevention is currently limited [26]. In high-income settings, reductions in the burden of preterm birth can largely be traced to improved care of preterm infants, which has yet to achieve major traction or wide-scale use even for simpler care such as feeding support, kangaroo mother care and infection prevention and treatment [27]. There is also considerable scope for impact through management of preterm birth, including ACS which is highly effective when provided by adequately trained health professionals in hospital settings where adequate maternal and neonatal follow-up and support are possible.

The important principle of "do no harm" and potential risks of ACS have been highlighted recently through the ACT trial. The benefits of ACS are dependent on high coverage in preterm babies <34 weeks; benefit is not expected or is marginal after 34 weeks, and risks increase close to term. Targeting based on gestational age and more accurate diagnosis of imminent preterm birth are therefore key aspects of effective, safe use as underscored in WHO guidelines. In addition, ACS alone cannot be a magic bullet; the preterm infant still requires a minimum of supportive care including warmth and feeding support, and if <32 weeks gestation is more likely to require oxygen therapy and respiratory support. Approximately half of the births in the ACT trial occurred at home or low-level primary care facilities [12].

Despite variation across the 11 countries that responded to the survey, the greatest barriers were consistent, highlighting three priority health system building blocks—health information systems, health service delivery and essential medical products and technologies—with the most critical common bottlenecks. Drawing from country programme experience, and evidence from literature (Table 2), this paper outlines potential solutions for programme managers and policymakers facing similar barriers.

Health information systems priority actions

Data on ACS coverage, use, and outcomes including safety were absent in nearly all countries. To enable continuous and quantitative assessment of ACS programmes, appropriate indicators need to be defined, and these data integrated into existing health information systems in order to allow tracking and comparison at facility, district, and national levels. ACS coverage data are one of the priority indicators identified in the Every Newborn Action Plan [28]. Coverage data are lacking and should also aim to assess false positives (women treated whose babies are born after 34 completed weeks).

Use of data for quality improvement would be aided if ACS were systematically included in safe childbirth checklists, partographs, clinical audits, and perinatal death reviews [29]. Data are also needed on process such as logistics and stock out. Two case studies of in-country implementation programmes provide examples of data collection and recordkeeping systems for ACS use, and how audit and feedback mechanisms using these records can be harnessed to improve quality of care for the management of preterm birth (Figure 4).

Health service delivery priority actions

Estimates suggest ACS coverage in LMICs is generally low even in tertiary facilities (Table 1), consistent with the poor grading of health service delivery among respondent country teams. All 11 countries in this analysis are among the 75 Countdown to 2015 countries with an estimate of 41% (weighted average) coverage of preterm births in secondary and tertiary facilities. Eight of 11 countries were also included in the WHO Multi-country Survey estimate of coverage in high-volume

facilities; these were DRC (16%), Kenya (32%), Nigeria (30%), Uganda (27%), India (69%), Nepal (20%), Pakistan (63%), and Vietnam (52%). These estimates are likely to be higher than the national average as the survey methodology sampled only large facilities from the capital city and two randomly selected provinces. National population coverage with ACS is likely to be much lower than facility coverage estimates, as a large proportion of births take place outside of high-volume facilities or outside any facility. In the 11 countries, institutional delivery rates (in any facility) ranged from 33% in Bangladesh to 92% in Vietnam, according to data compiled by UNICEF in 2015 [30].

Available evidence supports focusing scale-up efforts in facilities with the capacity for gestational age assessment and diagnosis of women at risk of imminent

---

Malawi

In Nkhoma Hospital, a new program of continuous quality improvement uses "improvement advisors" to engage midwives in identifying facility-specific bottlenecks and improving coverage and quality of care.

Improvement advisors first surveyed midwives on their self-reported use of antenatal corticosteroids (ACS). Advisors and midwives, clinicians, and data clerks then worked together to first compile data, then review patient records to quantify actual use and identify cases where more mothers and babies could benefit from treatment. Midwives, clinicians, and data clerks then discussed barriers and potential strategies for increasing use, identified the most promising solutions, and agreed together to implement them. Pharmacy technicians were additionally involved in quantifying use of dexamethasone from pharmacy to the maternity ward and contributed to a solution in relocating drug storage.

In an ongoing process, midwives, clinicians, and data clerks meet every two weeks to review new patient records, evaluate the impact of the changes implemented, and repeat their discussion of further improvements.

Thus far, solutions have included stickers in patient records to flag eligible mothers and track doses of ACS, moving drug storage into the room where high risk of preterm birth is diagnosed to eliminate delays in going to the pharmacy, and estimating gestational age with two different methods rather than relying on patients' own estimates. Midwives have also been empowered to prescribe and administer dexamethasone at admission instead of referring to a clinician for a prescription.

Uganda

An intervention in five high-volume maternity hospitals and two health centres aims to increase correct ACS use. Each month, quality improvement teams established at each facility: track gestational age estimation, identification of women with high risk of preterm birth, use of dexamethasone, correct use of dexamethasone, preterm newborn mortality, and stillbirths. They then identify bottlenecks and test changes through Plan-Do-Study-Act (PDSA) cycles. Three coaches with quality improvement experience visit each facility twice monthly.

The quality improvement process has pinpointed weak gestational age estimation as a major difficulty in identifying women with high risk of preterm birth. A shortage of health workers results in insufficient time to perform calculations, and providers lack measuring tapes and clarity on how to proceed when fundal height and last menstrual period (LMP) estimates differ. Solutions being tested include gestational age calculation wheels, posted job aids, and distribution of measuring tapes. Coloured chart stickers indicating 24-37 weeks gestational age (yellow) and high risk of preterm birth (red) are also being piloted to improve tracking of eligible women.

Figure 4 The use of continuous quality improvement for antenatal corticosteroid use in Malawi and Uganda. ACS: antenatal corticosteroids. PDSA: Plan-Do-Study-Act

preterm birth, as well as ongoing support for preterm infants and well-functioning maternity wards [4]. The recent study (ACT) which extended ACS to include non-hospital facilities in six countries (including Kenya, India, and Pakistan) found increased perinatal mortality as well as increased rates of presumed maternal infection [12]. The specific cause(s) of newborn mortality were not ascertainable, but service delivery challenges included limited ability to estimate gestational age and accurately diagnose high risk of preterm birth. As a consequence, ACS was under prescribed for preterm and early preterm babies likely to benefit from treatment and overprescribed to babies born at or near term, when ACS may have increased risks.

With clear evidence for use in hospitals in HICs with adequate neonatal support and reason for caution at lower-level facilities in LIC settings, programmatic scale-up is best focused on higher-level and high-volume facilities, where resources can also be used to produce significant impact cost-effectively and also improve targeting and safety tracking. Increased population coverage will then depend on increased and timely identification and referral of at-risk women, both in lower-level facilities and in homes. Systemic improvements are needed to encourage institutional deliveries with skilled birth attendants and to strengthen referral systems, while guidelines and training at lower levels of care will be critical to building capacity for timely identification. Expanded care such as a pre-referral dose may also improve care by allowing a longer time for ACS to take effect. However, such steps must be considered cautiously by each country based on the capacity of lower-level facilities to provide adequate care to ensure safety.

Human resource and skills for service delivery

Within hospitals, coverage is often limited by inadequate numbers of physicians or other providers present and also adequately trained to assess gestational age, diagnose high risk of preterm birth, and authorised to prescribe and administer ACS. The majority of countries reported both a shortage of health workers at higher cadres and a mismatch between provider cadres allowed to prescribe ACS and those cadres likely to be caring for women at risk of preterm birth (Table S2, additional file 2).

Expanded prescribing authority for midwives providing care to pregnant women could greatly increase the capacity of hospitals to manage preterm birth with ACS. However, any change in policy must be considered based on the capability to correctly diagnose conditions, which lead to preterm birth and provide adequate supportive care to both mother and baby. Currently WHO only recommends administration of ACS by doctors and advanced level associate clinicians and recommends against use by nurses and auxiliary nurses. Prescription and administration of ACS by non-advanced associate

clinicians has not been evaluated by the WHO due to lack of rigorous evaluation of this question [31]. The WHO recommends cautious consideration of ACS administration by midwives and auxiliary nurse-midwives (ANMs) in LMICs with shortages of physicians-those settings described by respondent countries. Consideration of expanded prescribing authority should be made in the context of rigorous research [31]. In the absence of prescribing authority, health workers providing care to mothers still have an important role in identifying potential risk of preterm birth and ensuring rapid and safe referral.

All countries reported a lack of training in assessing gestational age, recognition of high risk of preterm birth and in management of preterm birth using ACS as well as inadequate supervision and mentoring systems. In-service training and increased support, both for cadres authorised to prescribe and administer ACS and for cadres involved in identification of risk and referral, are also critical to any scale-up effort.

Guidelines implementation and quality improvement

For any policy to reach every mother and every newborn, clear guidelines and adequate training must reach all relevant cadres of health worker and levels of care. As indicated by the country teams' responses to leadership and governance questions, it is critical both to develop clear guidelines and to ensure active dissemination. An active model of dissemination should ideally integrate systems of supervision, mentoring, and monitoring of quality improvement - all areas reported as inadequate by all 11 country teams.

A study of active dissemination in the United States showed that use of local opinion leaders, technical updates, reminders, interactive small-group learning, and audit and feedback were effective in accelerating facility uptake of ACS. These five elements were also effective in increasing use of a maternal health intervention in LMICs, with a structure reflecting the differing needs of low-resource settings. Figure 5 shows the five-component structure of the interventions in these two RCTs and details their implementation in each setting. Figure 6 outlines a program with similar features currently being studied in a facility in Cambodia. In particular, the audit and feedback component provides one model for continuous quality monitoring and improvement, an essential part of quality implementation of guidelines. This pilot model also provides a further example of the role of the continuous use of outcome data in improving safety and quality of care.

Essential medical products and technologies priority actions

Corticosteroids for ACS treatment are inexpensive (often under 1 USD for a full course) and are often assumed to

In the United States, acceptance and use of antenatal corticosteroids (ACS) increased rapidly following publication of National Institute of Health recommendations and the American Congress of Obstetricians and Gynecologists endorsement in 1994. Leviton *et al.* [45] detailed a model of active dissemination which accelerated uptake using five key components: opinion leaders, lectures and information, reminders, interactive group learning, and audit and feedback. A year-long program of active dissemination in 13 hospitals increased coverage by 108% over baseline, compared with an increase in 14 hospitals with usual dissemination (information only) of 75%.

A 2008 overview of systematic reviews of quality improvement strategies for low and middle income countries (LMICs) identified each of these components as applicable to facilities in LMICs and highlighted considerations specific to low-resource settings, particularly a training of trainers model to limit the number of health workers diverted from providing care during educational meetings [46]. An intervention for increasing use of oxytocin for postpartum haemorrhage in Argentina and Uruguay employed active dissemination with the same five components over 18 months. Median oxytocin use increased from 2.1% to 83.6% in 10 intervention hospitals, compared to a change from 2.6% to 12.3% in nine control hospitals, with stable results at one-year follow-up [47].

These two models of active dissemination are summarised below:

Program component	Implementation for increased use of ACS in the United States	Implementation for increased use of oxytocin in Argentina and Uruguay
1. Opinion leaders	One influential physician and one nurse coordinator per facility, recommended by director of obstetrics or of maternal and fetal medicine.	Team of 3-6 birth attendants (physicians, residents, and/or midwives) identified by peers using a validated sociometric questionnaire.
2. Technical update	Grand rounds lecture by nationally respected expert; distribution of printed materials, sample sticker prompt, and sample chart reminder.	Guidelines dissemination by opinion leader teams. One computer per hospital with guidelines, World Health Organization Reproductive Health Library, *BMJ Clinical Evidence.*
3. Reminders	Chart reminder system to prompt physician consideration: Nurse coordinators inserted large, brightly coloured reminders into eligible charts as soon as possible after admission.	Reminders placed in labour and delivery wards, birth attendant surgical packages, and clinical records.
4. Interactive group learning	Group discussion of case scenarios led by influential physicians: 1-hour, informal groups of obstetricians and residents discussing four case scenarios in which ACS might be administered: • ideal case of spontaneous preterm labour • preterm premature rupture of membranes (PPROM) • early gestational age and no prenatal care • complicated pregnancy (maternal chronic hypertension and diet-controlled diabetes).	Training for opinion leader teams: • 5-day workshop: Training to develop and disseminate evidence-based guidelines in a 5-day workshop focused on critical evaluation of medical literature, development of clinical-practice guidelines, communication skills, and methods of conducting one-on-one academic detailing visits with hospital birth attendants to discuss facility implementation. • 1-day workshop in training skills at facility. Training and visits for birth attendants.
5. Audit and feedback	Monitoring and feedback to physicians: Nurse coordinators kept logs of preterm admissions and deliveries, use of chart reminders, and use of ACS; influential physicians received and shared reports on use of chart reminders, use of ACS, and timing of ACS administration.	Monthly reports on rates of use based on hospital clinical data.

Figure 5 An adaptable model for active dissemination of guidelines on the use of antenatal corticosteroids. ACS: antenatal corticosteroids. LMICs: low and middle income countries

be widely available. Yet most respondents indicated shortages at the country level, primarily attributed to a lack of supporting policy or effective logistics systems. NEML listing for the fetal lung maturation indication is essential to prioritisation for procurement as well as integration into supply chain, from forecasting to distribution.

Adequate procurement further depends on development and dissemination of guidelines on ACS use, including clarity on the choice of corticosteroid and appropriate regimen. Two corticosteroids, dexamethasone and betamethasone, have been shown to be safe and effective to manage preterm birth. Betamethasone is sometimes preferred in HICs due to limited evidence suggesting better outcomes (44% reduction in RDS and 33% reduction in neonatal mortality versus placebo or no treatment, compared with 20% reduction in RDS and 28%

An ongoing intervention at Phnom Penh National Maternal Child Health Centre offers a model for increasing antenatal corticosteroid (ACS) use applying program components similar to those described in Figure 5:

Technical updates
- Initial 2-day technical update for facility leaders including current evidence and guidelines as well as standardised gestational age assessment.
- Replication of 2-day technical update by facility leaders *for entire maternity unit staff.*

Interactive group learning
Routine group discussion during morning handover meetings for care providers and Friday meetings for medical staff.

Focused data collection and reminders
- Midwives record use of dexamethasone (amount, number, and timing of doses) and time for next dose.
- Dexamethasone use recorded on maternity unit whiteboard used to track high-risk patients.

Audit and feedback
- Monthly audit of rates of preterm birth and provision of dexamethasone.
- Monthly feedback call with the head of the clinical team to identify challenges, address misconceptions, and reinforce good practices.

Figure 6 Active dissemination of guidelines on the use of antenatal corticosteroids in Phnom Penh, Cambodia. ACS: antenatal corticosteroids. LMIC: Low and middle income countries

reduction in neonatal mortality for dexamethasone versus placebo or no treatment) and potentially lower risk of maternal infection [4].

However, evidence on dexamethasone still conclusively supports its overall safe and effective use for management of preterm birth. A meta-analysis of 9 studies directly comparing dexamethasone with betamethasone further found no statistically significant differences apart from a greater reduction in intraventricular haemorrhage using dexamethasone (RR 0.44, 95% CI 0.21 to 0.92, 4 studies, 549 infants). A large RCT directly comparing dexamethasone to betamethasone is currently underway [32].

Critically, only dexamethasone is a feasible choice for scale-up in most LMICs. While dexamethasone is widely available from international suppliers for a variety of indications, the formulation of betamethasone supported by most evidence (a suspension of betamethasone acetate in betamethasone phosphate, rather than betamethasone phosphate alone) has been subject to global shortages [33] and costs 25 times as much as dexamethasone per course of ACS [34].

Dexamethasone also faces fewer policy hurdles to increased use for management of preterm birth. With a variety of uses, dexamethasone in the recommended formulation is already registered, listed on the NEML, and included in procurement and supply chain in all 11 countries, for other indications. Dexamethasone is the only ACS listed on the WHO EML with a fetal lung maturation indication [35].

National policies, in line with the current WHO guideline, should therefore focus on promoting appropriate use of dexamethasone through procurement policy, clear guidelines, and integration into forecasting, procurement, and supply chain.

Key messages

- Antenatal corticosteroids (ACS) are effective at reducing deaths and serious complications in preterm infants <34 weeks gestation if administered to mothers at risk of imminent preterm birth in order to stimulate fetal lung maturation. World Health Organization guidelines strongly recommend use in the context of adequate obstetric care and appropriate newborn care.

- Coverage of ACS for management of preterm birth remains low in high-burden countries.

- Bottlenecks to scaling up ACS were reported across all health system building blocks, and identified the greatest barriers in health information systems (including data on gestational age), health service delivery, and essential medicines.

Key action points

- Health information systems: Establish indicators and collect data within routine hospital and national data collection systems on ACS coverage, quality of care, and outcomes after ACS treatment for delivery <34 weeks, or for women with infections. Incorporate indicators for ACS into audit and feedback systems to track quality especially regarding safety. Improve gestational age assessment and recording.

- Essential medicines: Include dexamethasone for the appropriate antenatal indication on national essential medicines lists, create needs-based forecasting and include dexamethasone in efforts to improve drug supply logistics.

- Research: Investigate, ideally in a mortality-powered randomised controlled trial, the effect and safety of use in hospital settings in low and middle income countries, including more accurate and feasible methods of assessing gestational age where first trimester ultrasound is unavailable, and minimum levels of maternal and neonatal care required. Other research questions include optimal dosage regimens for dexamethasone, the feasibility and safety of pre-referral ACS dose, and validity and feasibility of improved coverage data.

Figure 7 Key messages and action points for scale-up of antenatal corticosteroids for management of preterm birth. ACS: antenatal corticosteroids

Limitations and implications for further research

Soliciting responses from a wide range of in-country partners and practitioners in maternal and newborn health captured context-specific challenges and generated collaborative solution ideas. The grading process also created consensus around priority bottlenecks and health system building blocks to be addressed. However, these consensus views are subjective. The quality and amount of information also varied depending on the level of knowledge of participants on health system issues and on workshop facilitation. In addition, bottlenecks were reported as perceived bottlenecks relative to the other health system building blocks. National-level assessment may mask regional disparities, particularly between urban and rural areas. This comprehensive questionnaire may have led to respondent fatigue, but this effect is least significant for ACS as the first intervention in the bottleneck analysis tool. For India and Pakistan, subnational responses may not mirror all national-level challenges. However, Pakistan submitted responses from all regions except two tribal territories, and although India returned data from only three of its 28 states, these areas are amongst the poorest states and include populations similar to those of Vietnam, Kenya, and DRC [36].

Further research is needed to establish the effectiveness of the solutions described here, especially in the context of ACS use in LMIC hospital settings where most of the world's births now occur. To date the evidence on ACS is primarily from HIC settings with neonatal intensive care [4] or the ACT trial from low-level settings with less-skilled workers [12]. The evidence base could be greatly advanced in LMIC settings, for instance through a multi-country, cluster-randomised trial in LMIC hospitals to assess the mortality impact and safety of a package optimising gestational age (where first trimester ultrasound is not routine) and clinical assessment of mothers, including risk of preterm birth and possible maternal infection, whilst providing appropriate maternal and newborn care. Given the lack of pharmacokinetic and dynamics data for both dexamethasone and betamethasone, other research questions include optimal dosage regimens. Data are now even more critically important and this gap is urgent to address, possibly for coverage and outcome data that could be tracked in routine health management information systems [29]. Further work is also needed to define signal functions for newborns by level of care. A signal function on ACS could be incorporated into existing monitoring systems, such as the signal functions for basic and comprehensive emergency obstetric care, to ensure consistent tracking of maternal and newborn interventions along the continuum of care [37].

Another important track of research is to improve the accuracy and also feasibility of gestational age assessment, including testing tools to improve accuracy of last menstrual period assessment, use of ultrasound dating in later pregnancy and ways to promote better recording in notes and use of the data by clinicians. Key messages and actions are summarised in Figure 7.

Conclusions

ACS for management of preterm birth has been a standard of care in wealthy countries for over 20 years, yet is greatly underused in low-resource countries, where complications of preterm birth have recently become the leading cause of death in children under 5. Preterm infants are over 12 times more likely to die in the poorest compared to the richest countries, and infants in the poorest countries have a survival rate at 32 weeks similar to that of infants born in the richest countries at 25 weeks. This systematic bottleneck analysis using data from 11 countries identifies critical areas of focus and suggests a set of actionable solutions for extending this inexpensive, high-impact intervention, whilst also promoting the tracking for safety, potentially saving hundreds of thousands of lives each year.

List of abbreviations

ACS: Antenatal corticosteroids; ANM: Auxiliary nurse-midwife; DRC: Democratic Republic of Congo; EML: Essential medicines list; FLM: Fetal lung maturation; HICs: High income countries; LIC: Low income country; LMIC: Low- or middle-income country; LMIS: Logistics management and information system; MIC: Middle-income country; MOH: Ministry of Health; NEML: National essential medicines list; NMR: Neonatal mortality rate; RCT: Randomised controlled trial; RDS: Respiratory distress syndrome; WHO: World Health Organization.

Competing interests

The authors have not declared any competing interests. The assessment of bottlenecks expressed during consultations reflects the perception of the technical experts and may not be national policy. The authors alone are responsible for the views expressed in this article and they do not necessarily represent the decisions, policy or views of the organisations listed, including WHO.

Authors' contributions

GL analysed data and drafted the manuscript in collaboration with JS. KED, AS-K JEL and SGM contributed to conceptualisation of the paper, data analysis and interpretation, and review of drafts. FA and MG and MM contributed to data interpretation and discussion and reviewed drafts. JMS, JH, PB, MJ, and EM contributed to country case studies. All authors reviewed drafts and approved the final manuscript.

Acknowledgements

This work would not have been possible without the country technical working groups and country workshop organiser and participants who carried out the bottleneck analyses. We would like to thank Helen Owen at LSHTM for her assistance with presentation of figures, and Fiorella Bianchi for her assistance with the submission process and the additional files. Finally, we would like to thank Jim Neilson and Jane Hirst for their helpful peer reviews of this paper.

Declarations

Publication costs for this supplement were funded by the Bill and Melinda Gates Foundation through a grant to US Fund for UNICEF (Grant ID: OPP1094117), and support from Save the Children's Saving Newborn Lives Programme. Additional funding for the bottleneck analysis was received from USAID (Grant ID: GHA-G-00-07-00007) through UNICEF. This article has been published as part of *BMC Pregnancy and Childbirth* Volume 15 Supplement 2, 2015: Every Woman, Every Newborn. The full contents of the supplement are available online at http://www. biomedcentral.com/bmcpregnancychildbirth/supplements/15/S2.

Authors' details

[1]Antenatal Corticosteroids Working Group of the UN Commodities Commission, Cambridge, MA, USA. [2]Antenatal Corticosteroids Working Group of the UN Commodities Commission, Oakland, CA, USA. [3]UNDP/UNFPA/UNICEF/WHO/World Bank Special Programme of Research,

Development and Research Training in Human Reproduction (HRP), Department of Reproductive Health and Research, World Health Organization, 20 Avenue Appia, 1211 Geneva 27, Switzerland. [4]Department of Maternal, Newborn, Child & Adolescent Health, World Health Organization, 20 Avenue Appia, 1211 Geneva 27, Switzerland. [5]Jhpiego, 1615 Thames St., Baltimore, MD, 21231, USA. [6]University Research Co., LLC, 7200 Wisconsin Avenue, Suite 600, Bethesda, MD 20814, USA. [7]Health Section, Programme Division, UNICEF Headquarters, 3 United Nations Plaza, New York, NY 10017, USA. [8]Institute for Healthcare Improvement, 20 University Road, Cambridge, MA 02138, USA. [9]Gillings School of Global Public Health, University of North Carolina at Chapel Hill, 135 Dauer Drive, Chapel Hill, NC 27599, USA. [10]MaiKhanda Trust, House number 14/56 Off Presidential Drive - Area 14, Private Bag B437, 265 Lilongwe, Malawi. [11]Maternal, Adolescent, Reproductive and Child Health (MARCH) Centre, London School of Hygiene and Tropical Medicine, London, WC1E 7HT, UK. [12]Saving Newborn Lives, Save the Children, 2000 L Street NW, Suite 500, Washington, DC 20036, USA. [13]Department of Infectious Disease Epidemiology, London School of Hygiene and Tropical Medicine, London, WC1E 7HT, UK. [14]Institute for Clinical Effectiveness and Health Policy (IECS), Dr. Emilio Ravignani 2024, Buenos Aires, C1414CPV, Argentina.

References

1. Blencowe H, Cousens S, Oestergaard MZ, Chou D, Moller AB, Narwal R, et al: National, regional, and worldwide estimates of preterm birth rates in the year 2010 with time trends since 1990 for selected countries: a systematic analysis and implications. Lancet 2012, 379:2162-72.
2. UN Inter-agency Group for Child Mortality Estimation: Levels & Trends in Child Mortality. Report 2014. New York; 2014.
3. Liu L, Oza S, Hogan D, Perin J, Rudan I, Lawn JE, Cousens S, et al: Global, regional, and national causes of child mortality in 2000-13, with projections to inform post-2015 priorities: an updated systematic analysis. Lancet 2015, 385(9966):430-440.
4. Roberts D, Dalziel S: Antenatal corticosteroids for accelerating fetal lung maturation for women at risk of preterm birth. Cochrane Db Syst Rev 2006, , 3: CD004454.
5. Vidyasagar D, Velaphi S, Bhat VB: Surfactant replacement therapy in developing countries. Neonatology 2011, 99:355-366.
6. Liggins GC, Howie RN: A controlled trial of antepartum glucocorticoid treatment for prevention of RDS in premature infants. Pediatrics 1972, 50:515-25.
7. Mwansa-Kambafwile J, Cousens S, Hansen T, Lawn JE: Antenatal steroids in preterm labour for the prevention of neonatal deaths due to complications of preterm birth. Int J Epidemiol 2010, 39(Suppl 1):i122-i133.
8. Sharma Gaurav, Mathai Matthews, Dickson Eva Kim, Weeks Andrew, Hofmeyr Justus G, Lavender Tina, Day Tina Louise, Mathews Elizabeth Jiji, Fawcus Sue, Simen-Kapeu Aline, de Bernis Luc: Quality care during labour and birth: a multi-country analysis of health system bottlenecks and potential solutions. BMC Pregnancy Childbirth 2015, 15(Suppl 2):S2.
9. Moxon GSarah, Lawn EJoy, Dickson EKim, Simen-Kapeu Aline, Gupta Gagan, Deorari Ashok, Singhal Nalini, New Karen, Kenner Carole, Bhutani Vinod, Kumar Rakesh, Molyneux Elizabeth, Blencowe Hannah: Inpatient care of small and sick newborns: a multi-country analysis of health system bottlenecks and potential solutions. BMC Pregnancy Childbirth 2015, 15(Suppl 2):S7.
10. Vesel Linda, Bergh Anne-Marie, Kerber Kate, Valsangkar Bina, Mazia Goldy, Moxon GSarah, Blencowe Hannah, Darmstadt LGary, de Graft Johnson Joseph, Dickson EKim, Ruiz Peláez Gabriel Juan, von Xylander Ritter Severin, Lawn EJoy, On behalf of the KMC Research Acceleration Group: Kangaroo mother care: a multi-country analysis of health system bottlenecks and potential solutions. BMC Pregnancy Childbirth 2015, 15(Suppl 2):S5.
11. Enweronu-Laryea Christabel, Dickson EKim, Moxon GSarah, Simen-Kapeu Aline, Nyange Christabel, Niermeyer Susan, Sobel LHoward, Lee CCAnne, von Xylander Ritter Severin, Lawn EJoy: Basic newborn care and neonatal resuscitation: a multi-country analysis of health system bottlenecks and potential solutions. BMC Pregnancy Childbirth 2015, 15(Suppl 2):S4.
12. Althabe F, Belizán JM, McClure EM, Hemingway-Foday J, Berrueta M, Mazzoni A, et al: A population-based, multifaceted strategy to implement antenatal corticosteroid treatment versus standard care for the reduction of neonatal mortality due to preterm birth in low-income and middle-income countries: the ACT cluster-randomised trial. Lancet 2015, 385(9968):629-639.
13. WHO: WHO recommendations on intervention to improve preterm birth outcomes. 2015, Available from: http://apps.who.int/iris/bitstream/10665/183037/1/9789241508988_eng.pdf?ua=1.
14. WHO: Integrated Management of Pregnancy and Childbirth - Managing Complications in Pregnancy and Childbirth: A guide for midwives and doctors. Geneva; 2000, Reprinted 2007.
15. NIH Consensus Development Panel: The Effect of Corticosteroids for Fetal Maturation on Perinatal Outcomes. NIH Consens Statement 1994, 12(2):1-24.
16. ACOG Committee on Obstetric Practice: ACOG Committee Opinion No. 475: Antenatal corticosteroid therapy for fetal maturation. Obstet Gynecol 2011, 117:422-4.
17. RCOG: Antenatal Corticosteroids to Reduce Neonatal Morbidity and Mortality., Green-top Guideline No. 7. https://www.rcog.org.uk/globalassets/documents/guidelines/gtg_7.pdf.
18. WAPM and Matres Mundi International: Recommendations and Guidelines for Perinatal Medicine. Barcelona; 2007.
19. FIGO, IPA: Joint FIGO and IPA statement on Prevention and Treatment of Preterm Births., August 3rd, 2012. http://ipa-world.org/Born%20Too%20Soon%20jul10%202012.pdf.
20. Stoll BJ, Hansen NI, Bell EF, Shankaran S, Laptook AR, Walsh MC, et al: Eunice Kennedy Shriver National Institute of Child Health and Human Development Neonatal Research Network: Neonatal outcomes of extremely preterm infants from the NICHD Neonatal Research Network. Pediatrics 2010, 126(3):443-456.
21. March of Dimes, PMNCH, Save the Children, WHO: Born Too Soon: the global action report on preterm birth. Geneva: World Health Organization; Howson C, Kinney M, Lawn J 2012.
22. Bhutta ZA, Das JK, Bahl R, Lawn JE, Salam RA, Paul VK, et al: Lancet Newborn Interventions Review Group; Lancet Every Newborn Study Group: Can available interventions end preventable deaths in mothers, newborn babies, and stillbirths, and at what cost? Lancet 2014, 384(9940):347-70.
23. McClure EM, de Graft-Johnson J, Jobe AH, Wall S, Koblinsky M, Moran A, et al: Maternal and Child Health Integrated Project (MCHIP) Antenatal Corticosteroid Conference Working Group: A conference report on prenatal corticosteroid use in low- and middle-income countries. Int J Gynaecol Obstet 2011, 115(3):215-9.
24. Dickson EKim, Kinney VMary, Moxon GSarah, Ashton Joanne, Zaka Nabila, Simen-Kapeu Aline, Sharma Gaurav, Kerber JKate, Daelmans Bernadette, Gülmezoglu Metin A, Mathai Matthews, Nyange Christabel, Baye Martina, Lawn EJoy: Scaling up quality care for mothers and newborns around the time of birth: an overview of methods and analyses of intervention-specific bottlenecks and solutions. BMC Pregnancy Childbirth 2015, 15(Suppl 2):S1.
25. Dickson KE, Simen-Kapeu A, Kinney MV, Huicho L, Vesel L, Lackritz E, et al: Every Newborn: health-systems bottlenecks and strategies to accelerate scale-up in countries. Lancet 2014, 384(9941):438-454.
26. Chang HH, Larson J, Blencowe H, Spong CY, Simpson JL, Lawn JE: Preterm births in countries with a very high human development index - Authors' reply. Lancet 2013, 381(9875):1356-7.
27. Lawn JE, Davidge R, Paul VK, von Xylander S, de Graft Johnson J, Costello A, et al: Born too soon: care for the preterm baby. Reprod Health 2013, 10(Suppl 1):S5.
28. Mason E, McDougall L, Lawn JE, Gupta A, Claeson M, Pillay Y, et al: Every Newborn: From evidence to action to deliver a healthy start for the next generation. Lancet 2014, 384(9941):455-67.
29. Moxon GSarah, Ruysen Harriet, Kerber JKate, Amouzou Agbessi, Fournier Suzanne, Grove John, Moran CAllisyn, Vaz MELara, Blencowe Hannah, Conroy Niall, Gülmezoglu Metin A, Vogel PJoshua, Rawlins Barbara, Sayed Rubayet, Hill Kathleen, Vivio Donna, Qazi Shamim, Sitrin Deborah, Seale CAnna, Wall Steve, Jacobs Troy, Ruiz Peláez Gabriel Juan, Guenther Tanya, Coffey SPatricia, Dawson Penny, Marchant Tanya, Waiswa Peter, Deorari Ashok, Enweronu-Laryea Christabel, Arifeen El Shams, Lee CCAnne, Mathai Matthews, Lawn EJoy: Count every newborn; a measurement improvement roadmap for coverage data. BMC Pregnancy Childbirth 2015, 15(S2):S8.
30. UNICEF: The State of the World's Children 2015: Maternal and Newborn Health. New York; 2015.

31. WHO: WHO recommendations: Optimizing health worker roles to improve access to key maternal and newborn health interventions through task shifting. WHO, Geneva; 2012.

32. Crowther CA, Harding JE, Middleton PF, Andersen CC, Ashwood P, Robinson JS: Australasian randomised trial to evaluate the role of maternal intramuscular dexamethasone versus betamethasone prior to preterm birth to increase survival free of childhood neurosensory disability (A*STEROID): study protocol. BMC Preg Childbirth 2013, 13(104).

33. Antenatal Corticosteroids Working Group: Dexamethasone versus betamethasone as an antenatal corticosteroid (ACS). Healthy Newborn Network; 2013 Available from: http://www.healthynewbornnetwork.org/sites/default/files/resources/ACS%20Beta%20vs%20Dexa%20130820.pdf.

34. Lawn JE, Althabe F: Proposal for the inclusion (as an additional purpose) on the WHO Model List of Essential Medicines of dexamethasone for accelerating lung maturation in preterm babies. 2012 [http://www.who.int/selection_medicines/committees/expert/19/applications/Dexamethasone_29_C_NI.pdf].

35. WHO: Model List of Essential Medicines. 18th List. Geneva; 2013 [http://www.who.int/medicines/publications/essentialmedicines/18th_EML_Final_web_8Jul13.pdf].

36. Data of Indian Population 2011 Census. [http://www.census2011.co.in/p/about.php].

37. Gabrysch S, Civitelli G, Edmond KM, Mathai M, Ali M, Bhutta ZA, et al: New signal functions to measure the ability of health facilities to provide routine and emergency newborn care. PLoS Med 2012, 9(11):e1001340.

38. Jones G, Steketee RW, Black RE, Bhutta ZA, Morris SS: How many child deaths can we prevent this year? Lancet 2003, 362(9377):65-71.

39. Vogel JP, Souza JP, Gulmezoglu AM, Mori R, Lumbiganon P, Qureshi Z, et al: Use of antenatal corticosteroids and tocolytic drugs in preterm births in 29 countries: an analysis of the WHO Multicountry Survey on Maternal and Newborn Health. Lancet 2014, 384(9957):1869-1877.

40. Bhutta ZA, Das JK, Bahl R, Lawn JE, Salam RA, Paul VK, et al: Can available interventions end preventable deaths in mothers, newborn babies, and stillbirths, and at what cost? Lancet 2014, 384(9940):347-370.

41. Tita AT, Selwyn BJ, Waller DK, Kapadia AS, Dongmo S: Evidence-based reproductive health care in Cameroon: population-based study of awareness, use and barriers. Bull World Health Organ 2005, 83(12):895-903.

42. Krauss Silva L, Pinheiro T, Franklin R, Oliveira N: Assessment of quality of obstetric care and corticoid use in preterm labor. Cadernos de Salude Publica 1999, 15(4):1-23.

43. Riganti AA, Cafferata ML, Althabe F, Gibbons L, Segarra JO, Sandoval X, et al: Use of prenatal corticosteroids for preterm birth in three Latin American countries. Int J Gynaecol Obstet 2010, 108:52-57.

44. Pattanittum P, Ewens MR, Laopaiboon M, Lumbiganon P, McDonald SJ, Crowther CA: Use of antenatal corticosteroids prior to preterm birth in four South East Asian countries within the SEA-ORCHID project. BMC Preg Childbirth 2008, 8:47.

45. Leviton LC, Goldenberg RL, Baker CS, Schwartz RM, Freda MC, Fish LJ, et al: Methods to encourage the use of antenatal corticosteroid therapy for fetal maturation: a randomized controlled trial. JAMA 1999, 281(1):46-52.

46. Althabe F, Bergel E, Cafferata ML, Gibbons L, Ciapponi A, Alemán A, et al: Strategies for improving the quality of health care in maternal and child health in low- and middle-income countries: an overview of systematic reviews. Paediatr Perinat Epidemiol 2008, 22(Suppl 1):42-60.

47. Althabe F, Buekens P, Bergel E, Belizán JM, Campbell MK, Moss N, et al: A behavioral intervention to improve obstetrical care. N Engl J Med 2008, 358(18):1929-40.

Time trends and risk factor associated with premature birth and infants deaths due to prematurity in Hubei Province, China from 2001 to 2012

Haiqing Xu[1], Qiong Dai[1], Yusong Xu[1], Zhengtao Gong[1], Guohong Dai[1], Ming Ding[2], Christopher Duggan[2,3], Zubin Hu[1] and Frank B. Hu[2*]

Abstract

Background: The nutrition and epidemiologic transition has been associated with an increasing incidence of preterm birth in developing countries, but data from large observational studies in China have been limited. Our study was to describe the trends and factors associated with the incidence of preterm birth and infant mortality due to prematurity in Hubei Province, China.

Methods: We conducted a population-based survey through the Maternal and Child Health Care Network in Hubei Province from January 2001 to December 2012. We used data from 16 monitoring sites to examine the trend and risk factors for premature birth as well as infant mortality associated with prematurity.

Results: A total of 818,481 live births were documented, including 76,923 preterm infants (94 preterm infants per 1,000 live births) and 2,248 deaths due to prematurity (2.75 preterm deaths per 1,000 live births). From 2001 to 2012, the incidence of preterm birth increased from 56.7 to 105.2 per 1,000 live births (P for trend < 0.05), while the infant mortality rate due to prematurity declined from 95.0 to 13.4 per 1,000 live births (P for trend < 0.05). Older maternal age, lower maternal education, use of assisted reproductive technology (ART), higher income, residence in urban areas, and infant male sex were independently associated with a higher incidence of preterm birth (all p values < 0.05). Shorter gestation, lower birth weight, and lower income were associated with a higher mortality rate, while use of newborn emergency transport services (NETS) was associated with a lower preterm mortality rate (all p values < 0.05).

Conclusion: An increasing incidence of preterm birth and a parallel reduction in infant mortality due to prematurity were observed in Hubei Province from 2001 to 2012. Our results provide important information for areas of improvements in reducing incidence and mortality of premature birth.

Background

Approximately 15 million infants are born prematurely each year, which is more than one tenth of all new-born infants globally [1]. Preterm infants have a high risk of birth complications, including infectious diseases, respiratory insufficiency, intraventricular hemorrhage, neurosensory deficits, and other organ system involvement [2]. Mortality due to complications of prematurity is the leading cause of neonatal death, and the second leading cause of death for children under age five [3]. Achieving Millenium Development Goal to reduce child mortality is therefore in large part dependent on reducing mortality related to premature birth [4].

For preterm infants who do survive, elevated risks for cognitive disorders and chronic non-communicable diseases exist [5, 6]. Preterm birth has been associated with elevated plasma insulin levels [7], altered growth

* Correspondence: nhbfh@channing.harvard.edu
[2]Department of Nutrition, Harvard School of Public Health, 655 Huntington Ave, Boston, MA 02115, USA
Full list of author information is available at the end of the article

patterns [5], and higher risk for cardiovascular diseases in adulthood [5]. The incidence of prematurity and subsequent risk of death due to prematurity-associated conditions is therefore an indicator of how women in a given country have access to safe and effective, pre- and post-natal medical care, as well as an indicator of the overall health of their society.

Large pooled analyses using data from multiple countries showed that the incidence of preterm birth has increased in recent years, with preterm birth an important risk factor for neonatal mortality [8, 9]. However, these analyses did not include data from China. One study analyzing the new-born information covering 2,377 monitoring sites in China showed that preterm birth complications are an important cause of child mortality in China [10]. The estimated number of preterm births (<37 weeks) was more than 250,000 in 2010 in China, ranking the second country behind India with the highest number of annual preterm births [11].

Economic development and government programs in China over the past two decades have together led to improved quantity and quality of maternal, child and newborn health care [11]. Secular trends in improved neonatal outcomes have not been well studied, however, including whether improved medical care has been evident in rural as well as rural settings [12]. Hubei Province is a large, economically, agriculturally and ethnically diverse province located in south-central China with approximately 57 million inhabitants. The aim of this study was therefore to describe secular trends in the incidence of premature birth as well as infant mortality linked with preterm birth in Hubei Province from 2001 to 2012, and to identify risk factors associated with these important health outcomes.

Methods
Study design
A random sampling stratified by urban and rural areas was conducted in Hubei Province, China. Sixteen counties were selected randomly by zip code from 9 urban areas and 13 rural areas as the monitoring sites, including 6 urban areas and 10 rural areas.

Data collection
The annual number of live infant births at each of the monitoring sites was recorded by trained staff of the Maternal and Child Health Care Network in Hubei Province from January 1, 2001 to December 31, 2012.The data were collected based on an electrical "three vertical level" health care system in Hubei Province. The "three vertical levels" include community/countryside, city, and province.

Upon the birth of each infant within the monitoring sites, the basic information of the mothers was collected

in face-to-face interview before hospital discharge by a licensed and trained health care provider in each county. The basic information was recorded electronically through the health care system, which included maternal age, education, income, occupation, pregnancy parity, birth parity, residence, use of Newborn Emergency Transport Service, infant gender, and use of assisted reproductive technology. The gestational week was assessed by trained doctors based on early pregnancy symptoms, pregnancy tests, and B-mode ultrasound tests. The birth weight was measured by trained doctors after the infant was delivered. Electronic weighing scales were used to weigh the infants, and the accuracy of weight was to 0.01 kg.

After the basic information was collected, health care providers in the city to which the counties belong reviewed and verified the total number of live births, preterm births, and preterm mortality. If the preterm infant was lost to follow-up within the first year after the infant's birth due to migration, the migrated infant was identified by the connected health care system of the monitoring sites in other provinces of China.

Finally, the data on annual births within each city was reported to the Hubei Provincial Maternity and Child Care Hospital (HBPMCCH). Validation studies on the underreport rate were conducted by randomly selecting one of the monitoring sites.

HBPMCCH doctors independently collected and verified the data collected from the county health providers, and compared the data to reported data in the health care system. The underreported rate of live births decreased from 4.5 % (4.67 % in rural areas and 0.23 % in urban areas) in 2001 to 0.54 % (0.69 % in rural areas and 0.11 % in urban areas) in 2012. Written informed consent was obtained from at least one parent, and the study was approved by the Ethics Committee of Hubei Maternal and Child Health Hospital.

Definition of preterm birth incidence and mortality of preterm birth
Live birth refers to the complete expulsion or extraction from its mother of a product of conception, irrespective of the duration of the pregnancy [13]. Preterm birth is defined as all births less than 37 whole weeks of gestation or fewer than 259 days since the first day of a woman's last menstrual period, according to the WHO standards [3]. In accordance with the International Statistical Classification of Diseases and Related Health Problems, 10th Revision (ICD-10), preterm death was defined as death in the first year of life resulting from any cause related to preterm birth, but not from accidental causes [14]. Incidence of preterm birth was calculated as the ratio of the number of preterm live births to the number

of total live births. Incidence of preterm mortality was calculated as the ratio of the number of preterm deaths to the number of preterm live infants.

Statistical Analysis

To compare the difference of proportions between groups, a Chi-Square test was used with $P < 0.05$ indicating significant difference. To identify factors significantly associated with incidence of preterm birth and mortality, we initially included all covariates into the model and used logistic regression with backward stepwise selection. Candidate variables in the logistic model included year (continuous), maternal age (<35 y vs. ≥ 35 y), education (>9 years vs. ≤ 9 years), occupation (physical labor vs. office job), birth weight (<2.5 kg vs. ≥ 2.5 kg), pregnancy parity (1 vs. ≥ 2), birth parity (1 vs. ≥ 2), assisted reproductive technology (yes vs. no), income (<500 USD/month vs. ≥ 500 USD/month), residence (rural vs. urban), Newborn Emergency Transport Service (yes vs. no), infant gender (female vs. male), and gestational week (<34 week vs. ≥ 34 week). The maternal age, gestational week, and birth weight were dichotomized based on the literature. Education, pregnancy parity, birth parity, and income were dichotomized, with the largest number of participants as the reference group. For the variables with missing values, a missing indicator was used. The data was analyzed using the Statistical Package for the Social Sciences (SPSS) version 11.5.

Results

The overall preterm incidence and mortality rates of preterm birth

A total of 818,481 live births were documented in the 16 survey areas in Hubei Province between 2001 and 2012. The incidence of preterm birth increased from 56.7 per 1,000 live births in 2001 to 105.2 per 1,000 live births in 2012, while the incidence of preterm mortality decreased from 95.1 per 1,000 live births in 2001 to 13.4 per 1,000 live births in 2012 (Fig. 1).

The incidence of preterm birth in urban and rural areas

Of the 76,923 preterm infants, 45,292 were in urban areas, and 31,631 were in rural areas. Preterm incidence increased steadily from 2001 to 2012 in both urban and rural areas. Preterm incidence rate in 2012 was almost 2 times the preterm incidence rate in 2001 in both urban and rural areas (Fig. 2). The incidence of preterm birth in the rural areas was lower than in the urban areas for each year. However, the trends between the rural and urban areas appeared to be similar.

The incidence of preterm birth for both genders increased steadily from 2001 to 2012. The trends for males and females appeared to be similar (Fig. 3).

The mortality of preterm birth in urban and rural areas

Of the 2,248 preterm deaths, 1,025 were in rural areas, and 1,123 were in urban areas. The mortality of preterm birth in rural areas decreased from 2001 to 2012, although an inverse V-shaped fluctuation pattern was observed. The mortality of preterm birth in 2012 was almost one-tenth the incidence in 2001. The mortality of preterm birth in urban areas also showed a downward trend with fluctuation from 2001 to 2012. The downward trend of mortality of preterm birth was steeper for rural areas than for urban areas, with the convergence of the two curves around 2012 (Fig. 4).

The overall trend and fluctuation patterns for both males and females were similar to Fig. 4. The preterm mortality rate was higher for males than females from 2001 to 2006 and converged thereafter (Fig. 5).

Factors significantly associated with the incidence and mortality of preterm births

Characteristics of the covariates of the study population were shown in Table 1. We firstly performed univariate

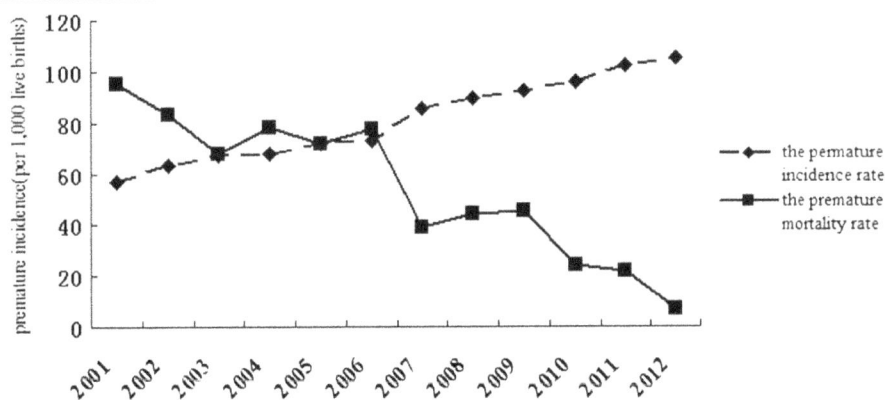

Fig. 1 Annual incidence and mortality of preterm birth in Hubei Province from 2001 to 2012. P value was obtained by fitting logistic models with year (continuous) as the independent variable

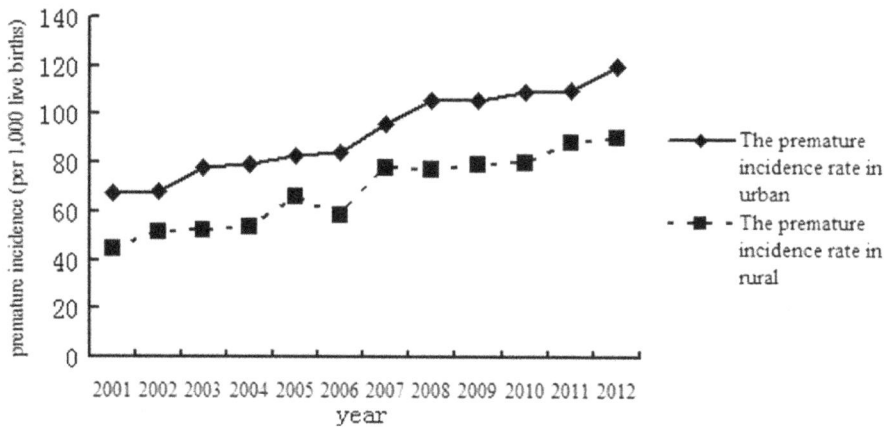

Fig. 2 The incidence rates of preterm birth in urban and rural areas in Hubei Province from 2001 to 2012

analysis to assess the associations between covariates shown in table 1 with risks of preterm birth and preterm mortality (Table 1, Table 2). After backward stepwise selection, older age of delivery, lower level of education, ART use, higher income, residence in urban areas, and being male were associated with significantly higher incidence of preterm birth (Table 2). Insufficient gestational week, lower birth weight, and lower income were associated with significantly higher mortality of preterm birth, while improved NETS were associated with significantly lower mortality of preterm birth (Table 3).

Sensitivity analysis

Given that plurality birth might be an important risk factor of preterm birth and preterm mortality [15], we conducted stratified analysis by singletons and multiples on the risk factors of preterm birth and preterm mortality. The risk factors identified by backward stepwise selection did not change within each stratum (Additional file 1: Table S1–S4).

Discussion

The incidence rate of preterm birth increased gradually from 56.7 to 105.2 per 1,000 live births, which was comparable to the overall preterm birth rate in China (7.1 %) in 2011 [16], while the incidence of preterm mortality decreased remarkably from 95.1 to 13.4 per 1,000 live births from 2001 to 2012 in Hubei Province, China. In this large sample, we identified significant predictors of incidence and mortality of preterm births.

Preterm birth occurs for a variety of reasons. Early induction of labor or cesarean birth, either for medical or non-medical reasons are causes of some of the preterm births. Most preterm births occur spontaneously [17]. Multiple pregnancies, infections, and chronic conditions such as diabetes and high blood pressure are common established causes. In addition, the use of ovulation inducing medications and intrauterine infections may also have contributed to the rise in the preterm birth rate.

Our study showed that the incidence and mortality of preterm birth differed in urban and rural areas. The

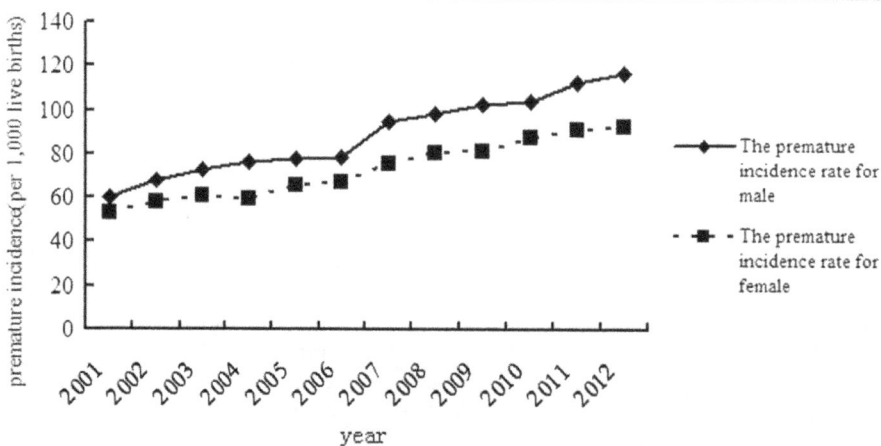

Fig. 3 The incidence of preterm birth for males and females in Hubei Province from 2001 to 2012

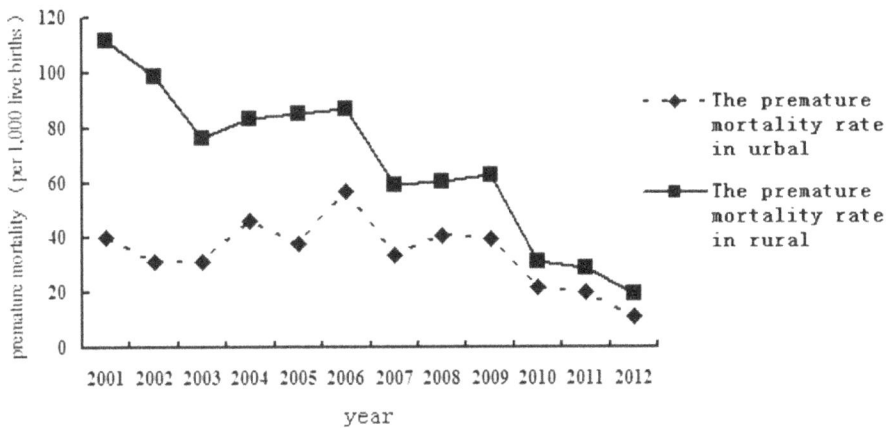

Fig. 4 Changes in infant mortality rate due to prematurity in urban and rural areas in Hubei Province from 2001 to 2012

regions in Hubei Province were divided into urban and rural areas according to the local economic development and population density of these areas. From 2001 to 2012, the incidence of preterm birth in urban areas was about 1.5 times that of rural areas, while the incidence of preterm mortality decreased faster in urban areas than in rural areas. The results of this study showed that premature incidence and mortality were associated with social-economic development of the area. Our results were similar to a study in North Carolina which found incidence of preterm birth was more pronounced in urban residents [18]. Economic development is not well balanced in Hubei Province. Our study found that higher income was a risk factor of preterm birth but a protective factor for the mortality of preterm birth. The shift to an urban lifestyle leads to increased work pressure, a delay of child-delivering age, and increased adolescent pregnancy (early marriage) risk, which are all factors associated with high rates of preterm births [19]. Previous studies have shown that preterm delivery often occurs in women aged <19 years old or >35 years old [20]. Our

study found that the incidence of preterm birth was positively associated with maternal age (years) ≥35. In addition, preterm incidence was significantly higher in women who used assisted reproductive technology for conception than women with natural conception [21]. Seven hospitals in urban areas were allowed to carry out human assisted reproductive technology in Hubei. This may explain the disparity of the incidence of preterm birth between urban and rural areas in the province.

In our study, except for in 2012, preterm mortality in urban areas was lower than rural areas. Although a great achievement has been made in reducing preterm mortality in Hubei Province, it is still relatively high in poor areas. Our study found that preterm mortality risk is lower for residents in urban areas. In fact, most preterm deaths and disabilities attributable to childbirth are avoidable, as there are medical solutions to prevent or manage preterm-related complications that cause preterm death. Thus, the establishment and improvement of the three-level health care network for women and children in China has proven to be

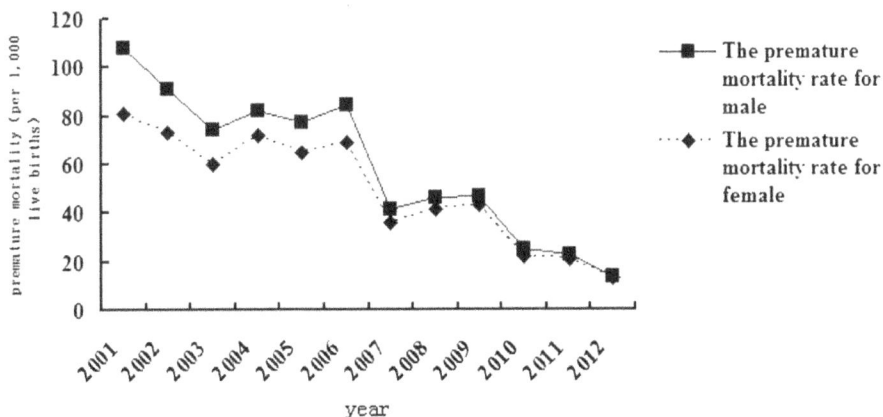

Fig. 5 Changes in infant mortality rate due to prematurity for males and females in Hubei Province from 2001 to 2012

Table 1 Characteristics of the covariates according to outcome status of preterm birth and preterm mortality

	Number of live birth	Number of preterm birth	Number of deaths due to prematurity	Preterm birth rate (%)	Preterm mortality rate (‰)
Number of participants	818481	76923	2248	9.40	2.75
Maternal age (years)					
<35	580486	27693	961	4.77	1.66
35+	237995	49230	1287	20.69	5.41
Gestational week (weeks)					
<34	189486	23077	1753	12.18	9.25
34+	628995	53846	495	8.56	0.79
Birth weight (kg)					
<2.5	344491	43994	1674	12.77	4.86
2.5+	473990	32929	574	6.95	1.21
Pregnancy parity					
1	94901	43808	1471	46.16	15.50
1+	723580	33115	777	4.58	1.07
Birth parity					
1	61375	31638	987	51.55	16.08
1+	757106	45285	1261	5.98	1.67
Assisted reproductive technology (Yes)					
Yes	30959	23469	756	75.81	24.40
No	787522	53454	1492	6.79	1.90
Income (USD/month)					
<500	418798	50392	1577	12.03	3.76
500+	399683	26531	671	6.64	1.68
Education					
College	74060	3315	68	4.48	0.91
Other	744421	73608	2180	9.89	2.93
Residence					
Urban	350154	45300	1123	12.94	3.21
Rural	468327	31623	1125	6.75	2.40
Newborn Emergency Transport Service					
Yes	12755	5562	48	43.60	3.75
No	805726	71361	2200	8.86	2.73
Infant gender					
Male	415496	44346	1348	10.67	3.24
Female	402985	32577	900	8.08	2.23
Occupation					
Office job	447921	20562	477	4.59	1.07
Other	370560	56361	1771	15.21	4.78
Single birth					
Yes	787168	73715	2229	9.36	2.83
No	31313	3208	19	10.24	0.60

effective and essential for immediate access to high-quality maternal health care both in rural and urban areas [22, 23].

From 2001 to 2012, premature incidence and mortality for males were higher than females, consistent with previous studies. Several mechanisms have been proposed

Table 2 Regression analysis identifying factors associated with preterm birth in Hubei Province, China (2001 – 2012)

Covariates	Univariate analysis OR (95 % CI)	Multivariable analysis* OR (95 % CI)
Year	1.01 (1.00 - 1.01)	——
Maternal age (<35 y vs. ≥ 35 y)	5.28 (5.04 - 5.45)	0.57 (0.55-0.58)
Gestational week(<34 week vs. ≥ 34 week)	2.21 (1.86 - 2.63)	——
Birth weight(<2.5 kg vs. ≥ 2.5 kg)	1.08 (1.05 -1.13)	——
Pregnancy parity (1 vs. ≥ 2)	2.80 (2.69 - 2.95)	——
Birth parity (1 vs. ≥ 2)	1.08 (1.01 - 1.10)	——
Assisted reproductive technology(yes vs. no)	1.97 (1.91 -2.05)	3.67 (3.56-3.78)
Income (<500 USD/month vs. ≥ 500 USD/month)	1.27 (1.22- 1.32)	0.63 (0.61-0.66)
Education (>9 years vs. ≤ 9 years)	0.71 (0.49 - 0.91)	1.04 (1.01-1.06)
Residence (rural vs. urban)	1.37 (1.35 - 1.39)	1.27 (1.24-1.30)
Newborn Emergency Transport Service (yes vs. no)	3.13 (3.02 - 3.23)	——
Infant gender (female vs. male)	0.59 (0.56 - 0.63)	3.31 (3.23 -3.39)
Occupation (physical labor vs. office job)	2.16 (2.09 - 2.23)	——
Single birth	0.91 (0.89 - 0.97)	——

*Multivariate logistic model was fit with all characteristics considered as predictors of preterm birth, and a backward-selection procedure was used to select significant variables included in the final model, with a P value < 0.05 indicating significance

Table 3 Regression analysis identifying factors associated with preterm mortality in Hubei Province, China (2001 – 2012)

Covariates	Univariate analysis OR (95 % CI)	Multivariable analysis* OR (95 % CI)
Year	1.00 (1.00 -1.01)	——
Maternal age (<35 y vs. ≥ 35 y)	1. 32 (1. 22–1.51)	——
Gestational week (<34 week vs. ≥ 34 week)	2.76 (1.92 -2.99)	1.01 (1.00-1.02)
Birth weight (<2.5 kg vs. ≥ 2.5 kg)	1.07 (1.02 - 1.11)	1.02 (1.00-1.03)
Pregnancy parity (1 vs. ≥ 2)	1.08 (1.08 -1.11)	——
Birth parity (1 vs. ≥ 2)	1.00 (1.00 - 1.01)	——
Assisted reproductive technology (yes vs. no)	1.13 (1.09-1.15)	——
Income (<500 USD/month vs. ≥ 500 USD/month)	1.31 (1.27 -1.39)	1.12 (1.01-1.22)
Education (>9 years vs. ≤ 9 years)	0.71 (0. 49–0. 89)	——
Residence (rural vs. urban)	1.14 (1.10 - 1.29)	——
Newborn Emergency Transport Service (yes vs. no)	2. 14 (2.00 - 3.02)	0.81 (0.77-0.99)
Infant gender (female vs. male)	0.67 (0.51 - 0.74)	——
Occupation (physical labor vs. office job)	1.18 (1.10 -1.23)	——
Single birth	0.97 (0.95 - 0.99)	——

*Multivariate logistic model was fit with all characteristics considered as predictors of preterm mortality, and a backward-selection procedure was used to select significant variables included in the final model, with a P value < 0.05 indicating significance

to explain why pregnancies carrying male fetuses could have a higher risk of preterm birth. First, heavier body weight of the male fetus increases the probability of using preterm labor [24]. Second, there is a greater susceptibility to gestational hypertension or infection which are associated with preterm birth. Third, male and female fetuses may have different sex-linked biochemical processes, including estrogen production from androgen precursors or by interleukin-1 [25]. In addition, male infants are more likely to have lower Apgar scores, and more likely to have respiratory distress syndrome or lung related injuries and disabilities [24].

Our study identified several factors that were associated with incidence and mortality of preterm birth. Unhealthy habits and lack of health knowledge are factors associated with preterm infant deaths [26]. It is essential that elementary obstetric and neonatology health providers are professionally trained in order to increase their capacity to successfully manage severe newborn complications such as intracranial hemorrhage [27]. Higher total expenditures on health per capita are

one of the factors associated with lower preterm mortality. Other important factors associated with low hospitalized delivery rates include inability to pay for expenditure of health care, and inconvenient transportation in rural and mountain areas, which delays the transfer of severely sick neonates among hospitals.

Our study found that higher preterm mortality risk is associated with lower per capita GDP. In poor areas, most of the preterm infants died at home immediately after leaving the delivery hospital. Some preterm infants born in low-income regions die within their first few days of life. In poor regions, even for those born in a clinic or hospital, primary neonatal care is often lacking [28]. The risk of a neonatal death due to complications of preterm birth is higher in poor than rich regions [29]. To reduce preterm birth, a priority system should be set up for tracking and providing emergency treatment to preterm children.

With rapid socio-economic development, as well as improvements in obstetrics and neonatal rescue technology, the neonatal transport network was set up to decrease preterm child mortality. Our study found that lower preterm mortality risk was associated with improved newborn emergency transport services. Essential newborn car includes thermal care, breastfeeding support, and infection prevention and management and, if needed, neonatal resuscitation. Extra care for small babies, such as Kangaroo Mother Care program (e.g., carrying the baby skin-to-skin, and additional support for breastfeeding), was estimated to save approximately 450,000 babies each year [30]. Care for preterm babies with complications includes treating infections with antibiotics, safe oxygen management, supportive care for respiratory distress syndrome, continuous positive airway pressure and/or surfactant, and neonatal intensive care for those regions with lower mortality and higher health system capacity [31].

There were several potential limitations in our study. First, we did not differentiate iatrogenic and spontaneous preterm birth. The higher rate of preterm birth over time might be due to the advanced technologies, such as induction of labour and cesarean section. It has been shown that in the United States, the increase of cesarean birth is in part responsible for the overall increase in the preterm birth rate from 1990 to 2007 and the decline in perinatal mortality [32]. Second, the ultrasound dating (USS) is more widely used to estimate gestational age nowadays instead of latest menopausal period (LMP), which has low accuracy due to the considerable variation in the length of menstrual cycle among women. A study conducted in Canada showed that the USS was associated with a higher rate of preterm birth than LMP [33]. However, we did not obtain detailed data on the estimation method of prematurity. Third, our preterm birth and infant mortality only included live births, and stillbirth was not taken into account [34]. Thus, the incidence and mortality rate of preterm birth might be underestimated in our study. Fourth, stillbirth in less developed areas might be turned into live birth in more developed areas, and this might contribute to the higher incidence of live birth in urban than rural areas. However, this phenomenon, even if true, could not explain the increasing trend of preterm birth in both urban and rural areas over time.

Conclusions

In summary, an increase in the incidence of preterm birth and a decrease in the mortality rate of preterm birth were observed in Hubei Province from 2001 to 2012. Our results showed that delivery at an advanced maternal age, use of ART, and the lack of NETS were associated with increased incidence and mortality of preterm birth. Our results provide important information for areas of improvements in reducing incidence and mortality of premature birth.

Additional file

Additional file 1: Table S1. Multivariable regression analysis identifying factors associated with preterm birth in Hubei Province, China from 2001 to 2012 among single birth infants. **Table S2.** Multivariable regression analysis identifying factors associated with preterm mortality in Hubei Province, China (2001 – 2012) among single birth infants. **Table S3.** Multivariable regression analysis identifying factors associated with preterm birth in Hubei Province, China from 2001 to 2012 among multiple birth infants. **Table S4.** Multivariable regression analysis identifying factors associated with preterm mortality in Hubei Province, China (2001 – 2012) among multiple birth infants.

Abbreviations
ART: Assisted reproductive technology; GDP: Gross domestic production; NETS: Newborn emergency transport services.

Competing interests
The authors declare that they have no competing interests.

Authors' contributions
FH, ZH, and HX conceived and designed the study. HX, QD, YX, ZG, GD, MD collected and analysed data and drafted the manuscript. FH and CD advised in the design of the study, data collection, analysis and interpretation of findings as well as critically commenting on the draft manuscript. All authors read and approved the final manuscript.

Acknowledgments
We sincerely thank all the staff for monitoring maternal mortality in the 16 areas of Hubei Province.

Author details
[1]Department of Child Health Care, Hubei Maternal and Child Health Hospital, Wuhan, China. [2]Department of Nutrition, Harvard School of Public Health, 655 Huntington Ave, Boston, MA 02115, USA. [3]Boston Children's Hospita, Boston, Massachusetts, USA.

Reference
1. The global burden of preterm birth. Lancet 2009, 374(9697):1214.
2. Rudan I, Chan KY, Zhang JS, Theodoratou E, Feng XL, Salomon JA, et al. Causes of deaths in children younger than 5 years in China in 2008. Lancet. 2010;375(9720):1083–9.
3. Beck S, Wojdyla D, Say L, Betran AP, Merialdi M, Requejo JH, et al. The worldwide incidence of preterm birth: a systematic review of maternal mortality and morbidity. Bull World Health Organ. 2010;88(1):31–8.
4. Hogan MC, Foreman KJ, Naghavi M, Ahn SY, Wang M, Makela SM, et al. Maternal mortality for 181 countries, a systematic analysis of progress towards Millennium Development Goal 5. Lancet. 1980–2008;375(9726): 1609–23.
5. Mwaniki MK, Atieno M, Lawn JE, Newton CR. Long-term neurodevelopmental outcomes after intrauterine and neonatal insults: a systematic review. Lancet. 2012;379(9814):445–52.
6. Goldenberg RL, Gravett MG, Iams J, Papageorghiou AT, Waller SA, Kramer M, et al. The preterm birth syndrome: issues to consider in creating a classification system. Am J Obstet Gynecol. 2012;206(2):113–8.
7. Wang G, Divall S, Radovick S, Paige D, Ning Y, Chen Z, et al. Preterm birth and random plasma insulin levels at birth and in early childhood. JAMA. 2014;311(6):587–96.
8. Blencowe H, Cousens S, Oestergaard MZ, Chou D, Moller AB, Narwal R, et al. National, regional, and worldwide estimates of preterm birth rates in the year 2010 with time trends since 1990 for selected countries: a systematic analysis and implications. Lancet. 2012;379(9832):2162–72.
9. Katz J, Lee AC, Kozuki N, Lawn JE, Cousens S, Blencowe H, et al. Mortality risk in preterm and small-for-gestational-age infants in low-income and middle-income countries: a pooled country analysis. Lancet. 2013;382(9890): 417–25.

10. Rudan I, Chan KY, Zhang JS, Theodoratou E, Feng XL, Salomon JA, et al. Causes of deaths in children younger than 5 years in China in. Lancet. 2008; 375(9720):1083–9.

11. World Health Organization. Born Too Soon: The Global Action Report on Preterm Birth. 2012.

12. Feng XL, Guo S, Hipgrave D, Zhu J, Zhang L, Song L, et al. China's facility-based birth strategy and neonatal mortality: a population-based epidemiological study. Lancet. 2011;378(9801):1493–500.

13. WHO: http://www.who.int/healthinfo/statistics/indmaternalmortality/en/.

14. World Health Organization. International statistical classification of disease and related health problem (ICD-10). 1993.

15. King JP, Gazmararian JA, Shapiro-Mendoza CK. Disparities in mortality rates among US infants born late preterm or early term, 2003–2005. Matern Child Health J. 2014;18(1):233–41.

16. Zou L, Wang X, Ruan Y, Li G, Chen Y, Zhang W. Preterm birth and neonatal mortality in China in 2011. Int J Gynaecol Obstet. 2014;127(3):243–7.

17. Ip M, Peyman E, Lohsoonthorn V, Williams MA. A case–control study of preterm delivery risk factors according to clinical subtypes and severity. J Obstet Gynaecol Res. 2010;36(1):34–44.

18. Miranda ML, Anthopolos R, Edwards SE. Seasonality of poor pregnancy outcomes in North Carolina. N C Med J. 2011;72(6):447–53.

19. McDonald SD, McKinney B, Foster G, Taylor V, Lutsiv O, Pullenayegum E. The combined effects of maternal depression and excess weight on neonatal outcomes. Int J Obes (Lond). 2015;39(7):1033–40.

20. Gavin LE, Catalano RF, David-Ferdon C, Gloppen KM, Markham CM. A review of positive youth development programs that promote adolescent sexual and reproductive health. J Adolesc Health. 2010;46(3 Suppl):S75–91.

21. Wang YA, Sullivan EA, Black D, Dean J, Bryant J, Chapman M. Preterm birth and low birth weight after assisted reproductive technology-related pregnancy in Australia between 1996 and 2000. Fertil Steril. 2005;83(6):1650–8.

22. Backman G, Hunt P, Khosla R, Jaramillo-Strouss C, Fikre BM, Rumble C, et al. Health systems and the right to health: an assessment of 194 countries. Lancet. 2008;372(9655):2047–85.

23. Anderson T. How can child and maternal mortality be cut? BMJ. 2010; 340:c431.

24. Zeitlin J, Saurel-Cubizolles MJ, De Mouzon J, Rivera L, Ancel PY, Blondel B, et al. Fetal sex and preterm birth: are males at greater risk? Hum Reprod. 2002;17(10):2762–8.

25. Stevenson DK, Verter J, Fanaroff AA, Oh W, Ehrenkranz RA, Shankaran S, et al. Sex differences in outcomes of very low birthweight infants: the newborn male disadvantage. Arch Dis Child Fetal Neonatal Ed. 2000;83(3):F182–5.

26. World Health Organization. Keeping promises, measuring results: Commission on Information and Accountability for Women's and Children's Health. 2011.

27. Lawn JE, Bahl R, Bergstrom S, Bhutta ZA, Darmstadt GL, Ellis M, et al. Setting research priorities to reduce almost one million deaths from birth asphyxia by 2015. PLoS Med. 2011;8(1), e1000389.

28. World Health Organization. WHO-UNICEF Joint Statement on home visits for the newborn child: a strategy to improve survival. 2009.

29. Lawn JE, Kinney M, Lee AC, Chopra M, Donnay F, Paul VK, et al. Reducing intrapartum-related deaths and disability: can the health system deliver? Int J Gynaecol Obstet. 2009;107 Suppl 1:S123–40. S140-122.

30. Lawn JE, Mwansa-Kambafwile J, Horta BL, Barros FC, Cousens S. Kangaroo mother care' to prevent neonatal deaths due to preterm birth complications. Int J Epidemiol. 2010;39 Suppl 1:i144–54.

31. Sweet D, Bevilacqua G, Carnielli V, Greisen G, Plavka R, Saugstad OD, et al. European consensus guidelines on the management of neonatal respiratory distress syndrome. J Perinat Med. 2007;35(3):175–86.

32. Ananth CV, Vintzileos AM. Epidemiology of preterm birth and its clinical subtypes. J Matern Fetal Neonatal Med. 2006;19(12):773–82.

33. Blondel B, Kaminski M. Trends in the occurrence, determinants, and consequences of multiple births. Semin Perinatol. 2002;26(4):239–49.

34. Evans DJ, Levene MI. Evidence of selection bias in preterm survival studies: a systematic review. Arch Dis Child Fetal Neonatal Ed. 2001;84(2):F79–84.

Neonatal and maternal outcomes following midtrimester preterm premature rupture of the membranes

Laura Aoife Linehan[1*], Jennifer Walsh[1], Aoife Morris[1], Louise Kenny[1,2], Keelin O'Donoghue[1], Eugene Dempsey[3] and Noirin Russell[1]

Abstract

Background: Preterm premature rupture of membranes (PPROM) complicates 1 % of all pregnancies and occurs in one third of all preterm deliveries. Midtrimester PPROM is often followed by spontaneous miscarriage and elective termination of ongoing pregnancies is offered in many countries. The aim of this retrospective descriptive cohort study was to investigate the natural history of midtrimester PPROM in a jurisdiction where termination of pregnancy in the absence of maternal compromise is unavailable.

Methods: Cases of midtrimester PPROM diagnosed between 14 and 23 + 6 weeks' gestation during April 2007 to June 2012 were identified following a manual search of all birth registers, pregnancy loss registers, annual reports, ultrasound reports, emergency room registers and neonatal death certificates at Cork University Maternity Hospital - a large (circa 8500 births per annum) tertiary referral maternity hospital in southwest Ireland. Cases where delivery occurred within 24 h of PPROM were excluded.

Results: The prevalence of midtrimester PPROM was 0.1 % (42 cases/44,667 births). The mean gestation at PPROM was 18 weeks. The mean gestation at delivery was 20 + 5 weeks, with an average latency period of 13 days.
Ten infants were born alive (23 %; 10/42). The remainder (77 %; 32/42) died in utero or intrapartum. Nine infants were resuscitated. Two infants survived to discharge. The overall mortality rate was 95 % (40/42).
Five women had clinical chorioamnionitis (12 %; 5/42) but 69 % demonstrated histological chorioamnionitis. One woman developed sepsis (2.4 %; 1/42). Other maternal complications included requirement of intravenous antibiotic treatment (38 %; 17/42), retained placenta (21 %, 9/42) and post-partum haemorrhage (12 %; 5/42).

Conclusions: This study provides useful and contemporary data on midtrimester PPROM. Whilst fetal and neonatal mortality is high, long-term survival is not impossible. The increased risk of maternal morbidity necessitates close surveillance.

Keywords: Preterm birth, Preterm premature rupture of membranes, Sepsis

* Correspondence: lauralinehan708@gmail.com
[1]The Department of Obstetrics and Gynaecology, University College Cork and Cork University Hospital, Cork, Ireland
Full list of author information is available at the end of the article

Background

Midtrimester preterm premature rupture of membranes (PPROM) is an uncommon complication, occurring in less than 1 % of pregnancies [1]. PPROM is an important contributor to perinatal mortality and morbidity; in pregnancies that continue following PPROM at early gestations, morbidity is high among surviving neonates with problems including respiratory distress syndrome, pulmonary hypoplasia, intraventricular haemorrhage and limb contractures [2]. Pregnancies complicated by PPROM early in pregnancy, when the risk of pulmonary hypoplasia is highest, present a counselling and management dilemma. It is difficult to predict the eventual outcome as many factors impact on this – the development of sepsis, the eventual gestational age at delivery and the degree of oligohydramnios. There is a wide variety in chorioamnionitis rates and survival rates quoted in the literature. Chorioamnionitis ranged from 28 to 42 % [3, 4], whilst survival rates quoted range from 6.25 [3] to 100 % [5], dependant on gestation. Advances in neonatal care, particularly intensive care to those at the threshold of viability, have dramatically enhanced survival rates. These changes, which reflect a multimodal approach to care, include advances in newborn stabilisation, surfactant administration, optimising respiratory support, the use of nitric oxide and reduction in associated morbidities such as infection and intraventricular haemorrhage and the use of probiotics to reduce necrotising enterocolitis (NEC) [6].

There is a paucity of contemporary evidence about the natural history of these pregnancies as therapeutic termination of pregnancy is routinely offered as standard care in many countries. Termination of pregnancy was not available in Ireland during the time period of this study. However, the publication of the Protection of Life during Pregnancy Act in 2013, provided clarification that termination of pregnancy may be performed if there is a "real and substantial risk of loss of the woman's life from a physical illness" [7]. There remains an absence of clear guidance if there is no imminent threat to maternal life or health, even in the case of fatal fetal abnormality or where prognosis for the fetus is poor.

Thus, in Ireland when PPROM occurs at a pre-viable gestation but the fetus remains alive, management is problematic. Parents are counselled regarding the guarded prognosis and a care plan is established to provide regular monitoring for the woman. This usually involves regular fetal heart checks via ultrasound and close surveillance for signs and symptoms of maternal sepsis. If there is evidence of developing infection, it may be necessary to induce delivery. This is generally done medically using mifepristone and misoprostol. There is a paucity of information with which to counsel parents regarding fetal and neonatal survival, long term health outcome of surviving infants and the risk of maternal complications, particularly chorioamnionitis and sepsis, in these cases following PPROM at less than 24 weeks' gestation.

Our objective was to establish the natural history of midtrimester PPROM. We aimed to establish how many women in our hospital experienced midtrimester PPROM and to establish the associated neonatal and maternal health outcomes. We aimed to provide information to assist clinicians to accurately counsel women about maternal and fetal risks associated with midtrimester PPROM.

Methods

This study was a retrospective descriptive cohort study. Ethical approval was obtained from The Clinical Research and Ethics Committee of the Cork Teaching Hospitals in November 2010, (ref no: ECM 4 (o) 07/12/10), prior to study commencement. The committee deemed that informed written or verbal consent was not required. All women who presented to Cork University Maternity Hospital between April 2007 and June 2012 with midtrimester PPROM were included. Midtrimester was defined as 14 + 0 to 23 + 6 weeks' gestation. Women who delivered within 24 h of rupture of membranes were not included as we wished to exclude those with preterm birth without prolonged rupture of membranes and those where a PPROM is rapidly followed by a miscarriage. We specifically wished to study those patients who experience a midtrimester prolonged PPROM but do not deliver rapidly so that we could best advise this cohort about the exact risks this poses for them and their baby. A manual search was performed of all birth registers, pregnancy loss registers, annual reports, ultrasound reports, emergency room registers and neonatal death certificates of Cork University Maternity Hospital from April 2007 to June 2012. Cases of midtrimester PPROM were identified and a retrospective chart review was performed. In order to complete data collection on these cases, laboratory and radiology databases were also reviewed.

Our primary outcome measures were gestation at PPROM, gestation at delivery, latency period, neonatal survival rate and neonatal and maternal morbidity. The study was adherent to the STROBE criteria as outlined in Additional file 1.

Results

We identified 42 cases of ongoing pregnancy after midtrimester PPROM during the study period, during which 44,667 births occurred. This gives a prevalence of 0.1 %. Maternal demographics are outlined in Table 1. A PPROM was diagnosed when a sterile speculum examination clearly demonstrated liquor to be present in the posterior fornix of the vagina. An ultrasound was also performed to confirm oligohydramnios.

The majority of women had no significant underlying medical conditions (n = 35). One woman had antiphospholipid antibodies, one had hypothyroidism, two women

Table 1 Maternal Demographics

Maternal age	Average: 32	(Range 19–42, n = 42)
Race	Caucasian 31	(n = 38)
	African 7	
BMI (kg/m²)	Underweight 4	Average BMI 28
	Normal 13	(n = 32, range 17–46)
	Overweight 8	
	Obese 5	
	Morbidly Obese 2	
Smoker	Pre-pregnancy 9	
	Pregnancy 4	
Alcohol	Pregnancy 7 (1–10units/wk.)	
Recreational Drug Use	None	

had type 2 Diabetes Mellitus with Body Mass Indices (BMI; kg/m²) of 40 and 45, one woman had multiple sclerosis, one woman had a PT20210 mutation (an inherited genetic mutation involving the prothrombin gene which increases the risk of thrombosis 2–3 fold) and one woman was HIV positive.

The majority of women (60 %, n = 26) had attended for a dating ultrasound scan prior to PPROM. The remainder had their first ultrasound scan at diagnosis of PPROM and dates were assigned via measurement of the bi-parietal diameter, head circumference and femur length. Obstetric history is outlined in Table 2. Of note, 7 % (3/42) had experienced prior PPROM, 9.5 % (4/42) had a prior preterm birth, 4.75 % (2/42) had a previous midtrimester miscarriage and 7 % (3/42) had a previous third trimester loss. Three further women experienced

Table 2 Obstetric History

Gravidity	Average 2.6 (range 1–7)
Parity	Average 1 (range 0–3)
Primigravidas	12 (29 %)
Prior Preterm Rupture of Membranes	3 (7 %)
	i. 21/40
	ii. 27/40
	iii. 36/40
Prior Preterm Birth	4 (9.5 %)
	i. 35/40 and 36/40 (IOL for IUD)
	ii. 28/40
	iii. 36/40
	iv. 36/40
Intrauterine Death	1 (36/40)
Stillbirth	1 (term)
Neonatal Death	1 (33/40)
Midtrimester Miscarriage	2 (Both at 18/40)
First Trimester Miscarriage	16 (38 %)
• 2 or More	5 (12 %)

consecutive midtrimester PPROM during the study period and are included twice.

All women in our study received oral antibiotics, usually in the form of oral erythromycin. This is in keeping with the Royal College of Obstetricians and Gynaecologists (RCOG) Green Top Guideline No. 44 "Preterm Prelabour Rupture of Membranes" [8] which recommends that erythromycin is given for 10 days following a diagnosis of PPROM. In this scenario, antibiotics were prescribed in the maternal interest due to the risk of sepsis. The majority of women (80 %; 37/42) remained as inpatients to receive this treatment, with 25 women (58 %) delivering in this time period. The average length of stay was 8 nights (range 1–36). Patients received a weekly ultrasound scan to assess fetal wellbeing. The average amniotic fluid index at diagnosis of PPROM was 1 cm (range 0–2, n = 12). Antenatal corticosteroids were routinely administered at 24 weeks gestation. Thirty women delivered before 24 weeks and did not receive corticosteroids (range 15 + 6–23 + 3 weeks). Twelve women received intramuscular dexamethasone (28 %) and 83 % of these women (10/12) delivered a live infant. Two of these infants delivered at 23 + 6 weeks. One infant was not actively resuscitated and the other infant lived for 21 days. The single long term surviving infant in this cohort delivered at 23 + 3 weeks after PPROM at 23 + 1 weeks and did not receive antenatal steroids.

One woman presented with symptoms of acute chorioamnionitis and sepsis having experienced PPROM at home 2 days prior to presentation. She was induced in the maternal interest at 20 + 5 weeks and remained an inpatient for intravenous treatment and observation for 3 days, going on to make an uneventful recovery. A placental swab later indicated Group B streptococcal infection. Sixteen other women required intravenous antibiotics but were managed at ward level, without complications.

Twelve percent (n = 5) of women suffered clinical chorioamnionitis, but histological chorioamnionitis was found in 69 % of examined placentas. Twenty-five women had recorded treatment with antibiotics. Fourteen had oral erythromycin only, 16 required intravenous antibiotics, namely benzylpenicillin, co-amoxiclav, metronidazole, clindamycin and gentamicin.

Over 20 % of mothers, (9/42), experienced a retained placenta following delivery, thus requiring manual removal. Additionally, 13.9 % (6/42) of women had retained products of conception, four were treated conservatively with antibiotics and two required a surgical uterine evacuation. Other maternal complications are outlined in Table 3. Two women required blood transfusion related to manual removal of placenta.

The mean gestation at PPROM was 18 weeks (range 15 + 5–23 + 6, n = 37). Five women were unsure of exact date of PPROM. The average interval from PPROM to

Table 3 Other Maternal Complications

Non-Substantial Ante-Partum Haemorrhage(NSAPH) Prior To PPROM	18 (42 %)
Haemorrhage Following PPROM	18 (42 %)
Suspected Abruption	1 (Emergency Caesarean Delivery At 23 + 3)
Post-Partum Haemorrhage	5 (12 %)
Blood Transfusion	3 (7 %)

delivery was 13 days (range 1.1–85 days, $n = 37$) and the average gestation at delivery was 20 weeks + 5 days (range 17 + 4–29 + 4, $n = 42$). The average birth weight was 614 g ($n = 19$). Twenty-seven infants had gender recorded, 19 male and eight female. Ten infants were born alive (23 %) with an average birth weight of 740 g (range 440–1100 g) and an average gestational age of 25 + 2 weeks (range 23 + 3–29 + 4). The remainder (76 %; 32/42) died in utero ($n = 4$), intrapartum or at birth due to previability ($n = 28$). No infants weighing less than 500 g were resuscitated. When the infants were grouped according to age, no infants in whom PPROM was recorded to have occurred at less than 17 weeks ($n = 11$) survived, three infants in the 17–21 + 6 group ($n = 17$) were born alive and seven of the infants where PPROM occurred after 22 weeks ($n = 9$) were born alive. Of those born alive, 90 % (9/10) were resuscitated and admitted to the neonatal intensive care unit (NICU). Seven received surfactant. Six required intravenous antibiotics. The average length of stay in NICU was 34.6 days (range 2 h–146 days).

Three infants died within 2 h of birth, including the infant not admitted. One of these infants had been a PPROM at 17 weeks gestation and delivered at 25 + 3 with pulmonary hypoplasia and limb contractures. The other two infants had low APGAR scores at delivery and were treated palliatively without active resuscitation. Complications affecting neonatal survivors are outlined in Table 4.

Seven infants survived at least 7 days. Two infants survived to discharge. Both were female infants. One female infant was born at 29 + 4 after a latency period of 85 days weighing 930 g. She was transferred to another paediatric

Table 4 Neonatal Complications

Respiratory Distress Syndrome	7 (70 %, 100 % of those surviving beyond 2 h)
Sepsis	3 (30 %)
Coagulase Negative Staphylococcal (CONS) Sepsis	2 (20 %)
Patent Ductus Arteriosus (PDA)	4 (40 %)
Necrotising Enterocolitis (NEC)	2 (20 %)
Intraventricular Haemorrhage(IVH)	3 (30 %)

surgical institution at 20 days of age but subsequently died of Necrotising Enterocolitis at 8 weeks of age. The surviving neonate was born to a 24 year old African woman who was HIV positive. Rupture of membranes occurred at 23 + 1 weeks and delivery was 2 days later at 23 + 3 weeks. The mother developed oligohydramnios and clinical chorioamnionitis. Treatment of this woman involved oral erythromycin, oral co-amoxiclav, intravenous gentamicin, intravenous metronidazole and intravenous ceftriaxone. A female infant weighing 580 g was delivered. Length of stay in the neonatal intensive care unit was 146 days. Complications following birth included respiratory distress syndrome, patent ductus arteriosus, patent foramen ovale, grade two intraventricular haemorrhage and multiple seizures. The infant was discharged home alive with a diagnosis of chronic lung disease but is currently a healthy 4 year old who had met all her developmental milestones on discharge from neonatology follow-up.

After delivery, women were investigated for potential underlying causes of second trimester loss and also screened for infection. These investigations included blood counts, high vaginal swabs, mid-stream urinalysis, placental swabs, serology for cytomegalovirus, toxoplasma, syphilis, rubella and parvovirus B19, thyroid function tests, thrombophilia and autoantibody screens. Cytogenetics, post mortem and placental histological examination were also offered. All women were followed up postnatally in the pregnancy loss clinic to discuss their pregnancy events and outcome, to follow up on investigations and to formulate a management plan for subsequent pregnancies. They were also supported by the specialist midwifes in bereavement and loss and offered formal counselling support where desired.

Placental histology was available in 32 cases. Although only five women had clinical symptoms of chorioamnionitis (12 %; 5/42) there was histological chorioamnionitis in 69 % of examined placentas (22/42). Two further placentas demonstrated retroplacental haemorrhage and one demonstrated haemorrhagic infarction. The remainder were reported as normal (17 %; 7/42). Nine infants had cytogenetic analysis which all demonstrated normal karyotypes. Three infants underwent post mortem examination. These demonstrated anatomically normal infants.

Twenty-eight women (67 %) had high vaginal swabs- two swabs cultured group B streptococcus. Twenty women (48 %) had mid-stream urine samples sent, none of which demonstrated significant infection. Seven women (17 %) had placental swabs taken – one cultured group B streptococcus. Only the woman who developed sepsis had blood cultures taken.

Discussion

The incidence of midtrimester PPROM was 1 in 1000 pregnancies. The mean gestational age at presentation was 18 weeks and the mean interval to delivery was 13 days. The average age at delivery in our study was 20 + 5, which is remote from viability. The average birth weight was 614 g. Thus survival in this cohort was very unlikely. Thirty-two infants (76 %) died in utero (4/42) or peripartum due to previability (28/42). Ten infants were born alive (23 %; 10/42) with an average birth weight of 740 g (range 440–1100 g) and an average gestational age of 25 + 2 weeks (range 23 + 3–29 + 4). Ninety percent (9/10) of these were actively managed and taken to the NICU. Six of these infants died in the NICU of sepsis, IVH or RDS, hence the overall survival to discharge was 4.76 % (2/42). No infants in whom PPROM was recorded to have occurred at less than 17 weeks (n = 11) survived, three infants in the 17–21 + 6 group (17 %, n = 17) were born alive and seven of the infants where PPROM occurred after 22 weeks (78 %, n = 9) were born alive. Maternal morbidity was low, despite the prolonged latency period and the lack of availability of termination or delivery on maternal request. The incidence of clinical chorioamnionitis was low (14 %; 6/42) but high histologically suggesting a high index of suspicion is required with these women. Whilst 17 women required antibiotics, only one woman developed sepsis. This suggests that it is reasonable to offer women conservative management of PPROM, once they are carefully monitored for signs of sepsis. Although neonatal survival rates are low, women may choose this as a more acceptable alternative to termination of pregnancy.

This study was distinctive in examining PPROM at early gestations. There are few studies examining the outcomes of these pregnancies. Additionally, we provide a unique perspective as elective termination of pregnancy is not routinely offered in Ireland for this indication in the absence of maternal compromise. This study provides significant information on the natural history of PPROM and vital information with which to counsel future affected women.

This is a small retrospective study that refers to a single institutional experience, thus our study is limited by the retrospective nature of data retrieval and the small number of cases available. Furthermore, a proportion of women in our study (5/42) were unsure as to the exact date of PPROM. Thus we must consider unrecognised PPROM may present as preterm labour or late miscarriage and may have been missed in our search. Similarly, late presentations close to viability may have been missed as duration of PPROM was not always well documented in this cohort. These groups may have yielded survivors.

Other studies have included women experiencing PPROM at much later gestations up to 34 weeks [9]. Indeed, this often accounts for their larger sample size (range 16–236) [3, 10]. Similarly as the infants in our study were born at earlier gestations, their survival rate

was also lower than other studies. A study by Manuck et al. also examined women experiencing PPROM between 14 and 23 + 6 weeks [11]. Their study was conducted over 6 years however with a larger cohort of 159 patients, presenting at a later mean gestational age (21 + 3) and delivering at a later mean gestation of 24 + 5 and included those delivering 12 h after PPROM. Indeed shorter latency periods and later gestational age may have contributed to the increased survival rate of 56 %. Holmgren et al. found a survival rate of 86 %, but included women who experienced PPROM between 14 + 0 and 32 + 0 weeks [12]. There were lower survival rates in all studies in the earlier PPROM cases but there was a wide variance in figures. Verma et al. had a survival rate of 18.3 % but examined pregnancies where PPROM occurred between 18 and 23 weeks only [13]. Conversely, Loeb et al. included pregnancies complicated by PPROM between 20 and 24 weeks gestation and found an overall survival rate of 6.25 % [3]. Survival was 40, 92 and 100 % of those experiencing PPROM at 14–19, 20–25 and 26–28 weeks respectively by Farooqi et al. [5]. Likewise, Newman et al. found a mortality of 98.8 % in PPROM occurring at 23–24 weeks which fell to 36.6 % in the 25–27week group [10]. Xiao reported a similarly high mortality rate of 82 % in their PPROM cases at less than 22 weeks gestation (14–21.9 weeks) [14]. Margato et al. also found that PPROM occurring at gestations less than 20 weeks had a lower survival rate [15]. This is consistent with our own findings which showed a 100 % mortality rate in those with PPROM at less than 17 weeks, but 78 % of infants experiencing PPROM after 22 weeks were born alive. Latency periods also varied widely (1.25 – 105 days) [2]. The consensus was that longer latency periods had a positive impact on survival, allowing time for corticosteroid administration and antibiotics, but equally increased the risk of chorioamnionitis [5, 13].

Chorioamnionitis rates in our study were lower than others at 13 %. Rates in other studies ranged from 28 to 42 % [4, 5]. Similarly, Loeb described a much higher incidence of histological versus clinical chorioamnionitis (85 % vs 39 %) [3]. There was a 20 % incidence of retained placenta. This is much higher than Verma et al. who reported an incidence of retained placenta of 9.09 % [13]. Of the women with retained placenta, four had histological chorioamnionitis (44 %, 4/9) and one had clinical signs of chorioamnionitis (11 %, 1/9). The remaining women (n = 4) did not have placental histology available. There appeared to be no association between latency period and retained placenta. With the exception of one woman with a latency period of 85 days, the remainder had an average latency of 4.2 days (n = 5, r = 2–7).

Neonatal complications were comparable to other studies. All infants transferred to the NICU had significant respiratory morbidity and were managed with mechanical ventilation, nitric oxide and surfactant. Verma et al. reported a similar finding with an incidence of RDS of 100 % [13]. Dinsmoor et al. reported sepsis among 34 % of subjects consistent with our rate of 30 % [1]. IVH occurred in 30 % of our cohort, two of which were grade 4. Other studies reported lower rates of severe IVH [1, 4, 13]. Most studies conceded that neonatal morbidity was high in this cohort and was often serious, with at least one major morbidity present in the range of 37 to 100 % [1, 2, 4, 11–14] of those infants surviving to discharge. Our single survivor had four major complications of prematurity and continues to have respiratory complications, emphasising the importance of antenatal steroids near viability. This places our survival rate of infants born alive at just 10 %, similar to Loeb but lower than other authors who found survival rates of 67–81 % [3, 12].

Conclusion

In summary our study shows that PPROM prior to viability is a rare complication of pregnancy, but one that carries significant fetal and maternal risks. By focusing on these women of earlier gestation we provide useful data for pregnant women and clinicians regarding these challenging cases. It is clear however that further work needs to be done in this area, involving larger numbers and a collaboration of experience from multiple institutions. There was an inconsistency of investigations, particularly in screening for infection on initial presentation. The introduction of a new national guideline on PPROM [16] and the Irish Maternity Early Warning System (I-MEWS) [17] should help to improve initial management as well as detection and prevention of sepsis. Future studies should focus on the impact of these measures.

Whilst our overall survival rate was 5 %, 78 % of foetuses in those pregnancies where the PPROM occurred after 22 weeks were born alive. Counselling must be frank regarding the poor prognosis of those remote from viability, but awareness of increasing fetal potential with enduring latency periods should encourage the clinician caring for this challenging cohort. Additionally, advances in neonatal care and therapies such as amnioinfusion or amniopatch may offer increased hope of survival in the future [18]. Acknowledging the risk to mother and fetus from infection should instigate due diligence in seeking signs and symptoms of sepsis. Recent changes to Irish legislation add another dimension to counselling and decisions surrounding delivery in the maternal interest in cases of acute chorioamnionitis [7, 16].

Abbreviations
PPROM: preterm premature rupture of membranes; RCOG: royal college of obstetricians and gynaecologists; NICU: neonatal intensive care unit; IVH: intraventricular haemorrhage; RDS: respiratory distress syndrome; NEC: necrotising enterocolitis; NSAPH: non-substantial antepartum haemorrhage; I-MEWS: Irish maternity early warning system.

Competing interests
The authors declare that they have no competing interests.

Authors' contributions
LAL was responsible for data interpretation and was the main author of manuscript. JW was responsible for data collection and drafting the manuscript. AGM was responsible for a significant proportion of data collection and participated in design and coordination of the study. KO'D participated in the design and coordination of the study and critical review of the manuscript. LK conceived of the study, and participated in its design and coordination and helped to draft and critically review the manuscript. ED was involved in critical review of the manuscript. NR was involved in the study design in addition to drafting and editing the manuscript. All authors read and approved the final manuscript.

Acknowledgements
None

Author details
[1]The Department of Obstetrics and Gynaecology, University College Cork and Cork University Hospital, Cork, Ireland. [2]The Irish Centre for Fetal and Neonatal Translational Research, Cork, Ireland. [3]The Department of Paediatrics and Child Health, University College Cork, Cork, Ireland.

References
1. Dinsmoor MJ, Bachman R, Haney EI, Goldstein M, MacKendrick W. Outcomes after expectant management of extremely preterm premature rupture of the membranes. Am J Obstet Gynecol. 2004;190(1):183–7.
2. Nourse CB, Steer PA. Perinatal outcome following conservative management of midtrimester pre-labour rupture of the membranes. J Paediatr Child Health. 1997;33(2):125–30.
3. Loeb LJ, Gaither K, Woo KS, Mason TC. Outcomes in gestations between 20 and 25 weeks with preterm premature rupture of membranes. South Med J. 2006;99(7):709–12.
4. Pristauz G, Bauer M, Maurer-Fellbaum U, Rotky-Fast C, Bader AA, Haas J, et al. Neonatal outcome and two-year follow-up after expectant management of second trimester rupture of membranes. Int J Gynecol Obstet. 2008; 101(3):264–8.
5. Farooqi A, Holmgren PA, Engberg S, Serenius F. Survial and 2 year outcome with expectant management of second-trimester rupture of membranes. Obstet Gynecol. 1998;92(6):895–901.
6. Salihu HM, Salinas-Miranda AA, Hill L, Chandler K. Survival of pre-viable preterm infants in the United States: a systematic review and meta-analysis. Semin Perinatol. 2013;37(6):389–400.
7. The Protections of Life During Pregnancy Act 2013, Chapter 1, section 7(1)(a)(i)
8. RCOG. Preterm Prelabour Rupture of Membranes, Green-Top 44, 2010. Available from: http://www.rcog.org.uk/womens-health/clinical-guidance/preterm-prelabour-rupture-membranes-green-top-44
9. Gopalani S, Krohn M, Meyn L, Hitti J, Crombleholme WR. Contemporary Management of Preterm Premature Rupture of Membranes: Determinants of Latency and Neonatal Outcome. Am J Perinatol. 2004;21(4):183–90.
10. Newman DE, Paamoni-Keren O, Press F, Wiznitzer A, Mazor M, Sheiner E. Neonatal outcome in preterm deliveries between 23 and 27 weeks' gestation with and without preterm premature rupture of membranes. Arch Gynecol Obstet. 2009;280(1):7–11.
11. Manuck TA, Eller AG, Esplin MS, Stoddard GJ, Varner MW, Silver RM. Outcomes of expectantly managed preterm premature rupture of membranes occurring before 24 weeks of gestation. Obstet Gynecol. 2009; 114(1):29–37.

12. Holmgren PA, Olofsson JI. Preterm premature rupture of membranes and the associated risk for placental abruption. Inverse correlation to gestational length. Acta Obstet Gynecol Scand. 1997;76(8):743–7.

13. Verma U, Goharkhay N, Beydoun S. Conservative management of preterm premature rupture of membranes between 18 and 23 weeks of gestation–Maternal and neonatal outcome. Eur J Obstet Gynecol Reprod Biol. 2006;128(1–2):119–24.

14. Xiao ZH, André P, Lacaze-Masmonteil T, Audibert F, Zupan V, Dehan M. Outcome of premature infants delivered after prolonged premature rupture of membranes before 25 weeks of gestation. Eur J Obstet Gynecol Reprod Biol. 2000;90(1):67–71.

15. Margato MF, Martins GL, Passini Júnior R, Nomura ML. Previable preterm rupture of membranes: gestational and neonatal outcomes. Arch Gynecol Obstet. 2012;285(6):1529–34.

16. Institute of Obstetricians and Gynaecologists, Royal College of Physicians of Ireland and Directorate of Strategy and Clinical Care, Health Service Executive Clinical Practice Guideline Preterm Prelabour Rupture of the Membranes Version 1.0 Date of publication: April 2013 Guideline No. 24

17. Institute of Obstetricians and Gynaecologists, Royal College of Physicians of Ireland and Directorate of Strategy and Clinical Care, Health Service Executive Clinical Practice Guideline The Irish Maternity Early Warning System (IMEWS) Version 1.0 Date of publication: July2014 Guideline No. 25

18. Hofmeyr GJ, Eke AC, Lawrie TA. Amnioinfusion for third trimester preterm premature rupture of membranes. Cochrane Database Syst Rev. 2014;3: CD000942. doi:10.1002/14651858.

Risk factors for small-for-gestational-age and preterm births among 19,269 Tanzanian newborns

Alfa Muhihi[1,2]*, Christopher R. Sudfeld[3], Emily R. Smith[3], Ramadhani A. Noor[2,3], Salum Mshamu[2], Christina Briegleb[4], Mohamed Bakari[2], Honorati Masanja[1], Wafaie Fawzi[3,4,5] and Grace Jean-Yee Chan[3,6]

Abstract

Background: Few studies have differentiated risk factors for term-small for gestational age (SGA), preterm-appropriate for gestational age (AGA), and preterm-SGA, despite evidence of varying risk of child mortality and poor developmental outcomes.

Methods: We analyzed birth outcome data from singleton infants, who were enrolled in a large randomized, double-blind, placebo-controlled trial of neonatal vitamin A supplementation conducted in Tanzania. SGA was defined as birth weight <10th percentile for gestation age and sex using INTERGROWTH standards and preterm birth as delivery at <37 complete weeks of gestation. Risk factors for term-SGA, preterm-AGA, and preterm-SGA were examined independently using log-binomial regression.

Results: Among 19,269 singleton Tanzanian newborns included in this analysis, 68.3 % were term-AGA, 15.8 % term-SGA, 15.5 % preterm-AGA, and 0.3 % preterm-SGA. In multivariate analyses, significant risk factors for term-SGA included maternal age <20 years, starting antenatal care (ANC) in the 3rd trimester, short maternal stature, being firstborn, and male sex (all $p < 0.05$). Independent risk factors for preterm-AGA were maternal age <25 years, short maternal stature, firstborns, and decreased wealth (all $p < 0.05$). In addition, receiving ANC services in the 1st trimester significantly reduced the risk of preterm-AGA ($p = 0.01$). Significant risk factors for preterm-SGA included maternal age >30 years, being firstborn, and short maternal stature which appeared to carry a particularly strong risk (all $p < 0.05$).

Conclusion: Over 30 % of newborns in this large urban and rural cohort of Tanzanian newborns were born preterm and/or SGA. Interventions to promote early attendance to ANC services, reduce unintended young pregnancies, increased maternal height, and reduce poverty may significantly decrease the burden of SGA and preterm birth in sub-Saharan Africa.

Keywords: Risk factors, Birth weight, Term-SGA, Preterm-AGA, Preterm-SGA, Tanzania

* Correspondence: selukundo@gmail.com
[1]Ifakara Health Institute, Kiko Avenue, Mikocheni, Dar es Salaam, Tanzania
[2]Africa Academy for Public Health, CM Plaza Building, Mwai Kibaki Road, Mikocheni, P.O.Box 79810, Dar es Salaam, Tanzania
Full list of author information is available at the end of the article

Background

Globally, more than 20 million infants (15.5 % of live births) each year are born low birthweight (LBW) or <2500 g [1], with the vast majority occurring in low and middle income countries (LMICs) [2]. LBW is due to preterm birth (PTB) and intrauterine fetal growth restriction (IUGR) or a combination of both [3, 4]. Small-for-gestational-age (SGA; weight less than 10th percentile for sex and gestational age) is the primary measure for IUGR. It is estimated that of the 135 million babies born in 2010 in LMICs, 21.9 % were term-SGA, 8.1 % were preterm-appropriate for gestational age (AGA) and 2.1 % were preterm-SGA [5].

Preterm and SGA births are both well documented to increase the risk of morbidity and mortality, and newborns who are both preterm and SGA have the highest risk [6, 7]. A multi-country analysis of mortality risk in preterm and SGA births from LMICs determined that, compared to babies born term-AGA, the relative risk for neonatal mortality was 2.44 for term-SGA births, 8.05 for preterm-AGA, and 15.4 for preterm-SGA births [6]. In addition to survival implications, preterm and SGA births have increased risk for malnutrition and life-long complications including impaired neurodevelopment, non-communicable diseases, and psychological or emotional distress [8–10].

Despite a significant body of literature that mortality, morbidity, growth and development outcomes vary for preterm and SGA births, few studies have identified risk factors for combinations of preterm and SGA births [11]. In this analysis we sought to differentiate risk factors for term-SGA, preterm-AGA and preterm-SGA births and to our knowledge this is the first study to do so in Sub-Saharan Africa.

Methods

Study design and data collection

This study consist of women and singleton infants enrolled in a randomized double-blind, placebo- controlled neonatal vitamin A supplementation trial conducted in Tanzania between August 2010 and March 2013. Trial recruitment and data collection procedures have been presented elsewhere [12]. Briefly, the trial enrolled participants from urban (Dar es Salaam) and rural (Morogoro) settings in Tanzania. In Dar es Salaam, participants were enrolled at antenatal clinics (ANC) and in labor wards of public health facilities in Kinondoni, Ilala, and Temeke districts. In Morogoro, the study recruited within the Health and Demographic Surveillance System (HDSS) of Ifakara Health Institute which covers approximately 2,400 km² and allowed for enrollment of both health facility and home births.

Newborns were eligible for randomization if they were able to feed orally, were born within the past 72 h, were not previously enrolled in other clinical trials, the family intended to stay in the study area for at least six months

post-delivery, and the parents provided written informed consent to participate. A total of 32,843 mothers and their newborns were screened for inclusion in the parent trial. A total of 844 (2.6 %) were excluded for the following reasons: 237 (0.7 %) were not age eligible (>72 h since birth), 38 (0.1 %) were not able to feed orally and 569 (1.7 %) did not plan to reside in the study area for the next six months after delivery. A total of 31,999 newborns were randomized in the trial of which 11,895 resided in Dar es Salaam and 20,104 in Morogoro. There were 30,891 singleton births, and 1,108 were of multiple gestation.

Trained study staff administered a baseline questionnaire to mothers in order to collect information on demographic, socioeconomic, and environmental factors as well as date of mother's last menstrual period (LMP). We assessed LMP twice, during pregnancy surveillance and at the time of Vitamin A dosing. All infants had their birthweight measured at the time of dosing (at health facility or home) by study staff using calibrated scales with digital screens. Scale calibration with standard weights and weight standardization for all study staff was completed regularly for quality assurance.

Statistical analysis

We restricted this analysis to 19,269 (62.4 %) singleton infants who had complete data on birth weight and gestational age. Gestational age was calculated from maternal last normal menstrual period (LMP) report and preterm birth was defined as delivery at <37 completed weeks of gestation. SGA was defined as birth weight <10th percentile for gestational age and sex using INTERGROWTH standards [13]. We combined preterm birth and SGA into four mutually exclusive categories; term appropriate-for-gestational age (term-AGA), term small-for-gestational age (term-SGA), preterm appropriate-for-gestational age (preterm-AGA), and preterm small-for-gestational age (preterm-SGA). In sensitivity analyses, we defined preterm as delivery <34 completed weeks of gestation and SGA as <3rd percentile for gestational age and sex using INTERGROWTH standards.

We then examined demographic, socioeconomic, and environmental risk factors of term-SGA, preterm-AGA, and preterm-SGA as compared to reference term-AGA using log-binomial regression models to obtain risk ratio estimates. Variables assessed in univariate and multivariate analyses included location (Dar es Salaam and Morogoro), maternal age (<20, 20–25, 25–30, 30–35 and ≥ 35 years), maternal and paternal education (no formal schooling, some primary, completed primary and secondary plus), wealth quintile, trimester of first ANC visit (1st, 2nd, 3rd trimester), maternal height (<150, 150.0-154.9, 155.0-159.9, and ≥160.0 cm), parity (first born, 2nd–4th, and 5th birth or greater), and infant sex. Home versus facility births were only examined in univariate analyses due to issues of causality (preterm births may lead to home births). Wealth index quintile was defined by a principal component analysis of household assets and characteristics (bicycle, radio, mobile phone, television, motorcycle, car, animal ownership, electricity, and roof type) stratified by Dar es Salaam and Morogoro residence. A *priori* we decided to examine potential effect modification of all predictors by location (Dar es Salaam vs. Morogoro). Effect modification was assessed through use of interaction terms with statistical significance determined by the log-rank test. If statistically significant effect modification by site was determined in the univariate model, the interaction term was automatically included in the multivariate model. Missing data were retained using the missing indicator method. All *p*-values were 2–sided with a $p < 0.05$ considered statistically significant. Statistical analyses were performed using SAS v 9.4 (SAS Institute Inc., Cary, NC, USA).

Results

Baseline characteristics of the 19,269 singleton newborns included in the analysis are presented in Table 1. Briefly, 13,166 newborns (68.3 %) were term-AGA, 3,051 (15.8 %) term-SGA, 2,989 (15.5 %) preterm-AGA, and 63 (0.3 %) were preterm-SGA. Further, 633 newborns (3.3 %) were born <34 weeks gestation and 1,494 newborns (7.8 %) were <3rd percentile for gestational age and sex. The majority of mothers and fathers of newborns in our cohort had at least completed primary school (79.5 and 84.9 % respectively) and most mothers attended their first ANC visit during the second trimester (58.9 %). A total of 1,707 (8.9 %) births took place in the home and there was no difference in mean birthweight for home (mean: 3085 ± 460 g) versus facility births (mean: 3083 ± 476 g) ($p = 0.87$). Baseline characteristics of singleton mothers unable to recall their LMP and who were excluded from the analysis, were similar to singleton mothers who were able to recall their LMP (Appendix 1).

In Table 2 we presented unadjusted risk factors for term-SGA, preterm-AGA, and preterm-SGA as compared to the reference of term-AGA. Significant risk factors for term-SGA include: younger maternal age, small stature, firstborns, and male sex ($p < 0.05$), with no formal paternal and maternal schooling showing slight protective associations in unadjusted analysis ($p < 0.05$). There was significant interaction between wealth quintile and study site in the crude analysis. Poverty (lowest wealth quintile) was a significant risk factor for term-SGA in Dar es Salaam (RR = 1.36, $p < 0.001$) but was slightly protective in Morogoro (RR = 0.94, $p = 0.044$) (*p*-value for interaction <0.001). Risk factors for preterm-AGA in unadjusted analysis included: younger maternal age, small stature, firstborns, and low maternal and paternal education ($p < 0.05$). We also found that decreased wealth was a significant risk factor for preterm-AGA in

Table 1 Baseline characteristics of study participants in total population and stratified by site

	Total Population (*n* = 19,269)
	Mean (SD) or *n* (%)
Residency	
Dar es Salaam region	7,667 (39.8)
Morogoro region	11,602 (60.2)
Maternal age (years)	25.8 ± 5.9
Maternal education	
No formal schooling	1,445 (7.5)
Some primary	1,311 (6.8)
Completed primary	13,294 (69.0)
Secondary and advanced	2,019 (10.5)
Paternal education	
No formal schooling	801 (4.2)
Some primary	926 (4.8)
Completed primary	13,148 (68.2)
Secondary and Advanced	3,209 (16.7)
Trimester of first ANC visit	
1st Trimester	1,858 (9.6)
2nd Trimester	11,339 (58.9)
3rd Trimester	1,630 (23.1)
Maternal height (cm)	155.3 ± 5.2
Infant Sex	
Male	9,963 (51.7)
Female	9,306 (48.3)
Parity	
First born	4,621 (24.0)
2nd-4th birth	8,918 (46.3)
5th or greater birth	1,996 (10.4)
Homebirths	1,707 (8.9)
Birth Outcome	
Term-AGA	13,166 (68.3)
Term-SGA	3,051 (15.8)
Preterm-AGA	2,989 (15.5)
Preterm-SGA	63 (0.3)

AGA Appropriate for gestational age, *ANC* Antenatal clinic, *SD* Standard deviation, *SGA* Small for gestational age

both Dar es Salaam and Morogoro (*p*-values 0.001 and <0.001 respectively), but the magnitude of association was significantly greater for Morogoro newborns (*p*-value for interaction: 0.008). In the unadjusted analysis risk factors for preterm-SGA included: both maternal age less than 25 years and older than 30 years as compared to the 25–30 year reference, being firstborn, and decreased maternal height ($p < 0.05$).

In the multivariate analysis, we identified several important risk factors for term-SGA, preterm-AGA, and

Table 2 Unadjusted predictors of term-SGA, preterm-AGA, and preterm-SGA as compared to term-AGA reference

Characteristic	Term-AGA	Term-SGA			Preterm-AGA			Preterm-SGA		
	% (n = 13,166)	% (n = 3,051)	Unadjusted RR (95 % CI)	p-value	% (n = 2,989)	Unadjusted RR (95 % CI)	p-value	% (n = 63)	Unadjusted RR (95 % CI)	p-value
Maternal age										
< 20 years	12.6	21.1	1.69 (1.54–1.86)	<0.001	16.8	1.37 (1.24–1.52)	<0.001	12.1	2.50 (0.88–7.11)	0.172
20–25 years	30.1	32.3	1.21 (1.11–1.32)	<0.001	33.9	1.20 (1.01–1.31)	<0.001	43.1	3.73 (1.61–8.61)	0.009
25–30 years	28.4	24.2	Ref.		25.5	Ref.		12.1	Ref.	
30–35 years	22.0	16.9	0.91 (0.82–1.02)	0.094	17.7	0.91 (0.82–1.01)	0.070	24.2	3.33 (1.35–8.24)	0.007
≥ 35 years	6.9	5.6	0.96 (0.82–1.12)	0.582	6.1	0.99 (0.85–1.15)	0.920	8.6	4.55 (1.74–11.94)	0.002
Maternal education										
No formal schooling	8.1	6.3	0.78 (0.68–0.90)	<0.001	9.2	1.11 (0.99–1.25)	0.073	9.1	1.22 (0.48–3.09)	0.682
Some primary	7.1	6.9	0.95 (0.83–1.08)	0.448	8.5	1.17 (1.04–1.32)	0.010	7.3	1.12 (0.40–3.14)	0.828
Completed primary	73.2	76.6	Ref.		72.4	Ref.		67.3	Ref.	
Secondary plus	11.6	10.2	0.86 (0.77–0.96)	0.009	10.0	0.89 (0.79–1.00)	0.045	16.4	1.52 (0.74–3.15)	0.255
Paternal education										
No formal schooling	4.4	3.4	0.78 (0.64–0.94)	0.009	5.8	1.23 (1.06–1.41)	0.005	1.8	0.42 (0.06–3.07)	0.394
Some primary	4.9	5.1	1.00 (0.86–1.16)	0.986	6.1	1.16 (1.01–1.34)	0.029	5.5	1.13 (0.35–3.64)	0.840
Completed primary	72.1	74.8	Ref.		73.2	Ref.		70.9	Ref.	
Secondary plus	18.6	16.7	0.89 (0.82–0.98)	0.012	15.0	0.83 (0.75–0.91)	<0.001	21.8	1.19 (0.62–2.28)	0.591
Dar es Salaam wealth quintile										
Q1 (Poorest)	15.9	16.3	1.36 (1.08–1.72)		15.9	1.35 (1.12–1.64)		28.6	3.02 (0.61–14.92)	
Q2	20.7	26.2	1.44 (1.16–1.79)		20.7	1.21 (1.01–1.45)		28.6	2.03 (0.41–10.01)	
Q3	14.9	17.2	1.27 (1.01–1.60)		14.9	1.16 (0.95–1.40)		4.8	0.44 (0.04–4.87)	
Q4	25.6	28.8	1.18 (0.95–1.46)		25.6	1.10 (0.92–1.31)		28.6	1.45 (0.29–7.15)	
Q5 (Richest)	11.1	11.5	Ref.	<0.001*	16.8	Ref.	0.001*	9.5	Ref.	0.464*
Morogoro wealth quintile										
Q1 (Poorest)	16.4	16.7	0.94 (0.83–1.07)		22.2	1.72 (1.49–1.99)		14.7	0.95 (0.30–2.99)	
Q2	21.3	19.2	0.86 (0.76–0.97)		26.7	1.62 (1.41–1.87)		17.7	0.88 (0.30–2.62)	
Q3	17.2	18.4	0.98 (0.87–1.11)		13.8	1.12 (0.95–1.32)		11.8	0.73 (0.21–2.48)	
Q4	20.1	21.7	0.99 (0.88–1.11)		19.2	1.30 (1.12–1.51)		35.2	1.86 (0.73–4.72)	
Q5 (Richest)	21.9	24.0	Ref.	0.044*	15.3	Ref.	<0.001*	20.6	Ref.	0.544*

Table 2 Unadjusted predictors of term-SGA, preterm-AGA, and preterm-SGA as compared to term-AGA reference *(Continued)*

		term-SGA			preterm-AGA			preterm-SGA		
Trimester of first ANC visit										
1st Trimester	12.9	11.9	0.96 (0.86–1.08)	0.513	11.4	0.90 (0.80–1.01)	0.074	16.0	1.40 (0.65–3.01)	0.393
2nd Trimester	76.5	76.0	Ref.		77.3	Ref.		68.0	Ref.	
3rd Trimester	10.7	12.2	1.09 (0.98–1.22)	0.125	11.3	1.03 (0.92–1.16)	0.567	16.0	1.68 (0.78–3.61)	0.187
Maternal height										
< 150 cm	7.7	12.7	1.90 (1.57–2.31)		9.9	1.48 (1.20–1.83)		23.3	6.36 (1.65–24.46)	
150.0–154.9 cm	33.1	33.5	1.31 (1.11–1.54)		36.8	1.33 (1.13–1.55)		36.7	2.35 (0.66–8.41)	
155.0–159.9 cm	37.9	38.2	1.31 (1.11–1.53)		36.5	1.18 (1.01–1.39)		30.0	1.69 (0.46–6.21)	
≥ 160.0 cm	21.3	15.6	Ref.	<0.001*	16.8	Ref.	<0.001*	10.0	Ref.	0.011
Parity										
First born	26.2	42.5	1.71 (1.59–1.84)	<0.001	31.9	1.25 (1.16 1.34)	<0.001	49.1	2.53 (1.51–4.22)	<0.001
2nd–4th birth	59.8	49.0	Ref.		55.9	Ref.		43.4	Ref.	
5th or greater	14.0	8.6	0.78 (0.68–0.89)	<0.001	12.2	0.95 (0.85–1.06)	0.386	7.6	0.73 (0.26–2.06)	0.553
Infant sex										
Male	51.0	54.0	1.10 (1.03–1.17)	0.004	52.4	1.05 (0.98–1.12)	0.168	50.8	0.99 (0.61–1.62)	0.971
Female	49.0	46.0	Ref.		47.6	Ref.		49.2	Ref.	
Place of birth										
Home	8.5	7.4	0.89 (0.79–1.01)	0.06	11.8	1.34 (1.22–1.48)	<0.001	12.7	1.56 (0.75–3.27)	0.236
Facility	91.5	92.6	Ref.		88.2	Ref.		87.3	Ref.	

*p-value for trend

AGA Appropriate for gestational age, *ANC* Antenatal clinic, *CI* Confidence interval, *SGA* Small for gestational age, *RR* Relative risk

preterm-SGA as compared to the term-AGA reference (Table 3). Significant, independent risk factors for term-SGA include: maternal age <20 years ($p = 0.002$), late ANC first visit in 3rd trimester as compared to 2nd trimester ($p = 0.025$), decreased maternal stature under 160 cm ($p < 0.001$), being firstborn ($p < 0.001$), and male sex ($p = 0.007$). Significant protective factors for term-SGA included maternal secondary education ($p = 0.018$) and no formal paternal schooling ($p = 0.028$). For preterm-AGA, significant risk factors included: maternal age <25 years, decreased maternal stature ($p < 0.001$), and being firstborn ($p = 0.003$). In addition, attending ANC for the first time in the first trimester as compared to second trimester ($p = 0.009$) and paternal secondary education were associated with significantly reduced risk of preterm-AGA. Decreased wealth was a significant risk factor for preterm-AGA in Morogoro ($p < 0.001$) and the results indicated a similar, but smaller in magnitude and not statistically significant trend in Dar es Salaam ($p = 0.076$) (p-value for interaction: 0.024). For preterm-SGA, significant independent risk factors included

maternal age >30 years, firstborns, and decreased maternal height ($p = 0.042$). Figure 1 illustrates the magnitude of risk of term-SGA, preterm-AGA, and preterm-SGA for maternal height. Women with short stature have an increased risk of all three adverse pregnancy outcomes.

Sensitivity analyses utilizing a preterm definition of <34 weeks and SGA as defined by <3rd percentile are presented in Appendix 2: Table 5 and Appendix 3: Table 6. We were unable to present risk factors for preterm-SGA in sensitivity analyses utilizing these more extreme definitions due to the small number of infants in this category ($n = 2$). Young maternal age, late ANC, short maternal stature, starting ANC in 3rd trimester, and firstborns remained significant risk factors for term-SGA (<3rd percentile) and were of similar magnitude (Appendix 2: Table 5). In addition, maternal secondary education was significantly associated with reduced risk of term-SGA (<3rd percentile). As for preterm (<34 weeks) –SGA, young maternal age and decreased wealth in Morogoro region remained significant predictors (Appendix 3: Table 6). In addition,

Table 3 Multivariate adjusted predictors of term-SGA, preterm-AGA, and preterm-SGA as compared to term-AGA reference

Characteristic	Term-SGA		Preterm-AGA		Preterm-SGA	
	Adjusted RR (95 % CI)	p-value	Adjusted RR (95 % CI)	p-value	Adjusted RR (95 % CI)	p-value
Maternal age						
< 20 years	1.19 (1.06–1.32)	0.002	1.24 (1.10–1.39)	<0.001	0.90 (0.29–2.80)	0.860
20–25 years	1.07 (0.98–1.17)	0.135	1.16 (1.06–1.27)	0.001	2.22 (0.93–5.29)	0.072
25–30 years	Ref.		Ref.		Ref.	
30–35 years	0.98 (0.89–1.09)	0.769	0.93 (0.83–1.03)	0.150	3.33 (1.33–8.35)	0.010
≥ 35 years	1.09 (0.93–1.28)	0.292	1.00 (0.86–1.18)	0.954	4.66 (1.39–15.67)	0.013
Maternal education						
No formal schooling	0.88 (0.76–1.02)	0.091	1.03 (0.91–1.17)	0.651	1.64 (0.61–4.41)	0.327
Some primary	1.01 (0.88–1.15)	0.913	1.11 (0.98–1.26)	0.108	1.38 (0.47–4.05)	0.559
Completed primary	Ref.		Ref.		Ref.	
Secondary plus	0.87 (0.77–0.98)	0.018	0.95 (0.84–1.07)	0.387	1.33 (0.58–3.01)	0.499
Paternal education						
No formal schooling	0.80 (0.66–0.98)	0.028	1.08 (0.93–1.26)	0.319	0.39 (0.05–3.06)	0.374
Some primary	0.98 (0.84–1.14)	0.799	1.07 (0.93–1.24)	0.334	1.15 (0.34–3.87)	0.826
Completed primary	Ref.		Ref.		Ref.	
Secondary plus	0.98 (0.89–1.08)	0.689	0.85 (0.77–0.95)	0.004	1.21 (0.57–2.55)	0.625
Dar es Salaam wealth quintile						
Q1 (Poorest)	1.26 (1.00–1.60)		1.21 (1.00–1.46)		3.00 (0.59–15.27)	
Q2	1.34 (1.08–1.67)		1.10 (0.92–1.32)		2.06 (0.41–10.39)	
Q3	1.18 (0.94–1.49)		1.08 (0.89–1.31)		0.43 (0.04–4.73)	
Q4	1.15 (0.93–1.42)		1.08 (0.90–1.29)		1.40 (0.28–6.97)	
Q5 (Richest)	Ref.	0.057*	Ref.	0.076*	Ref.	0.827*
Morogoro wealth quintile						
Q1 (Poorest)	1.00 (0.90–1.12)		1.49 (1.32–1.68)		1.67 (0.67–4.25)	
Q2	0.95 (0.86–1.06)		1.39 (1.24–1.56)		1.34 (0.54–3.29)	
Q3	1.00 (0.90–1.11)		1.13 (1.00–1.28)		0.66 (0.22–1.99)	
Q4	0.95 (0.86–1.05)		1.23 (1.09–1.37)		1.64 (0.73–3.67)	
Q5 (Richest)	Ref.	0.432*	Ref.	<0.001*	Ref.	0.842*
Trimester of first ANC visit						
1st Trimester	0.98 (0.88–1.09)	0.712	0.86 (0.76–0.96)	0.009	1.33 (0.61–2.89)	0.475
2nd Trimester	Ref.		Ref.		Ref.	
3rd Trimester	1.13 (1.02–1.26)	0.025	1.06 (0.94–1.19)	0.323	1.83 (0.84–9.98)	0.127
Maternal height						
< 150 cm	1.60 (1.33–1.94)		1.34 (1.09–1.66)		5.92 (1.50–23.30)	
150.0–154.9 cm	1.24 (1.06–1.46)		1.22 (1.04–1.43)		2.58 (0.72–9.32)	
155.0–159.9 cm	1.17 (1.00–1.37)		1.13 (0.97–1.33)		1.64 (0.44–6.08)	
≥ 160.0 cm	Ref.	<0.001*	Ref.	<0.001*	Ref.	0.042
Parity						
First born	1.56 (1.42–1.70)	<0.001	1.15 (1.05–1.26)	0.003	3.21 (1.63–6.33)	0.001
2nd–4th birth	Ref.		Ref.		Ref.	
5th or greater	0.75 (0.64–0.86)	<0.001	0.99 (0.87–1.12)	0.869	0.45 (0.14–1.42)	0.174
Infant sex						
Male	1.09 (1.02–1.16)	0.007	1.05 (0.98–1.12)	0.134	1.02 (0.62–1.67)	0.947
Female	Ref.		Ref.		Ref.	

*p-value for trend

AGA Appropriate for gestational age, *ANC* Antenatal clinic, *CI* Confidence interval, *SGA* Small for gestational age, *RR* Relative risk

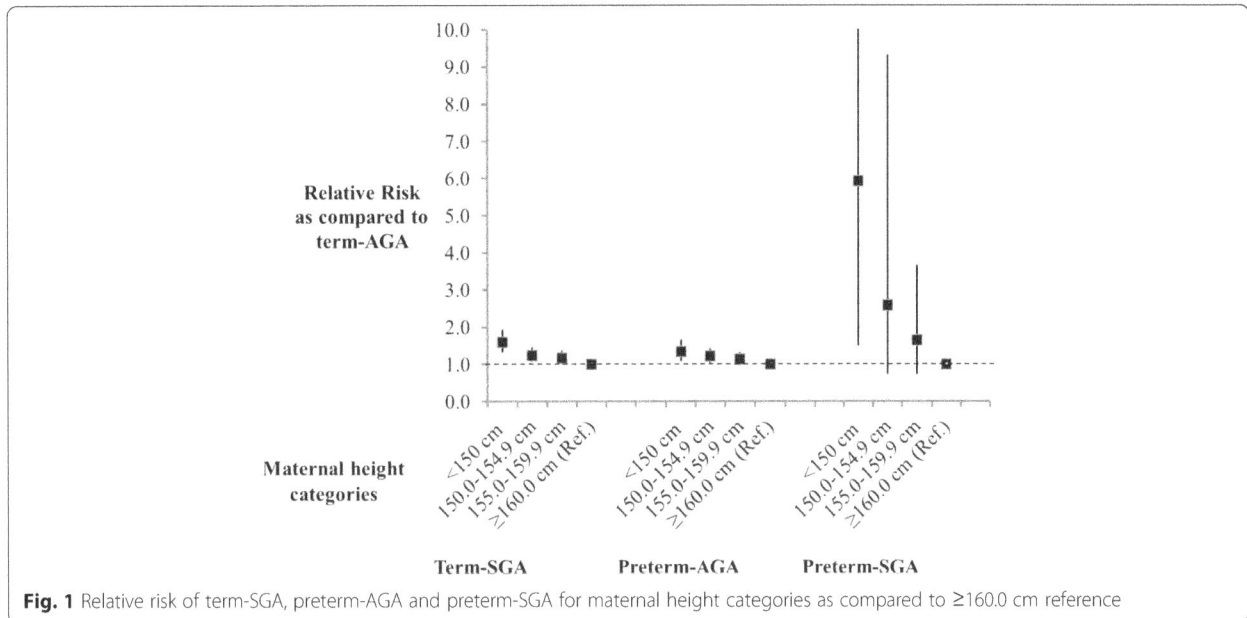

Fig. 1 Relative risk of term-SGA, preterm-AGA and preterm-SGA for maternal height categories as compared to ≥160.0 cm reference

decreased wealth in Dar es Salaam approached statistical significance as a predictor of preterm (<34 weeks) –SGA.

Discussion

In this analysis we found both common and distinct risk factors for term-SGA, preterm-AGA, and preterm-SGA births. Short maternal stature and being firstborn were significant risk factors for all three pregnancy outcomes. Young maternal age was a risk factor for both term-SGA and preterm-AGA, while advanced maternal age over 30 years was associated with increased risk for preterm-SGA. Additional risk factors for term-SGA were starting ANC late in the third trimester of pregnancy and male sex. Poor socioeconomic status for women residing in the rural setting increased the risk for preterm-AGA, while starting ANC early in the first trimester of pregnancy was protective.

We determined that young maternal age was associated with an increased risk of term-SGA and preterm-AGA, whereas maternal age >30 years was associated with increased risk of preterm-SGA. A similar pattern was also seen in a study differentiating risks of preterm and SGA births in Nepal, but results were not statistically significant [14]. The leading biological mechanisms to explain the high risk of adverse birth outcomes of young mothers include maternal-fetal competition for nutrients or incomplete physical maturation which might contribute to adverse neonatal outcomes [15]. As for the relationship of maternal age above 30 years, older women have increased risk for congenital abnormalities and pregnancy comorbidities including hypertension and gestational diabetes which can increase the risk of preterm and

SGA [16, 17]. Family planning interventions to prevent unintended early pregnancies may reduce the risk of preterm-AGA and term-SGA births and their consequences, while access to essential newborn care is critical for pregnant women of advanced maternal age due to risk of preterm-SGA births, which carry the highest risk of mortality.

Consistent with other studies which examined the association of maternal anthropometry with pregnancy outcomes [18, 19], we found that short maternal stature, an indicator of chronic malnutrition, was independently associated with increased risk for term-SGA, preterm-AGA and preterm-SGA. The association of short maternal stature and adverse pregnancy outcomes is likely to be due to a combination of increased risk of cephalo-pelvic disproportion and an indicator of poor supply of nutrients to the fetus due to maternal malnutrition [20, 21]. Our results also confirm the association between short maternal stature and pregnancy outcomes appears to be stronger for SGA as compared to PTB [22].

Being firstborn was associated with risk of all combinations of preterm and SGA birth outcomes. This finding matches with findings from rural Nepal and a meta-analysis examining parity and maternal age as risk factors for PTB and SGA [11, 14]. From the meta-analysis, it was suggested that the association with PTB was largely driven by young maternal age and/or its interaction with null parity. Starting ANC late in the third trimester of pregnancy was associated with increased risk for term-SGA as compared to the second trimester, while starting ANC early in the first trimester of pregnancy reduced risk of preterm-AGA. The mechanism leading to this association may be a combination of early detection and management of pregnancy related health conditions and increased duration of standard pregnancy interventions like iron and folic acid supplementation and sulphadoxine pyrimethamine (SP) for prevention of malaria in pregnancy [23].

There are few limitations to our analysis. First, exclusion of newborns that were unable to feed orally in the parent trial may have underestimated the burden of PTB and SGA, as well as biased associations determined in this paper. Nevertheless, only 38 infants were excluded from the trial due to inability to feed orally, which is likely to have a negligible effect on our estimates based on 19,269 births. In addition, we were limited by data collected in the primary neonatal vitamin A supplementation trial and did not have information to evaluate or control for other known risk factors for adverse birth outcomes including: pre-pregnancy BMI, weight gain during pregnancy, history of chronic diseases like hypertension and diabetes, birth intervals, and previous history of PTB and SGA [24, 25]. Lastly, preterm and SGA were defined using maternal report of LMP, which likely lead to some misclassification. Nevertheless, errors in maternal report of LMP are likely not systematically related to both birth outcomes and risk factors of interest which would lead to underestimation of the associations of interest.

Conclusion
This study identified common and unique risk factors for term-SGA, preterm-AGA and preterm-SGA ranging from anthropometric, economic, demographic and behavioral factors. Some of the risk factors like late ANC attendance, young maternal age at conception, short maternal stature, and poverty are potentially modifiable, and provide an opportunity to improve birth outcomes. In addition, due to high burden of preterm and SGA births in both urban and rural settings in Tanzania, it is vital to advocate for universal access to essential newborn care within the country and similar settings. Overall, targeted combinations of prevention and treatment interventions during pregnancy may decrease the burden of preterm and SGA births and provide substantial reductions in child mortality, morbidity, growth and developmental delay in resource-limited settings.

Ethics approval and consent to participate
The study protocol was approved by the Institutional Review Boards of the Harvard T.H. Chan School of Public Health, Ifakara Health Institute, Medical Research Coordinating Council of Tanzania, and by the WHO Ethical Review Committee. Individual informed consent was sought from at least one parent of every infant who was enrolled in the trial.

Consent for publication
Not applicable.

Appendix 1

Table 4 Comparison of baseline characteristics of singleton trial participants who were able to recall LMP versus those who were not able to recall LMP

	Able to Recall LMP (n = 19,269)	Unable to recall LMP (n = 11,622)
Maternal age (years)	25.8 ± 5.9	26.0 ± 5.9
Maternal education		
No formal schooling	1,445 (7.5)	1,111 (9.6)
Some primary	1,311 (6.8)	920 (7.9)
Completed primary	13,294 (69.0)	8,054 (69.3)
Secondary and advanced	2,019 (10.5)	882 (7.6)
Paternal education		
No formal schooling	801 (4.2)	607 (5.2)
Some primary	926 (4.8)	787 (6.8)
Completed primary	13,148 (68.2)	8,149 (70.1)
Secondary and Advanced	3,209 (16.7)	1,446 (12.4)
Wealth quintile		
Q1 (Poorest)	3,073 (16.0)	2,451 (21.1)
Q2	4,085 (21.2)	2,582 (22.2)
Q3	3,124 (16.2)	1,807 (15.6)
Q4	4,440 (23.0)	2,301 (19.8)
Q5 (Richest)	3,432 (17.8)	1,631 (14.0)
Trimester of first ANC visit		
1st Trimester	1,858 (9.6)	817 (7.0)
2nd Trimester	11,339 (58.9)	7,730 (66.5)
3rd Trimester	1,630 (23.1)	1,186 (10.2)
Maternal height (cm)	155.3 ± 5.2	155.7 ± 4.5
Infant Sex		
Female	9,306 (48.3)	5,390 (46.4)
Male	9,963 (51.7)	6,232 (53.6)
Parity		
First born	4,621 (24.0)	2,953 (25.4)
2nd-4th birth	8,918 (46.3)	5,287 (45.4)
5th or greater birth	1,996 (10.4)	1,618 (13.9)

ANC Antenatal clinic, LMP Last Menstrual period

Appendix 2

Table 5 Unadjusted and multivariate adjusted predictors of term (≥37 weeks) -SGA (<3rd percentile)

Characteristic	Term-AGA (>3 %)	Term (≥37 weeks) -SGA (<3rd percentile)				
	% (n = 14,738)	% (n = 1,479)	Unadjusted RR (95 % CI)	p-value	Multivariate adjusted RR (95 % CI)	p-value
Maternal age						
< 20 years	13.4	21.7	1.78 (1.54–2.05)	<0.001	1.21 (1.02–1.43)	0.027
20–25 years	30.3	32.9	1.25 (1.09–1.43)	<0.001	1.07 (0.94–1.23)	0.304
25–30 years	28.0	23.8	Ref.		Ref.	
30–35 years	21.5	17.1	0.94 (0.80–1.10)	0.428	1.00 (0.85–1.17)	0.979
≥ 35 years	6.8	4.4	0.78 (0.60–1.00)	0.054	0.86 (0.65–1.13)	0.270
Maternal education						
No formal schooling	8.0	5.5	0.68 (0.54–0.85)	0.001	0.78 (0.62–0.99)	0.042
Some primary	7.0	7.1	0.97 (0.80–1.18)	0.787	1.09 (0.89–1.33)	0.406
Completed primary	73.5	77.1	Ref.		Ref.	
Secondary plus	11.5	10.3	0.87 (0.74–1.03)	0.100	0.84 (0.70–1.00)	0.054
Paternal education						
No formal schooling	4.2	3.7	0.85 (0.65–1.11)	0.235	0.94 (0.71–1.25)	0.679
Some primary	5.0	4.8	0.93 (0.73–1.18)	0.541	0.95 (0.75–1.21)	0.668
Completed primary	75.8	72.3	Ref.		Ref.	
Secondary plus	15.7	18.5	0.82 (0.72–0.95)	0.007	0.83 (0.71–0.97)	0.016
Dar es Salaam wealth quintile						
Q1 (Poorest)	15.0	16.3	1.16 (0.82–1.64)		1.02 (0.71–1.45)	
Q2	22.3	29.1	1.36 (1.00–1.86)		1.24 (0.90–1.70)	
Q3	17.2	14.5	0.91 (0.64–1.31)		0.85 (0.59–1.22)	
Q4	31.0	26.6	0.92 (0.67–1.27)		0.91 (0.67–1.26)	
Q5 (Richest)	14.5	13.5	Ref.	0.020*	Ref.	0.717*
Morogoro wealth quintile						
Q1 (Poorest)	16.9	17.0	0.96 (0.79–1.15)		1.22 (1.00–1.49)	
Q2	21.8	18.2	0.81 (0.67–0.97)		0.94 (0.77–1.13)	
Q3	17.8	19.3	1.03 (0.86–1.23)		1.19 (1.00–1.44)	
Q4	20.9	21.5	0.98 (0.82–1.16)		1.08 (0.90–1.29)	
Q5 (Richest)	22.7	24.0	Ref.	0.153*	Ref.	0.324*
Trimester of first ANC visit						
1st Trimester	12.9	11.6	0.91 (0.77–1.09)	0.300	0.89 (0.74–1.05)	0.169
2nd Trimester	76.4	76.0	Ref.		Ref.	
3rd Trimester	10.8	12.5	1.15 (0.97–1.36)	0.100	1.23 (1.00–1.55)	0.014
Maternal height						
< 150 cm	8.1	13.5	1.94 (1.47–2.57)		1.65 (1.25–2.19)	
150.0–154.9 cm	33.4	31.2	1.17 (0.92–1.48)		1.09 (0.86–1.38)	
155.0–159.9 cm	37.8	39.0	1.18 (1.02–1.61)		1.18 (0.94–1.49)	
≥ 160.0 cm	20.7	16.3	Ref.	0.001*	Ref.	0.005*
Parity						
First born	27.6	45.1	1.87 (1.69–2.07)	<0.001	1.79 (1.57–2.05)	<0.001
2nd–4th birth	58.9	46.2	Ref.		Ref.	
5th or greater	13.4	8.7	0.81 (0.67–0.99)	0.039	0.88 (0.71–1.10)	0.267
Infant sex						
Male	52.1	46.4	0.81 (0.75–0.90)	<0.001	0.82 (0.74–0.90)	<0.001
Female	47.9	53.6	Ref.		Ref.	

*p-value for trend
AGA Appropriate for gestational age, ANC Antenatal clinic, CI Confidence interval, SGA Small for gestational age, RR Relative risk

Appendix 3

Table 6 Unadjusted and multivariate adjusted predictors of preterm (<34 weeks)-SGA (<10th percentile)

Characteristic	Term-AGA (>10 %) % (n = 15,522)	Preterm (<34 weeks)-SGA (<10th percentile) % (n = 633)	Unadjusted RR (95 % CI)	p-value	Multivariate adjusted RR (95 % CI)	p-value
Maternal age						
< 20 years	13.1	19.1	1.66 (1.31–2.10)	<0.001	1.46 (1.11–1.92)	0.007
20–25 years	30.6	35.4	1.33 (1.08–1.64)	0.006	1.27 (1.02–1.57)	0.029
25–30 years	28.0	24.1	Ref.		Ref.	
30–35 years	21.5	15.3	0.84 (0.65–1.08)	0.174	1.00 (0.85–1.17)	0.979
≥ 35 years	6.8	6.1	1.05 (0.74–1.50)	0.787	0.86 (0.65–1.13)	0.270
Maternal education						
No formal schooling	8.3	8.1	0.99 (0.74–1.33)	0.942	0.92 (0.67–1.26)	0.599
Some primary	7.3	6.9	0.96 (0.70–1.32)	0.789	0.86 (0.62–1.20)	0.382
Completed primary	73.1	72.0	Ref.		Ref.	
Secondary plus	13.0	11.3	1.16 (0.91–1.47)	0.233	1.24 (0.95–1.61)	0.114
Paternal education						
No formal schooling	4.6	4.9	1.06 (0.73–1.54)	0.774	0.96 (0.64–1.43)	0.838
Some primary	5.1	6.5	1.26 (0.91–1.76)	0.161	1.15 (0.82–1.61)	0.430
Completed primary	72.3	72.0	Ref.		Ref.	
Secondary plus	18.0	16.7	0.94 (0.75–1.17)	0.565	0.94 (0.74–1.20)	0.626
Dar es Salaam wealth quintile						
Q1 (Poorest)	15.1	21.9	1.76 (1.16–2.68)		1.73 (1.11–2.69)	
Q2	22.5	20.1	1.11 (0.73–1.71)		1.07 (0.69–1.68)	
Q3	17.0	16.4	1.20 (0.77–1.88)		1.15 (0.73–1.82)	
Q4	30.7	29.9	1.21 (0.81–1.81)		1.20 (0.79–1.80)	
Q5 (Richest)	14.7	11.7	Ref.	0.028*	Ref.	0.053*
Morogoro wealth quintile						
Q1 (Poorest)	17.1	27.1	2.22 (1.56–3.16)		1.82 (1.23–2.68)	
Q2	22.3	21.8	1.40 (0.97–2.02)		1.20 (0.81–1.78)	
Q3	16.7	13.6	1.17 (0.77–1.76)		1.05 (0.69–1.62)	
Q4	19.9	19.6	1.40 (0.96–2.04)		1.24 (0.84–1.84)	
Q5 (Richest)	21.0	14.5	Ref.	<0.001*	Ref.	0.006*
Trimester of first ANC visit						
1st Trimester	12.7	10.7	0.86 (0.65–1.14)	0.293	0.81 (0.61–1.08)	0.153
2nd Trimester	76.6	76.2	Ref.		Ref.	
3rd Trimester	10.7	13.0	1.21 (0.93–1.57)	0.152	1.24 (0.96–1.61)	0.803
Maternal height						
< 150 cm	7.9	12.9	1.57 (1.01–2.42)		1.42 (0.92–2.20)	
150.0–154.9 cm	33.8	34.6	1.01 (0.71–1.42)		0.95 (0.67–1.34)	
155.0–159.9 cm	37.9	31.7	0.83 (0.58–1.17)		0.80 (0.56–1.13)	
≥ 160.0 cm	20.5	20.8	Ref.	0.099*	Ref.	0.613*
Parity						

Table 6 Unadjusted and multivariate adjusted predictors of preterm (<34 weeks)-SGA (<10th percentile) *(Continued)*

First born	26.9	34.6	1.36 (1.15–1.62)	<0.001	1.12 (0.90–1.39)	0.318
2nd–4th birth	59.2	55.1	Ref.		Ref.	
5th or greater	13.8	10.3	0.80 (0.61–1.07)	0.130	0.85 (0.62–1.17)	0.333
Infant sex						
Male	51.3	52.1	1.03 (0.89–1.21)	0.663	1.04 (0.90–1.22)	0.572
Female	48.8	47.9	Ref.		Ref.	

*p-value for trend

AGA Appropriate for gestational age, *ANC* Antenatal clinic, *CI* Confidence interval, *SGA* Small for gestational age, *RR* Relative risk

Abbreviations
AGA: appropriate-for-gestational age; ANC: antenatal care clinic; HDSS: Health and demographic surveillance system; IUGR: intrauterine fetal growth restriction; LBW: low birthweight; LMICs: low and middle income countries; LMP: last normal menstrual period; PTB: preterm birth; RR: relative risk; SGA: small-for-gestational age; WHO: World health organization.

Competing interests
The authors declare that they have no competing interests.

Authors' contributions
AM, ERS, HM and WF drafted the article with contributions from all authors. AM, SM, CB, RN, and MB participated in data collection. All authors participated in monitoring field implementation of the primary trial and quality of data. AM, ERS, CRS and GC contributed to statistical analyses. All authors read and approved the final version of the paper.

Acknowledgements
We thank the mothers and their newborns for participating voluntarily in this study and the communities where the primary trial was carried out for their support and cooperation. We also thank the administrative authorities of Kinondoni, Ilala and Temeke districts in Dar es Salaam region; Kilombero, Ulanga and Kilosa districts in Morogoro region for their unlimited support. Special thanks to administrative staff of hospitals, health centers and dispensaries where the study was conducted. We acknowledge coordinators, supervisors, research assistants, field supervisors, interviewers and HDSS staff at Ifakara Health Institute for their tireless efforts that made the primary trial successful.

Funding
The primary trial was funded through a grant from Bill and Melinda Gates Foundation to the World Health Organization (WHO). Bill and Melinda Gates Foundation did not have any role in the design of study, data collection, analysis and interpretation of the findings as well as in the writing of the manuscript.

Author details
[1]Ifakara Health Institute, Kiko Avenue, Mikocheni, Dar es Salaam, Tanzania. [2]Africa Academy for Public Health, CM Plaza Building, Mwai Kibaki Road, Mikocheni, P.O.Box 79810, Dar es Salaam, Tanzania. [3]Department of Global Health and Population, Harvard T. H. Chan School of Public Health, Boston, USA. [4]Department of Nutrition, Harvard T. H. Chan School of Public Health, Boston, USA. [5]Department of Epidemiology, Harvard T. H. Chan School of Public Health, Boston, USA. [6]Department of Medicine, Boston Children's Hospital, Boston, USA.

References
1. UNICEF and WHO. Low Birth Weight: Country, Regional and Global Estimates. New York. 2004. http://www.unicef.org/publications/index_24840.html. Accessed 15 Jun 2015.
2. Blencowe H, Cousens S, Oestergaard MZ, Chou D, Moller A-B, Narwal R, et al. National, regional, and worldwide estimates of preterm birth rates in the year 2010 with time trends since 1990 for selected countries: a systematic analysis and implications. Lancet. 2012;379:2162–72.
3. Berkowitz GS, Papiernik E. Epidemiology of preterm birth. Epidemiol Rev. 1993;15:414–43.
4. Kramer MS. Determinants of low birth weight: methodological assessment and meta-analysis. Bull World Health Organ. 1987;65:663–737.
5. Lee ACC, Katz J, Blencowe H, Cousens S, Kozuki N, Vogel JP, et al. National and regional estimates of term and preterm babies born small for gestational age in 138 low-income and middle-income countries in 2010. Lancet Glob Heal. 2013;1:e26–36.
6. Katz J, Lee ACC, Kozuki N, Lawn JE, Cousens S, Blencowe H, et al. Mortality risk in preterm and small-for-gestational-age infants in low-income and middle-income countries: a pooled country analysis. Lancet. 2013;382:417–25.
7. Sania A, Spiegelman D, Rich-Edwards J, Okuma J, Kisenge R, Msamanga G, Urassa W, Fawzi WW. The contribution of preterm birth and intrauterine growth restriction to infant mortality in Tanzania. Paediatr Perinat Epidemiol. 2014;28:23–31.
8. Blencowe H, Cousens S, Chou D, Oestergaard M, Say L, Moller A-B, Kinney M, Lawn J. Born too soon: the global epidemiology of 15 million preterm births. Reprod Health. 2013;10 Suppl 1:S2.
9. Christian P, Lee SE, Angel MD, Adair LS, Arifeen SE, Ashorn P, et al. Risk of childhood undernutrition related to small-for-gestational age and preterm birth in low- and middle-income countries. Int J Epidemiol. 2013;42:1340–55.
10. Hernández MI, Mericq V. Metabolic syndrome in children born small-for-gestational age. Arq Bras Endocrinol Metabol. 2011;55:583–9.
11. Kozuki N, Lee AC, Silveira MF, Victora CG, Adair L, Humphrey J, et al. The associations of birth intervals with small-for-gestational-age, preterm, and neonatal and infant mortality: a meta-analysis. BMC Public Health. 2013;13 Suppl 3:S3.
12. Masanja H, Smith ER, Muhihi A, Briegleb C, Mshamu S, Ruben J, et al. Effect of neonatal vitamin A supplementation on mortality in infants in Tanzania (Neovita): a randomised, double-blind, placebo-controlled trial. Lancet. 2014; 385(9975):1324–32.
13. Papageorghiou AT, Ohuma EO, Altman DG, Todros T, Cheikh Ismail L, Jaffer YA, Bertino E, Gravett MG, Purwar M, Noble JA, Pang R, Victora CG, Barros FC, Carvalho M, Salomon LJ, Bhutta ZA, Kennedy SH, Villar J. International standards for fetal growth based on serial ultrasound measurements: the Fetal Growth Longitudinal Study of the INTERGROWTH-21st Project. Lancet. 2014;384:869–79.
14. Kozuki N, Katz J, LeClerq SC, Khatry SK, West KP, Christian P. Risk factors and neonatal/infant mortality risk of small-for-gestational-age and preterm birth in rural Nepal. J Matern Fetal Neonatal Med. 2015;28(9):1019-25.
15. Kramer K, Lancaster J. Teen Motherhood in cross-cultural perspective. Ann Hum Biol. 2010;37:613–28.
16. Carolan M, Frankowska D. Advanced maternal age and adverse perinatal outcome: a review of the evidence. Midwifery. 2011;27:793–801.
17. Yogev Y, Melamed N, Bardin R, Tenenbaum-Gavish K, Ben-Shitrit G, Ben-Haroush A. Pregnancy outcome at extremely advanced maternal age. Am J Obs Gynecol. 2010;203(558e):558e-1–558-e.7.
18. Panaretto K, Lee H, Mitchell M, Larkins S, Manessis V, Buettner P, Watson D. Risk factors for preterm, low birth weight and small for gestational age birth in urban Aboriginal and Torres Strait Islander women in Townsville. Aust N Z J Public Health. 2006;30:163–70.
19. Rodrigues T, Barros H. Comparison of risk factors for small-for-gestational-age and preterm in a Portuguese cohort of newborns. Matern Child Health J. 2007;11:417–24.
20. Van Roosmalen J, Brand R. Maternal height and the outcome of labor in rural Tanzania. Int J Gynaecol Obs. 1992;37:169–77.

21. Rush D. Nutrition and maternal mortality in the developing world. Am J Clin Nutr. 2000;72 Suppl 1:212S–40.

22. Heaman M, Kingston D, Chalmers B, Sauve R, Lee L, Young D. Risk factors for preterm birth and small-for-gestational-age births among Canadian women. Paediatr Perinat Epidemiol. 2013;27:54–61.

23. Rijken MJ, De Livera AM, Lee SJ, Boel ME, Rungwilailaekhiri S, Wiladphaingern J, et al. Quantifying low birth weight preterm birth and small-for-gestational-age effects of malaria in pregnancy: a population cohort study. PLoS One. 2014;9:e100247.

24. Kogan MD. Social causes of low birth weight. J R Soc Med. 1995;88:611–5.

25. Esimai O, Ojofeitimi E. Pattern and determinants of gestational weight gain an important predictor of infant birth weight in a developing country. Glob J Heal Sci. 2014;6:34808.

5

Is maternal trait anxiety a risk factor for late preterm and early term deliveries?

Margarete Erika Vollrath[1,2*], Verena Sengpiel[3], Markus A. Landolt[4,5], Bo Jacobsson[6,7] and Beatrice Latal[8]

Abstract

Background: Anxiety is associated with preterm deliveries in general (before week 37 of pregnancy), but is that also true for late preterm (weeks 34/0–36/6) and early term deliveries (weeks 37/0–38/6)? We aim to examine this association separately for spontaneous and provider-initiated deliveries.

Methods: Participants were pregnant women from the Norwegian Mother and Child Cohort Study (MoBa), which has been following 95 200 pregnant women since 1999. After excluding pregnancies with serious health complications, 81 244 participants remained. National ultrasound records were used to delineate late preterm, early term, and full-term deliveries, which then were subdivided into spontaneous and provider-initiated deliveries. We measured trait anxiety based on two ratings of the anxiety items on the Symptom Checklist-8 (Acta Psychiatr Scand 87:364–7, 1993). Trait anxiety was transformed into categorizing the score at the mean and at ± 2 standard deviations.

Results: Trait anxiety was substantially associated with late preterm and early term deliveries after adjusting for confounders. In the whole sample, women with the highest anxiety scores (+2 standard deviations) were more likely [(odds ratio (OR) = 1.7; 95 % confidence-interval (CI) 1.3-2.0)] to delivering *late preterm* than women with the lowest anxiety scores. Their odds of delivering *early term* were also high (OR = 1.4; CI 1.3-1.6). Women with spontaneous deliveries and the highest anxiety scores had higher odds (OR = 1.4; CI 1.1-1.8) of delivering late preterm and early term (OR = 1.3; CI = 1.3-1.5). The corresponding odds for women with provider-initiated deliveries were OR = 1.7 (CI = 1.2-2.4) for late preterm and OR = 1.3 for early term (CI = 1.01-1.6). Irrespective of delivery onset, women with provider-initiated deliveries had higher levels of anxiety than women delivering spontaneously. However, women with high anxiety were equally likely to have provider-initiated or spontaneous deliveries.

Conclusions: This study is the first to show substantial associations between high levels of trait anxiety and late preterm delivery. Increased attention should be given to the mechanism underlying this association, including factors preceding the pregnancy. In addition, acute treatment should be offered to women displaying high levels of anxiety throughout pregnancy to avoid suffering for the mother and the child.

Keywords: Anxiety, Mental health, Personality, Pregnancy, Preterm, Prospective, Longitudinal, Women

Background

Research on preterm deliveries has been devoted to deliveries occurring before week 37 of gestation, with a focus on the earliest births. However, very early deliveries remain relatively rare. The substantial increase in shortened gestations noted in the last decades occurred late in the preterm period, between 34 and 36 weeks (*late preterm*), and in deliveries in weeks 37 and 38 (*early term*). These two forms of delivery onset together reach a share of up to 30 % of births in the United States [1, 2]. Not only newborns delivered late preterm but also newborns delivered early term have a higher risk for neonatal morbidity and later neurodevelopmental and behavioral problems [3, 4], as confirmed also recently in the Norwegian Mother and Child Cohort Study (MoBa) study [5, 6].

Therefore, there has been a continuous quest to find modifiable risk factors that could be treated or

---

* Correspondence: mavo@fhi.no
[1]Domain of Mental and Physical Health, Norwegian Institute of Public Health, Oslo, Norway
[2]Psychological Institute, University of Oslo, Oslo, Norway
Full list of author information is available at the end of the article

prevented to reduce the number of preterm deliveries. An important risk factor for spontaneous preterm deliveries in general is anxiety [7, 8]. Recently, there has also been a focus on birth anxiety, which involves fears concerning pregnancy and birth. However, we find this approach too narrow. Women experiencing fear of childbirth often have a history of anxiety disorders [8]. A way to approximate this history is to assess trait anxiety, which is a disposition to feel anxious, excessively worried, and nervous [9]. Trait anxiety lies on a continuum with anxiety disorders and increases the individual's risk of feeling fearful and stressed in both harmless and harmful conditions. Feeling anxious and worried in turn triggers the biological stress response, which again activates neuroendocrinological mechanisms involving the hypothalamic-pituitary-adrenal axis [10].

Anxiety also increases the propensity to use psycho-active substances such as alcohol and tobacco, both before and during pregnancy, which again increases the risk for preterm births [11–13]. Moreover, shared genes for anxiety and addiction have been discovered [14]. Beyond the physiologically mediated risks, women experiencing anxiety may seek increased medical attention by requesting additional diagnostics or even demanding cesarean sections that are not medically indicated. Also, in a life course perspective, anxiety during pregnancy is probably an extension of dispositional anxiety before the pregnancy, which in turn may result in poorer reproductive health even before the first pregnancy [10, 15, 16].

This study addresses the association of trait anxiety with late preterm and early term delivery, both in the population of all pregnant women and in the subgroups of spontaneous and provider-initiated deliveries. We hypothesize that trait anxiety is associated with both gestational length, and that the association is higher in provider-oriented deliveries.

Methods
Study population
The Norwegian Institute of Public Health conducts a nationwide study of pregnant women, the Norwegian Mother and Child Cohort Study (MoBa). The study included 95 200 mothers recruited between 1999 and 2008 at about 100 hospitals and birth clinics across Norway, who were scheduled for a routine ultrasound examination [17, 18]. Among these, 40.6 % consented to participate [11] and completed questionnaires about their health and lifestyle at pregnancy weeks 17 and 30, and at 6, 18, and 36 months after childbirth. The MoBa study is linked to pregnancy and birth records in the Medical Birth Registry of Norway.

Sample inclusion and exclusion criteria
MoBa releases updates every year; this study used the complete quality-assured MoBa dataset made available for research in 2013 (version 7). We included women who conceived spontaneously, gave birth to a singleton live-born infant, had a pre-pregnancy body mass index (BMI) from 14 to 50 [19], and provided valid information on anxiety on the week 17 and week 30 questionnaires. This reduced the sample to 90,083 women. We excluded women with deliveries before week 34/0 days and after week 40/6 days, women who participated with a second or third pregnancy in MoBa, and women with serious pre-pregnancy disorders (rheumatoid arthritis, kidney disease, chronic hypertension, heart disease, epilepsy, and diabetes type 1 or type 2). We also excluded women with infants who had Apgar scores less than 7 or had serious malformations. After we applied all the inclusion and exclusion criteria, 81,244 pregnant women remained in the sample.

Measures
Preterm delivery
The length of all pregnancies in Norway is determined by second trimester ultrasound examination and recorded in days [20, 21]. If ultrasound information is missing, which applied to 1.7 % of deliveries in this study, pregnancy length was determined according to the date of the last menstruation. We distinguished three groups of gestational length in accordance with the recent criteria of the American College of Obstetrics and Gynecology [2]: *late preterm deliveries* (34/0–36/6 weeks), *early term deliveries* (37/0–38/9 weeks), and *full term deliveries* (39/0–40/6 weeks). Further, we subdivided the gestational age groups into spontaneous deliveries (delivery starting by spontaneous labor or spontaneous rupture of the membranes) and provider-initiated deliveries (induced labor or primary cesarean section) [20, 21]. All information was available from the Medical Birth Registry of Norway [18].

Trait anxiety
We used anxiety items completed on both questionnaires during pregnancy. We derived the items from a scale that was included in all MoBa questionnaires, the eight-item Symptom Checklist (SCL-8). The SCL-8 was specifically developed for medical patients and validated in seven European countries including Norway [22]. To avoid confounding with somatic symptoms, it only records emotional symptoms of anxiety and depression (four items for each construct). The four anxiety questions ask respondents about: (1) 'feeling fearful', (2) 'feeling nervousness or shakiness inside', (3) 'worrying too much about things', and (4) 'feeling sudden fear for no reason.' The response categories ranged from 'not at all bothered' (1) to 'very bothered' (4). We pooled the anxiety items into one average score for both time points, which had an excellent reliability

(Cronbach's alpha = 0.84) and high longitudinal stability ($r = 0.83$) with the identically constructed anxiety score measured at child age 3 years. We divided the pooled anxiety scale into four categories by means of cut-off points at the mean and ±2 standard deviations. The categories were: 'very low' = 1.0–1.25, 'low to mean' = 1.26–1.95, 'mean to high' =1.96–2.30, and 'high' = 2.31–4.00.

Confounders

Confounders are variables that are associated with both the exposure and the outcome. Therefore, we included only confounders that correlated with both gestational length and trait anxiety in preliminary analyses. We examined the variables maternal education, civil status, age, BMI before pregnancy, parity, daily smoking, alcohol consumption at least 1–3 times per month, urinary tract infections, gestational diabetes, and hypertension in pregnancy. We obtained information on most of these confounders from the Medical Birth Register of Norway, complemented by information from the questionnaires.

Data analyses

All analyses were carried out with IBM SPSS Statistics, version 22 [23] As recommended for longitudinal data, we imputed erroneous and missing values by means of maximum likelihood estimation, taking into account auxiliary, correlated data and information from later waves of the study [24]. For instance, missing maternal education was estimated by information on maternal age, income, and spouse's/partner's education and income. Missing data on smoking was imputed from information registered in the Medical Birth Register of Norway.

Second, we explored the associations of the confounders with gestational age group by means of univariate and multivariate multinomial regressions [23] separately for spontaneous and provider-initiated deliveries. In the two delivery onset groups, and the whole sample, neither gestational length nor anxiety was significantly associated with women's alcohol use or urinary tract infections in bivariate associations. Hence, both variables were excluded. In multivariate analyses in the entire sample, marriage status, smoking, and planned pregnancy were not significantly associated with gestational length group. They were therefore excluded as well; education, parity, gestational diabetes, and hypertension remained in the multivariate analyses.

Third, to calculate associations of anxiety with gestational age group, we computed multinomial regression analyses with full term deliveries and 'very low anxiety' as reference. To determine whether anxiety and delivery onset interacted, we examined both main and interaction effects in the whole sample.

Results

Women's trait anxiety was distributed as follows in the whole sample: 2.3 % had very high anxiety, 3.3 % had high anxiety, 33.5 % had low anxiety, and 60.9 % had very low anxiety (numbers not shown in the table). The low frequencies in the high anxiety classes reflect that all traits tapping negative emotions show a reverse J-shaped form, with most individuals clustering on the 'no negative emotions' side.

Table 1 presents trait anxiety according to type of delivery (spontaneous vs. provider initiated) and gestation

Table 1 Characteristics of mothers with late preterm, early term and full term deliveries by delivery onset

Gestational length[b]	Spontaneous deliveries[a]			Provider-initiated deliveries			All deliveries		
	Late preterm	Early term	Full term	Late preterm	Early term	Full term	Late preterm	Early term	Full term
N	1812	9701	56 527	1 007	4535	7824	2819	14054	64351
Anxiety Groups[c]	%	%	%	%	%	%	%	%	%
Very high	2.8	2.6	2.0	4.6	3.6	2.9	3.4	2.9	2.1
High	3.5	3.1	3.1	3.4	4.1	4.1	3.4	3.4	3.2
Low	36.6	33.7	32.6	38.2	37.9	35.8	37.2	35.0	33.0
Very low	57.1	60.6	62.3	53.8	54.5	57.1	55.9	58.7	61.7
Age, y; mean ± SD	29.6±5.0	29.7± 3.6	29.9±4.5	30.4±5.0	31.1±4.8	30.8±4.8	29.9 ± 5.0	30.1±4.7	30.1±4.5
Body Mass Index; mean ±SD	24.0±4.4	23.6±4.1	23.7±4.0	24.7±4.9	25.0±4.9	25.1±4.8	24.2 ± 4.6	24.1±4.4	23.9±4.1
Education less than college	43.6	39.8	37.4	42.2	43.1	39.7	43.1	40.9	37.7
Primiparous	53.9	44.9	42.8	48.6	34.2	45.3	52.0	41.6	43.1
Gestational diabetes	0.9	0.8	0.4	1.7	2.9	2.5	1.2	1.5	0.7
Gestational hypertension	5.7	3.9	2.7	37.9	15.9	16.4	17.2	7.6	4.3
Cesarean section	4.9	6.6	9.2	55.0	60.4	41.9	25.6	23.2	9.4

[a]Spontaneous deliveries (SD) = delivery onset by spontaneous labor or spontaneous rupture of the membranes
[b]Late preterm: weeks 34-36; early term: weeks 37-38; full term: weeks 39-41
[c]Cut-points at mean and ± 2 standard deviations. 'Very low' = 1.0-1.25; 'low to mean' = 1.26-1.95; 'mean to high' = 1.96-2.30; 'high' = 2.31-4.00

length within these categories. Data for gestation length is also given for the whole sample. In addition, the table shows demographic and pregnancy-related characteristics of the women according to delivery period and type. Looking at the 'very high' and 'high' anxiety categories, we find small proportions overall, ranging from 2.0 % to maximal 4.6 %. Women with provider-initiated deliveries have very high and high trait anxiety in all delivery periods more frequently than women with spontaneous deliveries (Chi^2 = 202 615; $p \leq 0.000$, phi = 0.05). For example, 4.6 % of women delivering late preterm by provider-initiation report high trait anxiety, versus 2.8 % in the corresponding spontaneous group. When we collapse the two highest anxiety classes, the percentage is 5.1 versus 7.0.

Further, Table 1 shows that women in all groups were on average from 30 to 32 years old, and only 37 % to 43 % showed educational levels below college. Women delivering late preterm were the most often primiparous; women delivering early term by provider-initiation were the least often primiparous. Of note, but to be expected, are the elevated levels of gestational diabetes and pregnancy-related hypertension in the group with provider-initiated deliveries.

Table 2 shows the multinomial regression findings among spontaneous deliveries, provider-initiated deliveries, and all deliveries. Beginning with the unadjusted analyses, the most noticeable finding is that women with

very high anxiety had odds of delivering *late preterm* OR = 1.5 and OR = 1.7 preterm in the spontaneous and provider-initiated groups, respectively. They had an OR = 1.8 in the entire sample. The odds of delivering early term were lower but still significant, ranging from 1.3 to 1.4 across women with spontaneous deliveries, provider-initiated deliveries and all deliveries. Women with high anxiety, the next category had no higher odds to deliver late preterm or early term. Women with low anxiety (compared to the reference group very low anxiety), had higher odds to deliver late preterm (OR = 1.2) and early term (OR = 1.1), but this finding was only significant in the entire sample. The adjustment for confounders did not reduce the associations of very high anxiety with late preterm and early term delivery remarkably.

Interaction analyses showed that the odds of delivering late preterm or early term for women with high anxiety were not greater in provider-initiated deliveries as compared to spontaneous deliveries (multinomial regression, interaction term anxiety*delivery onset; $Chi2$ = 4.34, df = 6, P = 0.59).

Discussion

In this study, high levels of trait anxiety predicted both late preterm and early term deliveries. Effect sizes were considerable: Women with very high trait anxiety had 80 % higher odds of delivering late preterm and 40 % higher odds of delivering early term. These associations

Table 2 Associations of trait anxiety with gestation length in women with sponteneous deliveries, provider-intitiated deliveries, and all deliveries

	Gestation length[b]	Spontaneous deliveries[a]			Provider-initiated deliveries			All deliveries		
		Late preterm	Early term	Full term (reference)	Late preterm	Early term	Full term (reference)	Late preterm	Early term	Full term (reference)
	N	1812	9701	56 527	1 007	4535	7824	2819	14054	64351
Unadjusted analyses		OR (95% CI)[c]	OR (95% CI)	OR (95% CI)	OR (95% CI)	OR (95% CI)	OR (95% CI)	OR (95% CI)	OR (95% CI)	OR (95% CI)
Anxiety groups[d]	Very high	1.5 (1.1-2.0)	1.3 (1.2-1.5)	-	1.7 (1.2-2.3)	1.3 (1.0-1.6)	-	1.8 (1.4-2.2)	1.4 (1.3-1.6)	-
	High	1.2 (0.9-1.6)	1.0 (0.9-1.2)	-	0.9 (0.6-1.2)	1.0 (0.9-1.3)	-	1,2 (1.0-1.5)	1.1 1.0-1.2)	-
	Low	1.2 (1.1-1.4)	1.1 (1.0-1.1)	-	1.1 (1.0-1.3)	1.1 (1.0-1.2)	-	1.2 (1.2-1.4)	1.1 (1.1-1.2)	-
	Very low (reference)	-	-	-	-	-	-	-	-	-
Adjusted analyses		OR (95% CI)	OR (95% CI)	OR (95% CI)	OR (95% CI)	OR (95% CI)	OR (95% CI)	OR (95% CI)	OR (95% CI)	OR (95% CI)
Anxiety groups	Very high	1.4 (1.0-1.8)	1.3 (1.1-1.5)	-	1.7 (1.2-2.4)	1.3 (1.0-1.6)	-	1.7 (1.3-2.0)	1.4 (1.3-1.6)	-
	High	1.1 (0.9-1.5)	1.0 (0.9-1.1)	-	0.9 (0.6-1.3)	1.0 (0.9-1.3)	-	1.1 (0.9-1-4)	1.1 (1.0-1.2)	-
	Low	1.2 (1.0-1.3)	1.0 (1.0-1.1)	-	1.1 (1.0-1.2)	1.1 (1.0-1.2)	-	1.2 (1.1-1.3)	1.1 (1.1-1.2)	-
	Very low (reference)	-	-	-	-	-	-	-	-	-

[a]Spontaneous deliveries = deliveries beginning by spontaneous labor or spontaneous rupture of the membranes
[b]Late preterm: weeks 34-36; early term: weeks 37-38; full term: weeks 39-41
[c]OR (95% CI): Odds Ratio and 95% Confidence Interval
[d]Cut-points at mean, and ± 2 standard deviations. 'Very low' = 1.0-1.25; 'low to mean = 1.26-1.95; 'mean to high' = 1.96-2.30; 'high' = 2.31-4.00

were the same for spontaneous and provider-initiated deliveries, although women with provider-initiated deliveries had higher trait anxiety than women with spontaneous deliveries. We consider these results important, because late preterm delivery and early term delivery are frequent in modern societies, affecting millions of women worldwide and posing considerable risks to the children [1, 3–7].

These results extend and strengthen previous research on the risks posed by high anxiety for preterm birth as demonstrated in recent meta-analyses [4, 7]. Different pathological pathways may explain the association between trait anxiety and preterm birth. The main focus in the literature has been the hypothesis that anxiety and depression during pregnancy lead to stress, which in turn activates the maternal hypothalamic-pituitary-adrenal (HPA) axis, triggering a cascade of endocrinological, immunological, and vascular reactions that may alter the fetal environment [10, 25].

However, in line with Wadhwa [10], we subscribe to the notion that negative consequences of anxiety on pregnancy outcomes must be understood from a life course perspective. Reproductive health may already have been reduced before the first pregnancy. Already in late adolescence and early adulthood, anxiety is associated with risky health behaviors and health conditions that negatively affect female reproduction outcome, such as smoking, drinking, risky sexual behaviors, unplanned pregnancies, and selective abortions [11–13, 26–28]. Further pathways may involve maladaptive reactions due to excessive worries, self-monitoring, and hypochondriac reactions, leading to frequent visits to antenatal care units, requests for extra diagnostic procedures or cesarean sections, and low compliance with antenatal health advice [29, 30]. We could not test these pathways in this study, but a previous study from the MoBa showed that anxiety and depression predicted higher rates of cesarean section—independent of gestation length [31].

The finding that women undergoing a provider-initiated delivery more often had high trait anxiety should alert obstetricians. Even if their anxiety may be a consequence of knowing that the pregnancy is riskier rather than a cause, these women need medical attention, and symptom relief should be attempted.

This study has limitations. The MoBa study is observational and thus precludes causal interpretations. Even randomized controlled trials cannot firmly confirm causal relations. The sample is biased, comprising more highly educated, older, married or cohabitating, non-smoking women compared to the total population of women delivering during the same decade in Norway. However, several studies in the MoBa examining the associations of important exposures with pregnancy outcomes showed findings similar to those in the entire Norwegian birthing population [17, 32]. Moreover, we did not have a standard scale for trait anxiety but had to make do with a short scale, which is a disadvantage that is typical with all multifocal, large epidemiological studies. The scale has been validated in Norway, however [33]. Also, we had no measures of anxiety levels during the life course of the women prior to pregnancy, but given the stability of personality dispositions, we trust that we captured a stable trait. Most importantly, however, we cannot exclude the possibility that unmeasured third factors may cause both higher trait anxiety and preterm delivery.

Conclusions

In conclusion, this study documented an association of high maternal trait anxiety with late preterm and early term delivery in one of the largest current mother and child cohort studies. Whether this association is mediated by stress, or other mechanisms, or can be explained largely by third variables may be examined by genetically informative studies such as family or twin studies or by molecular genetic linkage studies [34, 35]. As for clinical implications, antenatal screening for anxiety—and depression—should be a part of antenatal health care. Many pregnant women may not be aware that their anxiety is not normal, particularly if they have been very anxious all their lives. Treatment decisions should then be taken by specialists. Even if treatment does not affect the risk of preterm birth [36, 37], treating the anxiety will provide a health benefit to the mothers that will also affect how she takes care of the child later on.

Abbreviations
BMI: Body mass index; MoBa: Norwegian Mother and Child Cohort Study; SCL: Symptom checklist; SCL-8: Symptom checklist with 8 items

Acknowledgements
The Norwegian Mother and Child Cohort Study is supported by the Norwegian Ministry of Health and the Ministry of Education and Research, NIH/NIEHS (Contract No. N01-ES-75558), NIH/NINDS (Grant Nos. 1 UO1 NS 047537–01 and 2 UO1 NS 047537-06A1). We are grateful to all the participating families in Norway who are taking part in this on-going cohort study.

Authors' contributions
MV conceived and designed the study, computed the analyses, interpreted them scientifically and wrote the paper. VS contributed to designing the analyses, interpreting them scientifically, and drafting the paper. BJ contributed to designing the analyses and interpreting them scientifically. ML contributed to interpreting the analyses and drafting the paper. BL conceived the study together with MV, contributed to analytic strategies, interpreting the findings, and drafting the paper. All authors approved the final submitted manuscript.

Competing interests

The authors declare that they have no competing interests.

Author details

[1]Domain of Mental and Physical Health, Norwegian Institute of Public Health, Oslo, Norway. [2]Psychological Institute, University of Oslo, Oslo, Norway. [3]Department of Obstetrics and Gynecology, Sahlgrenska University Hospital, Gothenburg, Sweden. [4]University Children's Hospital Zurich, Zurich, Switzerland. [5]Department of Child and Adolescent Health Psychology, Institute of Psychology, University of Zurich, Zurich, Switzerland. [6]Department of Obstetrics and Gynaecology, Sahlgrenska Academy, Gothenburg University, Gothenburg, Sweden. [7]Department of Genes and Environment, Norwegian Institute of Public Health, Oslo, Norway. [8]Child Development Center, University Children's Hospital Zurich, Zurich, Switzerland.

References

1. Ananth CV, Friedman AM, Gyamfi-Bannerman C. Epidemiology of moderate preterm, late preterm and early term delivery. Clin Perinatol. 2013;40:601–10.
2. ACOG. ACOG committee opinion no. 579: definition of term pregnancy. Obstet Gynecol. 2013;122:1139–40.
3. Engle WA. Morbidity and mortality in late preterm and early term newborns: a continuum. Clin Perinatol. 2011;38:493–516.
4. Dong Y, Chen SJ, Yu JL. A systematic review and meta-analysis of long-term development of early term infants. Neonatology. 2012;102:212–21.
5. Stene-Larsen K, Brandlistuen RE, Lang AM, Landolt MA, Latal B, Vollrath ME. Communication impairments in early term and late preterm children: a prospective cohort study following children to age 36 months. J Pediatr. 2014;165(6):1123–8.
6. Zambrana IM, Vollrath ME, Sengpiel V, Jacobsson B, Ystrom E. Preterm delivery and risk for early language delays: a sibling-control cohort study. Int J Epidemiol. 2016;45(1):151–9.
7. Ding X, Wu YL, Xu SJ, et al. Maternal anxiety during pregnancy and adverse birth outcomes: a systematic review and meta-analysis of prospective cohort studies. J Affect Disord. 2014;159:103–10.
8. Rubertsson C, Hellström J, Cross M, Sydsjö G. Anxiety in early pregnancy: prevalence and contributing factors. Arch Womens Ment Health. 2014;17(3):221–8.
9. Gaudry E, Vagg P, Spielberger CD. Validation of the state-trait distinction in anxiety research. Multivariate Behav Res. 1975;10(3):331–41.
10. Wadhwa PD, Entringer S, Buss C, Lu MC. The contribution of maternal stress to preterm birth: issues and considerations. Clin Perinatol. 2011;38:351–84.
11. Stene-Larsen K, Torgersen L, Strandberg-Larsen K, Normann PT, Vollrath ME. Impact of maternal negative affectivity on light alcohol use and binge drinking during pregnancy. Acta Obstet Gynecol Scand. 2013;92(12):1388–94.
12. Hauge LJ, Aarø LE, Torgersen L, Vollrath ME. Smoking during consecutive pregnancies among primiparous women in the population-based Norwegian Mother and Child Cohort Study. Nicotine Tob Res. 2013;15(2):428–34.
13. Savitz DA, Murnane P. Behavioral influences on preterm birth: a review. Epidemiology. 2010;21:291–9.
14. Hodgson K, Almasy L, Knowles EE, Kent JW, Curran JE, Dyer TD, et al. Genome-wide significant loci for addiction and anxiety. Eur Psychiatry. 2016;36:47–54. doi:10.1016/j.eurpsy.2016.03.004. Epub 2016 Jun 16.
15. Jokela M, Hintsa T, Hintsanen M, Keltikangas-Järvinen L. Adult temperament and childbearing over the life course. Eur J Pers. 2010;24:151–66.
16. World Health Organization. Mental health aspects of women's reproductive health: a global review of the literature. Geneva: WHO Press; 2009.
17. Nilsen RM, Vollset SE, Gjessing HK, et al. Self-selection and bias in a large prospective pregnancy cohort in Norway. Paediatr Perinat Epidemiol. 2009;23:597–608.
18. Norwegian Institute of Public Health. Norwegian Mother and Child Cohort Study: end of enrolment. Revised protocol. Protocol II. Norway: Norwegian Institute of Public Health; 2012. https://www.fhi.no/globalassets/dokumenterfiler/usortert/moba-cohort-update-ije-april-2016.pdf. Accessed 31 July 2016.
19. Haugen M, Brantsaeter AL, Winkvist A, et al. Associations of pre-pregnancy body mass index and gestational weight gain with pregnancy outcome and postpartum weight retention: a prospective observational cohort study. BMC Pregnancy Childbirth. 2014;14:201.
20. Morken N-H, Källen K, Jacobsson B. Predicting risk of spontaneous preterm delivery in women with a singleton pregnancy. Paediatr Perinat Epidemiol. 2014;28:11–22.
21. Morken NH, Magnus P, Jacobsson B. Subgroups of preterm delivery in the Norwegian Mother and Child Cohort Study. Acta Obstet Gynecol Scand. 2008;87:1374–7.
22. Fink P, Ornbol E, Huyse FJ, et al. A brief diagnostic screening instrument for mental disturbances in general medical wards. J Psychosom Res. 2004;57:17–24.
23. IBM Corp. IBM SPSS Statistics for Windows, Version 22.0. Armonk: IBM Corporation; 2013.
24. Schafer JL, Graham JW. Missing data: our view of the state of the art. Psychol Methods. 2002;7:147–77.
25. Buss C, Entringer S, Swanson JM, Wadhwa PD. The role of stress in brain development: the gestational environment's long-term effects on the brain. Cerebrum. 2012;2012:4.
26. Stotland NL. Psychiatric aspects of induced abortion. J Nerv Ment Dis. 2011;199(8):568–70.
27. Cooper ML, Agocha VB, Sheldon MS. A motivational perspective on risky behaviors: the role of personality and affect regulatory processes. J Personality. 2000;68:1059–88.
28. Kelly RH, Russo J, Katon W. Somatic complaints among pregnant women cared for in obstetrics: normal pregnancy or depressive and anxiety symptom amplification revisited? Gen Hosp Psych. 2001;23:107–13.
29. Fuglenes D, Aas E, Botten G, Oian P, Kristiansen IS. Why do some pregnant women prefer cesarean? The influence of parity, delivery experiences, and fear of birth. Am J Obstet Gynecol. 2011;205:45.e1-9.
30. Kringeland T, Daltveit AK, Moller A. How does preference for natural childbirth relate to the actual mode of delivery? A population-based cohort study from Norway. Birth. 2010;37(1):21–7.
31. Nilsen RM, Suren P, Gunnes N, et al. Analysis of self-selection bias in a population-based cohort study of autism spectrum disorders. Paediatr Perinat Epidemiol. 2013;27:553–63.
32. Kaprio J, Pulkkinen L, Rose RJ. Genetic and environmental factors in health-related behaviors: studies on Finnish twins and twin families. Twin Res. 2002;5:366–71.
33. Tambs K, Moum T. How well can a few questionnaire items indicate anxiety and depression? Acta Psychiatr Scand. 1993;87:364–7.
34. Cordell HJ, Clayton DG. Genetic association studies. Lancet. 2005;366:1121–31.
35. Yonkers KA, Blackwell KA, Glover J, Forray A. Antidepressant use in pregnant and postpartum women. Annu Rev Clin Psychol. 2014;10:369–92.
36. Sydsjo G, Sydsjo A, Gunnervik C, Bladh M, Josefsson A. Obstetric outcome for women who received individualized treatment for fear of childbirth during pregnancy. Acta Obstet Gynecol Scand. 2012;91:44–9.
37. Khianman B, Pattanittum P, Thinkhamrop J, Lumbiganon P. Relaxation therapy for preventing and treating preterm labour. Cochrane Database Syst Rev. 2012;8:Cd007426.

6

Maternal intake of seafood and supplementary long chain n-3 poly-unsaturated fatty acids and preterm delivery

Anne Lise Brantsæter[1*], Linda Englund-Ögge[2], Margareta Haugen[1], Bryndis Eva Birgisdottir[3], Helle Katrine Knutsen[1], Verena Sengpiel[2], Ronny Myhre[4], Jan Alexander[5], Roy M. Nilsen[6], Bo Jacobsson[4,7] and Helle Margrete Meltzer[1]

Abstract

Background: Preterm delivery increases the risk of neonatal morbidity and mortality. Studies suggest that maternal diet may affect the prevalence of preterm delivery. The aim of this study was to assess whether maternal intakes of seafood and marine long chain n-3 polyunsaturated fatty acids (LCn-3PUFA) from supplements were associated with preterm delivery.

Methods: The study population included 67,007 women from the Norwegian Mother and Child Cohort Study. Maternal food and supplement intakes were assessed by a validated self-reported food frequency questionnaire in mid-pregnancy. Information about gestational duration was obtained from the Medical Birth Registry of Norway. We used Cox regression to estimate hazard ratios (HR) with 95% confidence intervals (CI) for associations between total seafood, lean fish, fatty fish, and LCn-3PUFA intakes and preterm delivery. Preterm was defined as any onset of delivery before gestational week 37, and as spontaneous or iatrogenic deliveries and as preterm delivery at early, moderate, and late preterm gestations.

Results: Lean fish constituted 56%, fatty fish 34% and shellfish 10% of seafood intake. Any intake of seafood above no/rare intake (>5 g/d) was associated with lower prevalence of preterm delivery. Adjusted HRs were 0.76 (CI: 0.66, 0.88) for 1–2 servings/week (20–40 g/d), 0.72 (CI: 0.62, 0.83) for 2–3 servings/week (40–60 g/d), and 0.72 (CI: 0.61, 0. 85) for ≥3 servings/week (>60 g/d), p-trend <0.001. The association was seen for lean fish (p-trend: 0.005) but not for fatty fish (p-trend: 0.411). The intake of supplementary LCn-3PUFA was associated only with lower prevalence of early preterm delivery (before 32 gestational weeks), while increasing intake of LCn-3PUFA from food was associated with lower prevalence of overall preterm delivery (p-trend: 0.002). Any seafood intake above no/ rare was associated with lower prevalence of both spontaneous and iatrogenic preterm delivery, and with lower prevalence of late preterm delivery.

Conclusions: Any intake of seafood above no/rare consumption was associated with lower prevalence of preterm delivery. The association was stronger for lean than for fatty fish. Intake of supplementary LCn-3PUFA was associated only with early preterm delivery. The findings corroborate the current advice to include fish and seafood as part of a balanced diet during pregnancy.

Keywords: Preterm delivery, Seafood consumption, Food frequency questionnaire, The Norwegian Mother and Child Cohort Study, MoBa

* Correspondence: AnneLise.Brantsaeter@fhi.no
[1]Department of Environmental Exposure and Epidemiology, Domain of Infection Control and Environmental Health, Norwegian Institute of Public Health, P.O. Box 4404Nydalen, NO-0403 Oslo, Norway
Full list of author information is available at the end of the article

Background

Preterm delivery, which is defined as spontaneous or iatrogenic delivery before gestational week 37, is the major cause of perinatal mortality and morbidity and is an important risk factor of long-term physical and mental disabilities [1–4]. In Scandinavia and some other European countries, the rate is around 5–7% of all deliveries, while in the United States it is as high as 12% [5].

Preterm delivery accounts for a high financial burden on healthcare and is a considerable trauma for those involved [6–8]. Several factors have been shown to be associated with preterm delivery, including maternal demographic characteristics, reproductive history, infection, and biological and genetic markers [1, 9–11]. However, the aetiologies for preterm delivery are largely unknown and currently there is no effective treatment to reduce the rate of preterm delivery. Hence, it is important to identify potential modifiable factors in order to prevent the complications and cost associated with preterm delivery.

Seafood is a rich source of essential nutrients including protein, selenium, iodine, vitamin D, and the marine long chain n-3 polyunsaturated fatty acids (LCn-3PUFA) which have important structural and physiological roles in the body, including neurological, immune, and cardiovascular systems [12–14].

In prospective observational studies, high levels of maternal fish consumption during pregnancy have been associated with longer gestation [15–17] and lower prevalence of preterm delivery [16, 18], but the results are not found in all studies [19–21]. The beneficial effects of fish consumption have primarily been attributed to the LCn-3PUFA eicosapentaenoic acid (EPA) and docosahexaenoic acid (DHA). Randomized controlled trials have shown lower risk of preterm delivery, and particularly early preterm delivery (<34 weeks) in women supplemented with EPA and DHA during pregnancy [22–25].

The current dietary advice to pregnant women in Norway and other countries is to include lean and fatty fish as part of a balanced diet and to limit or avoid consumption of contaminated species [26–28]. In Norway there is a long tradition not only for eating seafood, but also for use of cod liver oil. More studies of maternal seafood and LCn-3PUFA intake in relation to preterm delivery are needed to disentangle, if possible, the role of different types of fish and supplementary LCn-3PUFA [29, 30]. In the Norwegian Mother and Child Cohort Study, women reported in detail their intakes of food and dietary supplements during pregnancy, making it possible to quantify their total seafood consumption and subcategories of lean and fatty fish, as well as LCn-3PUFA contributed by use of dietary supplements and LCn-3PUFA contributed by food (i.e., fish) [31–34].

The aim of the present study was to examine associations of maternal seafood and LCn-3PUFA supplement intakes with the risk of preterm delivery. We hypothesized that higher intake of seafood is associated with lower risk of preterm delivery and that associations vary by seafood categories. We investigated the associations with all preterm deliveries and with the outcome stratified as spontaneous and iatrogenic preterm delivery and as early, moderate and late preterm delivery.

Methods
Population and study design

The Norwegian Mother and Child Cohort Study (MoBa) is a prospective population-based pregnancy cohort study conducted by the Norwegian Institute of Public Health [35]. Participants were recruited from across Norway from 1999 through 2008, and 40.6% of the invited women participated. The cohort now includes 114,500 children, 95,200 mothers and 75,200 fathers. Women were recruited to the study by postal invitation before the routine free ultrasound examination around gestational week 18. The women were asked to provide blood and urine samples at baseline and to answer questionnaires at regular intervals during pregnancy and after birth. Follow-up is conducted by questionnaires at regular intervals and by linkage to national health registries [35, 36].

The data included in this study were from two questionnaires answered around gestational weeks 17 (questionnaire 1) [37] and 22 (questionnaire 2) [38]. Questionnaire 1 was a general questionnaire covering lifestyle, background, illness and health-related factors. Questionnaire 2 was a semi-quantitative food frequency questionnaire (FFQ), in which women reported their dietary habits from the start of the pregnancy. The response rates for the questionnaires during pregnancy were 95% for questionnaire 1 and 92% for questionnaire 2 [39]. Pregnancy and birth records from the Medical Birth Registry of Norway (MBRN) are linked to the MoBa database [36].

The current study is based on version 5 of the quality-assured data files released for research in 2010 ($n = 108,264$). To be included in the study, participants had to have delivered a live, singleton baby and to have answered both the first general questionnaire and the FFQ. They also had to have a valid energy intake between 4.5 and 20 MJ/day, resulting in $n = 83,386$ eligible for analysis. We excluded women with a duration of pregnancy less than 22^{+0} or more than 41^{+6} weeks (+days) ($n = 6798$), those with missing information about parity ($n = 51$) and those with missing information about previous preterm delivery ($n = 42$). To avoid the use of multiple dependent observations in our analyses, women who participated in the cohort more than once ($n = 9488$)

were only included with their first participation, resulting in a final study sample of 67,007 mother-infant pairs (Fig. 1).

Dietary assessment

The MoBa FFQ was completed around the 22nd week of gestation, and the dietary data were collected from February 2002 and onwards [32]. The MoBa FFQ is a semi-quantitative questionnaire designed to capture dietary habits during the first 4 to 5 months of pregnancy [38]. The FFQ included questions about intake of 255 food items with special emphasis on various seafood items. There were 10 questions about cold cuts and spreads made of fish or shellfish, 16 questions about fish or shellfish eaten for dinner, and four questions about cod liver oil, cod liver oil capsules or fish oil capsules.

Nutrient calculations were performed with the use of FoodCalc [40] and the Norwegian food composition table [41]. In the FFQ, the women were asked to record the use of dietary supplements. We have developed a database for nutrient content in more than 1000 dietary supplements reported by MoBa participants. For calculating intake of LCn-3PUFA from supplements we used name and brand name combined with reported frequency and amount. The FFQ has been thoroughly validated with regard to nutrients, foods and dietary supplements [31, 33, 42].

Definition of fish and seafood variables and LCn-3PUFA intake

The daily intakes (g/day) of fish items were grouped as lean fish or fatty fish and included items eaten as bread spread, in salad, as dinner or as part of a mixed dish such as fish fingers or fish au gratin. In composite fish dishes, only the fish part of the dish was included in the calculated fish intake. Lean fish species included cod, saithe, haddock, pollock, halibut, plaice, flounder, tuna, perch, pike, Atlantic cat fish and fish roe (0.3–6.0% fat). Fatty fish species included mackerel, herring, salmon and trout (10–24% fat). We also calculated the intakes of shellfish (shrimp, crab and mussels (0.8–2.5% fat) and fish liver. Total seafood was the combined intake of lean fish, fatty fish, shellfish, and fish liver.

When evaluating the association between seafood consumption and preterm delivery, seafood intake was treated both as a continuous variable (g/d) and divided into the following categories: 0–5 g/d, >5- ≤ 20 g/d, >20- ≤ 40 g/ d, >40- ≤ 60 g/d, and ≥60 g/d. The same categories were used in two previous studies that examined seafood intake in relation to infant size at birth [34, 43]. Assuming a serving size of 140 g, these categories correspond to; never/rare intake, <1 serving/week, 1to <2 servings/week, 2 to <3 servings/week and 3 or more servings/week. When seafood was eaten as bread spread, a serving size was estimated to be 20–25 g. Lean and fatty fish variables were examined as continuous variables and divided into the five categories described above. In adjusted analyses, these variables were mutually adjusted (i.e., both entered in the same models). Lean and fatty fish intakes correlated with $r_s = 0.22$ ($p < 0.001$), while correlations for lean and fatty fish with shellfish and fish liver were weaker.

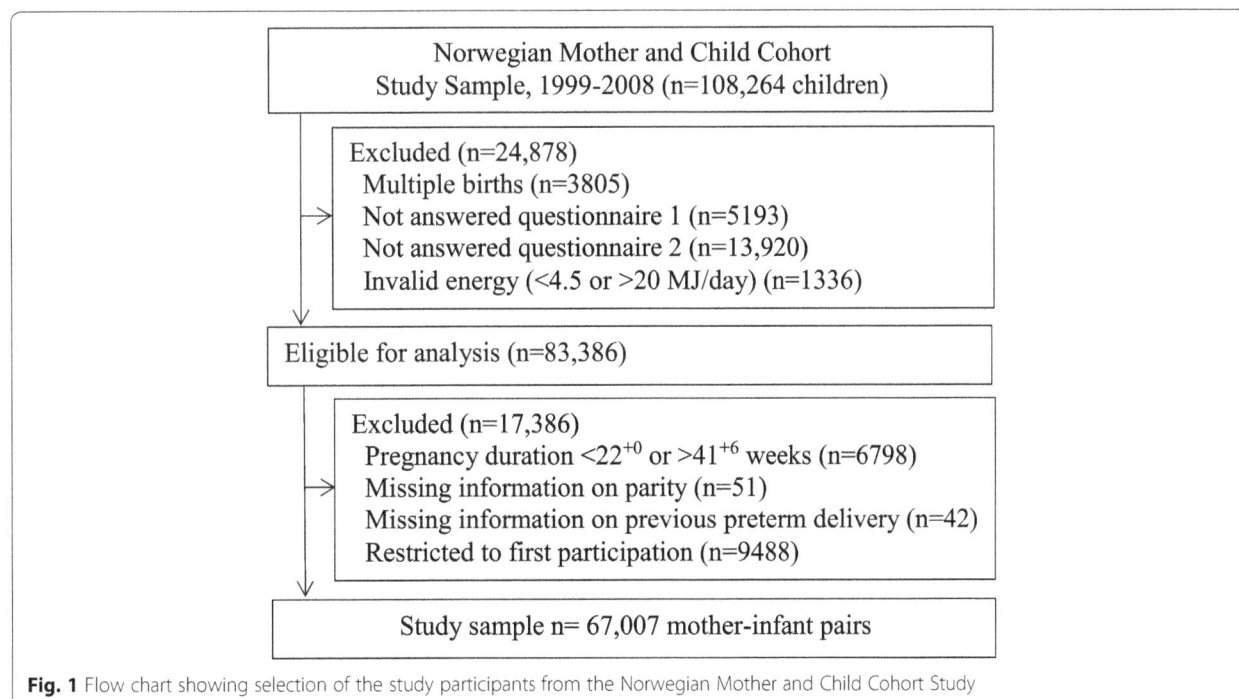

Fig. 1 Flow chart showing selection of the study participants from the Norwegian Mother and Child Cohort Study

Norwegian Mother and Child Cohort
Study Sample, 1999-2008 (n=108,264 children)

Excluded (n=24,878)
Multiple births (n=3805)
Not answered questionnaire 1 (n=5193)
Not answered questionnaire 2 (n=13,920)
Invalid energy (<4.5 or >20 MJ/day) (n=1336)

Eligible for analysis (n=83,386)

Excluded (n=17,386)
Pregnancy duration <22^{+0} or >41^{+6} weeks (n=6798)
Missing information on parity (n=51)
Missing information on previous preterm delivery (n=42)
Restricted to first participation (n=9488)

Study sample n= 67,007 mother-infant pairs

LCn-3PUFA in the current study was defined as the sum of eicosapentaenoic acid (EPA) and docosahexaenoic acid (DHA). The amount (mg/d) of LCn-3PUFA contributed by dietary supplements (EPA and DHA in cod liver oil, fish oil, cod liver oil capsules and fish oil capsules) and the amount of LCn-3PUFA contributed by fish (EPA and DHA) was estimated from the FFQ. The variables for LCn-3PUFA (i.e., amount contributed from food and amount contributed from supplements) were examined as continuous and as ranked variables. LCn-3PUFA from food and the total sum of LCn-3PUFA from food and supplements were divided into quintiles. In all models with seafood intake as the exposure, we adjusted for the amount of LCn-3PUFA from supplements divided into three categories with non-users as one group and consumers ranked into two groups divided by median.

Preterm delivery

We defined preterm delivery as delivery before gestational week 37^{+0} and used this as the primary outcome. Gestational age in days was obtained from the MBRN and determined by second-trimester ultrasound in 98.2% of pregnancies and based on the last menstrual period in the remaining cases [36]. Preterm delivery was categorised based on delivery initiation, i.e., spontaneous preterm delivery (preterm labour or preterm prelabour rupture of the membranes) or iatrogenic preterm delivery (induced or primary caesarean delivery on maternal or foetal indications). Preterm delivery was also categorised into late (34^{+0} to 36^{+6} weeks), moderately (32^{+0} to 33^{+6} weeks) and early preterm (22^{+0} to 31^{+6} weeks).

Other variables

We included a range of potential covariates and examined their association with seafood intake and preterm delivery. Information about maternal age at delivery and previous preterm delivery was obtained from the MBRN. We treated maternal age as a continuous variable. History of previous preterm delivery was analysed as a dichotomous variable (yes/no). Body mass index (BMI) was calculated from prepregnancy weight and height that women had reported in questionnaire 1. We only included women with pre-pregnancy weight in the range 35–180 kg and height above 1.40 m. BMI was divided into four categories (<18.5, 18.5–24.9, 25–29.9, $\geq$ 30 kg/m^2) and a missing category ($n = 1723$). Height was divided into quartiles. Information about parity came from questionnaire 1 and from MBRN and was divided into two categories (nulliparous or parous). Information about marital status, smoking in pregnancy, maternal education and household income was obtained from questionnaire 1. Marital status was divided into living alone or cohabiting and smoking into yes (occasional or daily smoker) or no.

Maternal education was divided into four categories: $\leq$12 years (high school or less), 13–16 years (3–4 years of college/university), 17 + years (4 years or more of college/university), or other/missing ($n = 1418$). Household income was expressed as a combination of the participant's and her partner's annual income and divided into three categories: both partners <300,000 NOK, one partner $\geq$300,000 NOK, both partners $\geq$300,000 NOK, or missing information ($n = 1936$). Information about alcohol intake and whether or not the pregnancy was planned was divided into yes or no. We used total energy intake (kJ) as a continuous variable.

Statistical methods

We used one-way analysis of variance for continuous variables, chi-square test for categorical variables and Mann-Whitney U test for nominal data to test differences between groups. The main exposure variables were total seafood, including the subcategories lean and fatty fish, and LCn-3PUFA from food and supplements. We used Cox regression to estimate hazard ratios (HR) for preterm delivery with 95% confidence intervals (CI). Preterm delivery was the defined event and gestational days the underlying time variable with day 153 as the entry time (22 completed weeks of gestation). Follow-up ended at the date of preterm delivery or at 259 days of gestation (36 completed weeks of gestation), whichever came first. In the separate analysis of spontaneous and iatrogenic preterm delivery, the other category was censored but kept in the analysis. P for trend was obtained by incorporating the categorical variables as linear terms in the models. Variables included in the adjusted models were: maternal age, education, history of previous preterm delivery, height, BMI, marital status, parity, smoking, household income and total energy intake.

Repeating the analyses using logistic regression resulted in odds ratios comparable to the hazard ratios obtained by Cox regression. Hazard ratios and odds ratios represent different association measures, but both approximate relative risks when the outcome is rare [44].

We examined the associations between seafood and preterm delivery separately in women with prepregnant BMI < 25 and those with prepregnant BMI $\geq$ 25 kg/m^2, and separately for nulliparous and parous pregnancies. We also conducted other sensitivity analyses, including complete case analysis.

We used visual inspection of the log-log plot to verify that the proportional-hazard assumption was essentially fulfilled All analyses were performed using PASW Statistics software version 19 for Windows (SPSS Inc., IBM Company, Chicago Ill., USA). All P values were two sided and values below 0.05 were considered statistically significant.

Results

Consumption of any seafood was reported by 97.7% of all women in this study, 5.7% reported no lean fish, 13% reported no fatty fish, 10.7% reported no shellfish and 91% reported no consumption of fish liver. The median intakes of total seafood, lean fish and fatty fish were 33.4, 18.5 and 8.3 g/day, respectively. Lean and fatty fish constituted on average 56 and 34% of the total seafood intake (Table 1). The median total seafood intake corresponds to 1–2 servings per week. The median amount of LCn-3PUFA from total seafood was 0.25 g/d (mean 0.37 g/d), with median 0.039 g/d from lean fish (mean 0.044 g/d)) and 0.188 g/d from fatty fish (mean 0.298 g/d). On average, fatty fish contributed 75% and lean fish 11% to the LCn-3PUFA intake from food (Table 1). Use of LCn-3PUFA supplements was reported by 67% of the women. The supplement users were divided into two groups based on the median intake of supplemental LCn-3PUFA (<0.30 g/d and ≥0.30 g/d). In the low group, LCn-3PUFA intakes ranged from 0.01 g/d-0.29 g/d (median 0.16 g/d) and in the high group from 0.30 g/d-8.8 g/d (median 0.80 g/d).

Maternal characteristics differed across increasing categories of seafood intake and between LCn-3PUFA non-supplement and supplement users (Table 2). Maternal age and energy intake increased with increasing seafood intake, while BMI decreased. Women in the lowest consumption categories included more nulliparous women and more women with low education and income than to those in the higher consumption categories. Increasing seafood intake was associated with not only increasing intakes of fish and shellfish, but also by increasing intakes of LCn-3PUFA from food and from supplements. LCn-3PUFA supplement users had lower BMI, included fewer first time mothers and fewer smokers, and included more women with high education and income than non-supplement users (Table 2).

The overall proportion of preterm delivery in the study population was 5.4% (n = 3630), comprising 3.1% (n = 2051) spontaneous and 2.2% (n = 1419) iatrogenic preterm deliveries, while information about delivery initiation was missing for 88 preterm cases (0.1%). Of all deliveries, 2659 (4.0%) were late preterm deliveries, 491 (0.7%) were moderately preterm and 480 (0.7%) were early preterm deliveries (Table 3). In crude analyses using continuous seafood intake variables, women with preterm deliveries had lower intakes of total seafood, lean fish and fatty fish than women with term deliveries. This was also found for LCn-3PUFA from food, while there was no difference in the amount of LCn-3PUFA from supplements between the groups. The differences in seafood intakes were seen particularly for the subcategories spontaneous and iatrogenic preterm delivery and for late preterm delivery (Table 3).

Examining seafood intake by categories with the never/rarely as the reference category, showed lower prevalence of preterm delivery for all other intake categories (Table 4). For total seafood intake, the lowest risk estimates were observed in the two highest intake categories with adjusted HR: 0.72 (95%CI: 0.62, 0.83) for 2-≤ 3 servings per week and HR: 0.72 (95%CI: 0.61, 0.85) for ≥3 servings per week, p-trend <0.001 (Table 3). When lean and fatty fish were examined as separate variables, significantly lower risk for preterm delivery was observed for lean fish intake in all intake categories except the highest category (p-trend: 0.005). For fatty fish, lower risk was seen only for the intake category corresponding to 1- ≤ 2 servings per week (p-trend 0.411). LCn-3PUFA from supplements was not associated with overall preterm delivery (Fig. 2 and Table 4).

We further examined whether the associations between LCn-3PUFA from supplements and preterm delivery differed between groups of women with low and high seafood intake. Low seafood intake was defined as no seafood intake and intakes below the 5th percentile. Total seafood intake was also ranked into tertiles, quintiles and deciles, and the association between LCn-3PUFA from supplements and preterm delivery examined in each strata separately. No significant association between LCn-3PUFA from supplements and preterm delivery was observed at any level of seafood intake (results not shown). Furthermore, we examined

Table 1 Calculated intake seafood and LCn-3PUFA from food and % contribution from subcategories in n = 67,007 women in the Norwegian Mother and Child Cohort Study 2002–2008

	Median, g/d	Mean, g/d	% of total seafood	LCn-3PUFA, median g/d	LCn-3PUFA, mean g/d	% of LCn-3PUFA
Total seafood	33.4	36.4		0.248	0.365	92
Lean fish	18.5	20.3	56	0.039	0.044	11
Fatty fish	8.3	12.2	34	0.188	0.298	75
Shellfish	2.4	3.6	10	0	0.009	2.2
Fish liver	0	0.3	0.7	0	0.014	3.7
Eggs[a]	7.8	11.4		0.014	0.019	4.8
Other food (poultry)[a]	18.8	22.4		0.010	0.012	3.0

[a]Eggs and other food contain LCn-3PUFA (eicosapentaenoic and docosahexaenoic acid) coming from marine feed ingredients

Table 2 Seafood consumption and LCn-3PUFA supplement use by maternal characteristics. $N = 67{,}007$ women in the Norwegian Mother and Child Cohort Study 2002–2008

	Seafood consumption (g/day)						LCn-3PUFA[b] supplement use		
	0–5 (4.4%)	>5–20 (18.4%)	>20–40 (40.4%)	>40–60 (24.5%)	>60 (12.3%)	p-value[a]	No (32.9%)	Yes (67.1%)	p-value[a]
Continuous Variables (mean and standard deviation)									
Maternal age at delivery (years)	28 (5)	29 (5)	30 (4)	31 (4)	31 (5)	<0.001	30 (5)	30 (4)	<0.001
Maternal height (m)[b]	1.67 (0.06)	1.68 (0.06)	1.68 (0.06)	1.68 (0.06)	1.68 (0.06)	<0.001	1.68 (0.06)	1.68 (0.06)	<0.001
Prepregnancy body mass index (kg/m^2)[c]	24.4 (4.6)	24.2 (4.4)	24.0 (4.2)	23.9 (4.2)	23.9 (4.3)	<0.001	24.6 (4.6)	23.7 (4.0)	<0.001
Total energy intake (MJ)	9.3 (2.8)	9.3 (2.5)	9.6 (2.5)	9.9 (2.5)	10.7 (2.9)	<0.001	9.7 (2.7)	9.7 (2.5)	0.216
Lean fish (g/day)	0.5 (1.1)	8.1 (4.5)	18.0 (7.3)	28.3 (10.5)	37.0 (17.3)	<0.001	20.4 (14.5)	20.2 (13.2)	0.196
Fatty fish (g/day)	0.5 (1.1)	4.0 (3.5)	8.6 (6.0)	15.4 (9.9)	34.4 (24.1)	<0.001	11.4 (14.1)	12.6 (14.1)	<0.001
Shellfish (g/day)	0.3 (0.8)	1.9 (2.4)	3.3 (4.5)	4.5 (5.2)	6.8 (10.9)	<0.001	3.6 (6.0)	3.7 (5.2)	0.405
LCn-3PUFA[b] from food (g/day)	0.09 (0.05)	0.21 (0.10)	0.36 (0.18)	0.57 (0.29)	1.18 (0.77)	<0.001	0.45 (0.45)	0.48 (0.44)	<0.001
LCn-3PUFA[b] from supplements (g/day)	0.29 (0.54)	0.32 (0.51)	0.37 (0.54)	0.40 (0.58)	0.44 (0.62)	<0.001	0	0.56 (0.60)	<0.001
Discrete characteristics (%)[b]									
Nulliparous mother (%)	38.4	41.7	48.1	52.7	52.5	<0.001	39.5	57.9	<0.001
Previous preterm delivery (%)	2.9	3.4	3.4	3.9	4.1	0.002	4.6	3.1	<0.001
Single mother (%)	5.8	3.8	3.3	3.9	4.9	<0.001	4.7	3.5	<0.001
Maternal smoking (%)[c]	14.2	8.8	7.3	7.5	8.9	<0.001	12.9	5.8	<0.001
Maternal education[c]									
≤ 12 years	48.3	34.7	28.3	28.5	34.4	<0.001	43.2	25.2	<0.001
13–16 years	33.2	40.2	43.3	42.8	38.2		37.4	43.6	
> 16 years	15.5	22.6	26.5	26.9	25.0		17.0	29.2	
Household income (annual)[c]									
Both partners < NOK 300,000	37.5	30.0	27.2	27.5	30.5	<0.001	34.3	24.2	<0.001
One partner ≥ NOK 300,000	42.3	42.3	41.9	42.3	42.8		41.9	40.6	
Both partners ≥ NOK 300,000	20.2	27.7	30.8	30.1	26.7		20.0	32.2	
Planned pregnancy[c]	74.6	80.6	81.4	80.7	77.8	<0.001	76.6	82.2	<0.001

[a]P value for difference: One-way analysis of variance for continuous variables, chi-square test for categorical variables

[b]LCn-3PUFA: marine long chain n-3 polyunsaturated fatty acids

[c]Missing information prepregnant body mass index: 2.6%, maternal education: 2.1%, household income: 2.9%, planned pregnancy:1.1%

Table 3 Maternal intake (g/day) of seafood and marine long chain n-3 polyunsaturated fatty acids (LCn-3PUFA) from food and dietary supplements in 67,007 women with and without preterm delivery (PTD) in the Norwegian Mother and Child Cohort Study (MoBa) 2002–2008

	N (%)	Total seafood Median (P5, P95)	Lean fish Median (P5, P95)	Fatty fish Median (P5, P95)	Food LCn-3PUFA Median (P5, P95)	Suppl. LCn-3PUFA Median (P5, P95)
Overall preterm delivery						
No	63,377 (94.6)	33.5 (6.2, 75.9)	18.5 (0, 45.2)	8.3 (0, 38.3)	0.35 (0.10, 1.27)	0.16 (0, 1.60)
Yes	3630 (5.4)	32.1 (3.5, 78.6)	17.7 (0, 44.8)	7.6 (0, 40.3)	0.34 (0.08, 1.32)	0.16 (0, 1.60)
Crude p-value[a]		<0.001	<0.001	<0.001	<0.001	0.936
Adjusted p-value[b]		0.004	0.008	0.349	0.171	0.879
Subcategories by delivery initiation[c]						
Spontaneous preterm deliveries						
No	63,377 (94.6)	33.5 (6.2, 75.9)	18.5 (0, 45.2)	8.3 (0, 38.3)	0.35 (0.10, 1.27)	0.16 (0, 1.60)
Yes	2051 (3.1)	31.7 (3.0, 78.4)	17.9 (0, 45.1)	7.6 (0, 39.3)	0.33 (0.08, 1.32)	0.16 (0, 1.60)
Crude p-value		<0.001	0.011	0.001	<0.001	0.680
Iatrogenic preterm delivery						
No	63,377 (94.6)	33.5 (6.2, 75.9)	18.5 (0, 45.2)	8.3 (0, 38.3)	0.35 (0.10, 1.27)	0.16 (0, 1.60)
Yes	1491 (2.2)	33.0 (4.1, 78.6)	17.5 (0, 45.3)	7.6 (0, 42.6)	0.35 (0.09, 1.33)	0.15 (0, 1.60)
Crude p-value		0.031	0.008	0.045	0.123	0.294
Subcategories by week of delivery						
Late PTD (35 to <37 w)						
No	63,377 (94.6)	33.5 (6.2, 75.9)	18.5 (0, 45.2)	8.3 (0, 38.3)	0.35 (0.10, 1.27)	0.16 (0, 1.60)
Yes	2659 (4.0)	31.8 (3.5, 78.3)	17.7 (0, 44.1)	7.6 (0, 39.6)	0.34 (0.09, 1.32)	0.16 (0, 1.60)
Crude p-value		<0.001	<0.001	0.002	0.001	0.720
Moderately PTD (32 to <34w)						
No	63,377 (94.6)	33.5 (6.2, 75.9)	18.5 (0, 45.2)	8.3 (0, 38.3)	0.35 (0.10, 1.27)	0.16 (0, 1.60)
Yes	491 (0.7)	33.6 (3.0, 81.0)	17.5 (0, 45.5)	8.1 (0, 44.1)	0.35 (0.08, 1.44)	0.15 (0, 1.60)
Crude p-value		0.530	0.155	0.378	0.712	0.386
Early PTD (22 to <32 w)						
No	63,377 (94.6)	33.5 (6.2, 75.9)	18.5 (0, 45.2)	8.3 (0, 38.3)	0.35 (0.10, 1.27)	0.16 (0, 1.60)
Yes	480 (0.7)	32.0 (3.3, 78.0)	18.1 (0, 45.8)	7.2 (0, 38.6)	0.33 (0.09, 1.23)	0.14 (0, 1.60)
Crude p-value		0.102	0.467	0.018	0.016	0.050

P5: 5th percentile, P95: 95th percentile
[a]Crude *P-values* from non-parametric Mann-Whitney *U* test
[b]Adjusted *P*-values from Cox regression with continuous seafood variables adjusted for the other seafood and LCn-3PUFA variables when relevant, maternal age, pre-pregnancy BMI, height, parity, energy intake, maternal education, smoking, marital status, household income and previous preterm delivery
[c]Missing data on delivery initiation for 88 preterm deliveries

LCn-3PUFA from supplements as a continuous variable and ranked into quintiles and deciles. No significant associations with preterm delivery were indicated (results not shown).

We repeated the analysis using the calculated LCn-3PUFA intake from food as the exposure and the lowest quintile as reference category. Lower risk estimates were seen in all the other quintiles (Additional file 1: Table S1), with the lowest HR observed in quintile 4 (HR 0.83, CI: 0.75, 0.92), *p*-trend 0.002. However, when we summed the intake of LCn-3PUFA from food and supplements, the association with preterm delivery was significant only in the third quintile

(Additional file 1: Table S1). When LCn-3PUFA from food was included in a model with seafood as the exposure, the hazard ratios for seafood and preterm delivery remained significant, but with wider confidence intervals (i.e., for 2–3 servings/week HR: 0.77 (95%CI: 0.64, 0.92) and for ≥3 servings/week HR: 0.75 (95%CI: 0.62, 0.92).

We further analysed associations between seafood intake and subcategories of preterm delivery. Any intake of seafood beyond no/rare intake was associated with lower prevalence of both spontaneous and iatrogenic preterm deliveries (Table 5), with HRs similar to those seen for any preterm (20–30% risk reduction). In these analyses, lean fish had a stronger influence on the

Table 4 Associations between total seafood intake, lean and fatty fish intake and marine long chain n-3 polyunsaturated fatty acids (LCn-3PUFA) from supplements and preterm delivery (PTD). $N = 67,007$ women in the Norwegian Mother and Child Cohort Study (MoBa) 2002–2008

	All	PTD	Unadjusted	Adjusted
	n	n (%)	HR[a] (95% CI)	HR[ab] (95% CI)
Total seafood				
≤ 5 g/d (never/rarely)	2966	220 (7.4)	1	1
> 5–20 g/d (<1 serving/week)	12,299	713 (5.8)	0.77 (0.66, 0.90)	0.80 (0.69, 0.93)
> 20–40 g/d (1–2 servings/week)	27,045	1440 (5.3)	0.71 (0.62, 0.82)	0.76 (0.66, 0.88)
> 40–60 g/d (2–3 servings/week)	16,432	824 (5.0)	0.67 (0.57, 0.77)	0.72 (0.62, 0.83)
> 60 g/d (≥3 servings/week)	8265	433 (5.2)	0.70 (0.59, 0.82)	0.72 (0.61, 0.85)
P for trend[c]			<0.001	<0.001
Lean fish				
≤ 5 g/d (never/rarely)	7453	492 (6.6)	1	1
> 5–20 g/d (<1 serving/week)	29,159	1578 (5.4)	0.82 (0.74, 0.90)	0.88 (0.79, 0.98)
> 20–40 g/d (1–2 servings/week)	24,834	1277 (5.1)	0.77 (0.70, 0.86)	0.86 (0.77, 0.95)
> 40–60 g/d (2–3 servings/week)	4799	236 (4.9)	0.74 (0.63, 0.86)	0.78 (0.67, 0.92)
> 60 g/d (≥3 servings/week)	762	47 (6.2)	0.93 (0.69, 1.26)	0.91 (0.67, 1.23)
P for trend[c]			<0.001	0.005
Fatty fish				
≤ 5 g/d (never/rarely)	22,035	1305 (5.9)	1	1
> 5–20 g/d (<1 serving/week)	33,297	1693 (5.1)	0.85 (0.80, 0.92)	0.91 (0.85, 0.98)
> 20–40 g/d (1–2 servings/week)	8654	448 (5.2)	0.87 (0.78, 0.97)	0.91 (0.81, 1.02)
> 40–60 g/d (2–3 servings/week)	1898	116 (6.1)	1.03 (0.85, 1.25)	1.06 (0.87, 1.28)
> 60 g/d (≥3 servings/week)	1123	68 (6.1)	1.03 (0.80, 1.31)	1.02 (0.80, 1.31)
P for trend[c]			0.088	0.411
LCn-3PUFA from supplements				
No supplement	22,018	1093 (5.4)	1	1
< 0.30 g/d (median 0.16 g/d)	22,493	1207 (5.4)	0.99 (0.92, 1.07)	1.00 (0.92, 1.09)
≥ 0.30 g/d (median 0.80 g/d)	22,496	1230 (5.5)	1.01 (0.93, 1.09)	1.02 (0.94, 1.11)
P for trend[c]			0.818	0.567

[a]HR: Hazard Ratio (Cox regression)
[b]Adjusted for the other seafood categories and LCn-3PUFA from supplements, maternal age, pre-pregnancy BMI, height, parity, energy intake, maternal education, smoking, marital status, household income and previous preterm delivery
[c]P for linear trend obtained by incorporating variable as linear term

association for iatrogenic than for spontaneous preterm delivery (*p*-trend: 0.012 for iatrogenic vs 0.219 for spontaneous), while fatty fish and LCn-3PUFA from supplements did not show a significant trend with either spontaneous or iatrogenic preterm delivery.

When preterm delivery was examined separately according to late, moderate or early onset, any increase in seafood beyond no/rare intake was associated with lower risk in the late preterm group, with HRs resulting in 20–30% risk reduction (*p*-trend <0.001) (Table 6). Although not statistically significant, the risk estimates for moderately and early preterm delivery were comparable to those for late preterm delivery. In these analyses LCn-3PUFA from supplements was not associated with late

or moderately preterm delivery, while a non-significant trend was indicated for early preterm delivery, HR 0.84 (CI: 0.67, 1.05) and HR 0.81 (CI: 0.65, 1.01) for the two supplement intake groups versus no LCn-3PUFA from supplements (*p*-trend 0.072) (Table 6).

Statistical significance of the adjusted associations was similar whether the seafood and LCn-3PUFA variables were modelled as continuous or categorical variables.

Obesity is a risk factor of preterm delivery, and we examined the associations between seafood intake and preterm delivery separately in women with pre-pregnant BMI <25 ($n = 45,119$) and those with BMI ≥ 25 kg/m^2 ($n = 20,165$). The prevalence of preterm delivery was 5.0% in the group with BMI <25 and 6.3% in the

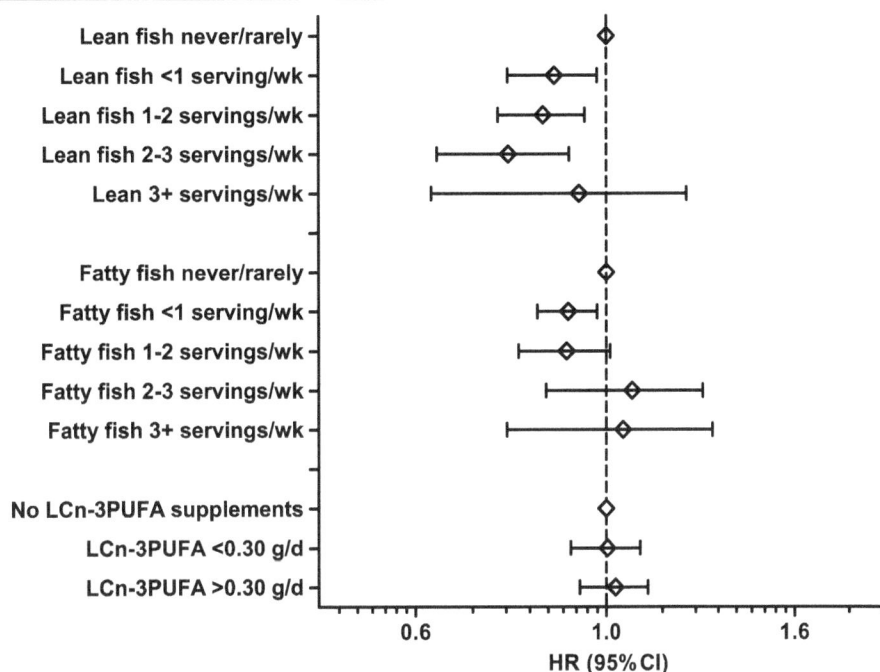

Fig. 2 Associations (hazard ratio (HR) and 95% confidence intervals (CI)) between intakes of lean fish, fatty fish and marine long chain n-3 polyunsaturated fatty acids (LCn-3PUFA) from supplements and preterm delivery. Intakes are mutually adjusted and adjusted for maternal age, pre-pregnancy BMI, height, parity, energy intake, maternal education, smoking, marital status, household income and previous preterm delivery. $N = 67,007$ women in the Norwegian Mother and Child Cohort Study (MoBa) 2002–2008

groups with BMI ≥ 25 kg/m^2. Lower risk of preterm delivery with seafood intake above 1 serving a week (20-30% risk reduction) was seen in both strata, although slightly stronger HRs were observed in women with BMI <25 than in those with BMI ≥ 25 kg/m^2 (Additional file 2: Table S2).

In our study sample, preterm delivery was more prevalent in nulliparous (6.3%) than in parous women (4.3%), and we also examined the associations between seafood intake and preterm delivery separately in nulliparous ($n = 34,731$) and parous women ($n = 32,276$). Lower HRs for preterm delivery were seen in both strata, but the effect size was smaller and the confidence intervals wider in parous than in nulliparous women (Additional file 2: Table S2). LCn-3PUFA from dietary supplements was not associated with preterm delivery in any of these analyses (Additional file 2: Table S2 and Additional file 3: Table S3).

Finally we tested whether the associations between seafood intake and preterm delivery were consistent in subcategories of maternal age, education and smoking. The risk estimates were comparable in all sub-strata, but in small groups e.g., smokers, the confidence intervals were wider (results not shown).

Excluding women who had a registered diagnosis of diabetes in the MBRN ($n = 1007$) or adjusting for diabetes as an independent variable did not change the

associations between seafood and LCn-3PUFA and preterm delivery (results not shown).

Discussion

The main finding in the present study was the significant association between maternal total seafood intake and lower likelihood of preterm delivery. The association was mainly explained by intake of lean fish. The results for the calculated intake of LCn-3PUFA from food reflected the results for seafood intake, while LCn-3PUFA from supplements was not associated with the outcome, with the exception of a borderline significant trend for early preterm delivery. Lower prevalence of preterm delivery with increasing seafood intake was observed for both the subcategories spontaneous and iatrogenic preterm delivery. Significantly lower HR was observed for moderately increased intakes relative to no/low intake, while we observed no additional risk reduction for the highest intake categories.

A beneficial relationship between seafood consumption and preterm delivery has been reported in several studies [15–18, 45]. In a previous study in nulliparous women in MoBa focusing on the Mediterranean diet, we found that eating fish at least twice weekly during pregnancy was associated with lower risk of preterm delivery [46]. We defined Mediterranean diet according to five

Table 5 Associations between seafood intake and marine long chain n-3 polyunsaturated fatty acids (LCn-3PUFA) from supplements and the subcategories spontaneous and iatrogenic preterm delivery. $N = 66,919$[a] women in the Norwegian Mother and Child Cohort Study (MoBa) 2002–2008

	All	Spontaneous	Adjusted	Iatrogenic	Adjusted
	n	PTD n (%)	HR[ab] (95% CI)	PTD n (%)	HR[bc] (95% CI)
		2051 (3.1)		1491 (2.2)	
Total seafood					
≤ 5 g/d (never/rarely)	2961	129 (4.4)	1	86 (2.9)	1
> 5–20 g/d (<1 serving/week)	12,275	405 (3.3)	0.79 (0.64, 0.96)	284 (2.3)	0.81 (0.63, 1.03)
> 20–40 g/d (1–2 servings/week)	27,010	802 (3.0)	0.73 (0.61, 0.89)	603 (2.2)	0.79 (0.63, 0.99)
> 40–60 g/d (2–3 servings/week)	16,416	469 (2.9)	0.71 (0.58, 0.86)	339 (2.1)	0.74 (0.58, 0.94)
> 60 g/d (≥3 servings/week)	8257	246 (3.0)	0.73 (0.58, 0.90)	179 (2.2)	0.71 (0.55, 0.92)
P for trend[d]			0.009		0.013
Lean fish					
≤ 5 g/d (never/rarely)	7437	278 (3.7)	1	198 (2.7)	1
> 5–20 g/d (<1 serving/week)	29,118	884 (3.0)	0.88 (0.77, 1.02)	653 (2.2)	0.89 (0.76, 1.05)
> 20–40 g/d (1–2 servings/week)	24,806	723 (2.9)	0.88 (0.76, 1.02)	526 (2.1)	0.84 (0.71, 0.99)
> 40–60 g/d (2–3 servings/week)	4797	139 (2.9)	0.85 (0.69, 1.04)	95 (2.0)	0.74 (0.57, 0.95)
> 60 g/d (≥3 servings/week)	761	27 (3.5)	0.99 (0.67, 1.47)	19 (2.5)	0.81 (0.50, 1.31)
P for trend[c]			0.219		0.012
Fatty fish					
≤ 5 g/d (never/rarely)	22,003	746 (3.4)	1	527 (2.4)	1
> 5–20 g/d (<1 serving/week)	33,257	949 (2.9)	0.89 (0.81, 0.99)	704 (2.1)	0.94 (0.84, 1.06)
> 20–40 g/d (1–2 servings/week)	8640	256 (3.0)	0.91 (0.79, 1.06)	178 (2.1)	0.89 (0.75, 1.06)
> 40–60 g/d (2–3 servings/week)	1897	59 (3.1)	0.94 (0.71, 1.23)	56 (3.0)	1.26 (0.95, 1.66)
> 60 g/d (≥3 servings/week)	1122	41 (3.7)	1.10 (0.80, 1.51)	26 (2.3)	0.94 (0.63, 1.39)
P for trend[c]			0.411		0.804
LCn-3PUFA from supplements					
No supplement	21,999	671 (3.1)	1	503 (2.3)	1
< 0.30 g/d (median 0.16 g/d)	22,456	671 (3.0)	0.97 (0.87, 1.09)	499 (2.2)	1.03 (0.90, 1.17)
≥ 0.30 g/d (median 0.80 g/d)	22,464	709 (3.2)	1.03 (0.92, 1.15)	489 (2.2)	1.01 (0.89, 1.15)
P for trend[d]			0.626		0.872

[a]Missing data on delivery initiation for 88 preterm deliveries
[b]HR: Hazard Ratio (Cox regression)
[c]Adjusted for the other seafood categories and LCn-3PUFA from supplements, maternal age, pre-pregnancy BMI, height, parity, total energy intake, maternal education, smoking, marital status, household income and previous preterm delivery
[d]P for linear trend obtained by incorporating variable as linear term

a-priori defined criteria, and associations with preterm delivery were examined for adherence to each criterion and for all criteria combined. Only the criterion 'eating fish at least twice weekly' was significantly associated with the outcome (adjusted OR: 0.84; 95% CI: 0.74, 0.95) [46]. A more recent study from MoBa examining maternal dietary patterns showed a reduced risk of preterm delivery associated with high adherence to a traditional dietary pattern characterised by i.e., potatoes, fish dishes and lean fish [47]. The present study complements the previous studies by including more detailed quantification of seafood intakes, by separating between lean and fatty fish

intakes, and by examining LCn-3PUFA from food and supplements as independent exposure variables.

Associations between fish consumption and LCn-3PUFA with increased length of gestation observed in previous studies have been explained by the anti-inflammatory properties of these fatty acids modulating the inflammatory pathways leading to cervical ripening and initiation of labour and delivery [48–51]. Klebanoff et al. (2011) studied fish consumption, erythrocyte fatty acids, and preterm delivery in a high-risk population of women with a prior preterm delivery. The women participated in a randomized controlled trial of n-3 supplementation [52]. Women were randomized to receive

Table 6 Associations between total seafood intake and the subcategories late preterm delivery (35 to <37 w), moderately preterm delivery (32 to <34 w) and early preterm delivery (22 to <32 w). $N = 67,007$ mothers in the Norwegian Mother and Child Cohort Study (MoBa) 2002–2008

	All	PTD n (%)	Unadjusted HR[a] (95% CI)	Adjusted HR[b] (95% CI)
Late PTD (35 to <37 w)		2659 (4.0)		
Total seafood intake				
≤ 5 g/d (never/rarely)	2903	157 (5.4)	1	1
> 5–20 g/d (<1 serving/week)	12,111	525 (4.3)	0.80 (0.67, 0.95)	0.82 (0.68, 0.98)
> 20–40 g/d (1–2 servings/week)	26,684	1079 (4.0)	0.74 (0.63, 0.88)	0.78 (0.66, 0.92)
> 40–60 g/d (2–3 servings/week)	16,194	586 (3.6)	0.66 (0.55, 0.79)	0.69 (0.58, 0.83)
> 60 g/d (≥3 servings/week)	8144	312 (3.8)	0.70 (0.58, 0.85)	0.71 (0.58, 0.86)
P for trend[c]			*<0.001*	*<0.001*
LCn-3PUFA from supplements				
No supplement	21,676	851 (3.9)	1	1
< 0.30 g/d (median 0.16 g/d)	22,203	917 (4.1)	1.05 (0.96, 1.16)	1.07 (0.97, 1.18)
≥ 0.30 g/d (median 0.80 g/d)	22,157	891 (4.0)	1.03 (0.93, 1.13)	1.04 (0.94, 1.15)
P for trend[c]			*0.609*	*0.450*
Moderately PTD (32 to <34w)		491 (0.7)		
Total seafood intake				
≤ 5 g/d (never/rarely)	2778	32 (1.2)	1	1
> 5–20 g/d (<1 serving/week)	11,680	94 (0.8)	0.70 (0.47, 1.04)	0.75 (0.50, 1.12)
> 20–40 g/d (1–2 servings/week)	25,784	179 (0.7)	0.60 (0.41, 0.88)	0.68 (0.47, 0.99)
> 40–60 g/d (2–3 servings/week)	15,730	122 (0.8)	0.67 (0.46, 0.99)	0.77 (0.52, 1.15)
> 60 g/d (≥3 servings/week)	7896	64 (0.8)	0.70 (0.46, 1.07)	0.78 (0.51, 1.20)
P for trend[c]			*0.432*	*0.792*
LCn-3PUFA from supplements				
No supplement	20,987	169 (0.8)	1	1
< 0.30 g/d (median 0.16 g/d)	21,424	138 (0.6)	0.83 (0.66, 1.05)	0.84 (0.66, 1.06)
≥ 0.30 g/d (median 0.80 g/d)	21,457	191 (0.9)	1.15 (0.94, 1.42)	1.19 (0.95, 1.48)
P for trend[c]			*0.158*	*0.093*
Early PTD (22 to <32 w)		480 (0.7)		
Total seafood intake				
≤ 5 g/d (never/rarely)	2777	31 (1.1)	1	1
> 5–20 g/d (<1 serving/week)	11,680	94 (0.8)	0.72 (0.48, 1.08)	0.77 (0.51, 1.16)
> 20–40 g/d (1–2 servings/week)	25,787	182 (0.7)	0.63 (0.43, 0.92)	0.71 (0.48, 1.04)
> 40–60 g/d (2–3 servings/week)	15,724	116 (0.7)	0.66 (0.44, 0.98)	0.75 (0.50, 1.12)
> 60 g/d (≥3 servings/week)	7899	57 (0.7)	0.65 (0.42, 0.99)	0.68 (0.43, 1.06)
P for trend[c]			*0.116*	*0.196*
LCn-3PUFA from supplements				
No supplement	21,005	180 (0.9)	1	1
< 0.30 g/d (median 0.16 g/d)	21,438	152 (0.7)	0.83 (0.67, 1.03)	0.84 (0.67, 1.05)
≥ 0.30 g/d (median 0.80 g/d)	21,414	148 (0.7)	0.81 (0.65, 1.00)	0.81 (0.65, 1.01)
P for trend[c]			*0.049*	*0.072*

[a]HR: Hazard Ratio (Cox regression)
[b]Adjusted for maternal age, pre-pregnancy BMI, height, parity, energy intake, maternal education, smoking, marital status, household income, previous preterm delivery and LCn-3PUFA from supplements
[c]P for linear trend obtained by incorporating variable as linear term

either an LCn-3PUFA supplement or placebo starting in mid-gestation (weeks 16–21). The results showed that women who reported the lowest fish consumption at gestational weeks 16–21 had higher risk of recurrent preterm birth than those who ate fish more frequently. The lowest occurrence of preterm birth was seen among women who ate fish approximately 2–3 times/week, while more frequent fish consumption was not associated with further risk reduction [52]. Interestingly, the lowest occurrence of preterm birth was observed among women in the second quartile of erythrocyte LCn-3PUFA concentrations, and no benefit of LCn-3PUFA supplementation was found, regardless of baseline fish consumption and erythrocyte n-3 concentration [52]. A multicentre randomized control trial in seven European countries comprising women with previous pregnancy complications found that fish oil supplementation (2.7 g LCn-3PUFA daily) delayed the onset of delivery for women with low (mean 16 g/d) and medium fish intake (mean 23 g/day), but not for women with high fish intake (mean 36 g/day) at baseline [53], suggesting that the effect of fish oil supplementation on timing of delivery depends on a woman's fish intake. In the current study, however, no association between LCn-3PUFA from supplements and overall preterm delivery was evident at any level of seafood intake. However, our finding of borderline significantly lower risk of early preterm delivery (<32 weeks) in women using LCn-3PUFA is in line with results from experimental studies in the US and Australia which found that supplementation with 0.6–0.8 g/d DHA reduced the prevalence of early preterm births in low risk pregnancies [22, 23]. Contrary to our findings, a prospective study in pregnant women in Massachusetts found no associations between intake of fish or LCn-3PUFA from food and preterm delivery [20]. Furthermore, another recent study from the US reported an increased risk of preterm in women with high intakes of lean fish [21].

In the present study, LCn-3PUFA from fish paralleled the results obtained for seafood, while LCn-3PUFA from supplements was not associated with overall preterm delivery. The association between seafood intake and preterm delivery remained significant also when adjusted for LCn-3PUFA from food, indicating that the observed associations between seafood consumption and lower prevalence of preterm delivery cannot be explained only by LCn-3PUFA. Alternative explanations could be other components in fish (e.g., proteins, iodine, and selenium) or other aspects of fish consumption (e.g., foods typically eaten with fish or foods displaced by fish) might modulate the inflammatory pathways leading to delivery. The effects of fatty fish, lean fish and LCn-3PUFA intake on inflammation have been studied in some intervention studies [54, 55]. In one study, participants were randomly

allocated to receive dietary advice plus either 300 g of fatty fish (salmon) or 300 g of lean fish (cod) per week for 6 months, or only dietary advice. Interestingly, the effect estimates did not differ between the lean and fatty fish groups, and a significantly lower concentration of the systemic inflammation marker C-reactive protein was found in both fish groups compared to the control group [54]. Another study investigated the effects of weight loss and seafood consumption in three intervention groups (salmon, cod, or LCn-3PUFA supplementation) and controls on inflammation parameters during energy restriction. The largest decrease in inflammation parameters was observed for salmon consumption, and no decrease was seen for LCn-3PUFA supplementation [55]. It could also be speculated that fish consumption may influence the gut microbiota which is crucial for optimal functioning of the digestive and immune systems [56]. Two experimental studies explored whether fish consumption influenced gut microbiota composition and local markers of gut inflammation without convincing results [54, 57]. However, in one of these studies a significant effect on the systemic inflammatory markers was observed for both lean and fatty fish [54].

An issue of particular concern when it comes to seafood consumption in women of childbearing age, is the concomitant exposure to environmental pollutants, e.g., methylmercury, polychlorinated biphenyls and perfluorinated alkylated substances, which may counteract the beneficial effects of fish consumption [28, 58–61]. However, a systematic review of environmental contaminant exposures and preterm birth found no consistent evidence for chemical exposure and increased risk of preterm delivery [62]. Likewise, studies in MoBa examining associations between maternal exposure to environmental pollutants primarily contributed by seafood and pregnancy outcomes showed no increased risk of preterm delivery [63, 64]. The result of the present study corroborates the current advice to pregnant women to include fish and seafood as part of a balanced diet and restricting the intake of species and items with known high concentrations of environmental pollutants [26, 65].

The strengths of this study include the prospective design and detailed information about maternal diet, demography, socioeconomic factors, and pregnancy outcomes. Thanks to the large sample size we were able to examine the associations between seafood intake and preterm delivery in subcategories. Participants in MoBa were recruited from urban and rural, coastal and inland regions and represented different socioeconomic groups. Dietary intake was assessed using an FFQ that was specifically developed and validated for use in this cohort [31, 32]. The FFQ included questions with special emphasis on various seafood items, and the validation study showed that the reported intakes of lean and fatty fish and LCn-3PUFA supplements were reflected by blood and urine samples [33]. The food frequency method challenges respondents with rather complex cognitive tasks and are more suitable for ranking participants according to high and low intakes than for precise intake calculations. Therefore, differential misclassification of seafood and n-3 supplement intakes cannot be excluded, but is as likely to occur in women with term delivery as in women with preterm delivery.

The somewhat low response rate in MoBa is a concern and participants are not representative of all pregnant women in Norway. The potential bias due to self-selection has been evaluated by comparison of eight exposure-outcome associations reported both in MoBa and in the MBRN. Significant differences in prevalence estimates were found for most variables, e.g., MoBa participants included less smokers than the general pregnant population. In spite of this, there were no statistically relative differences in association measures, e.g., prenatal smoking and low birthweight [66]. It is a strength that the women who do participate remain in the study, illustrated by a response rate of more than 90% for the three extensive questionnaires answered during pregnancy [39]. However, the study is observational and we cannot rule out the possibility that residual or unmeasured confounding may still exist.

Conclusions

This study showed that maternal seafood consumption was associated with reduced risk of preterm delivery. The association was mainly explained by intake of lean fish. The association was seen for subcategories spontaneous, iatrogenic and late preterm delivery. Intake of LCn-3PUFA from seafood was associated with preterm delivery, while intake of LCn-3PUFA from supplements was associated only with early preterm delivery. The association between supplementary LCn-3PUFA and preterm delivery did not differ between women with low or high seafood intake. Furthermore, the association between seafood intake and reduced risk of preterm delivery remained significant when adjusted for LCn-3PUFA from food, indicating that the observed associations cannot be explained only by LCn-3PUFA and that other properties related to fish and seafood consumption may also be of importance. The findings corroborate the current advice to include fish and seafood as part of a balanced diet during pregnancy. Preterm delivery is a serious public health problem resulting in high societal costs, and no effective preventive strategies for the general population exist. Dietary changes have low cost and low risk compared with medical interventions and even moderate changes may be of public health importance.

Additional files

Additional file 1: Table S1. Associations between estimated intake of polyunsaturated fatty acids (LCn-3PUFA) from food and total LCn3-PUFA (food and supplements) and preterm delivery.

Additional file 2: Table S2. Associations between total seafood intake and marine long chain polyunsaturated fatty acids (LCn-3PUFA) from supplements and preterm delivery in women stratified according to pre-pregnant BMI <25 ($n = 45,119$) or pre-pregnant BMI ≥ 25 kg/m2 ($n = 20,165$) in the Norwegian Mother and Child Cohort Study (MoBa) 2002–2008.

Additional file 3: Table S3. Associations between total seafood intake and marine long chain polyunsaturated fatty acids (LCn-3PUFA) from supplements and preterm delivery in women stratified according to nulliparous ($n = 34,731$) and parous women ($n = 32,276$) in the Norwegian Mother and Child Cohort Study (MoBa) 2002–2008.

Abbreviations

BMI: Body Mass Index; CI: Confidence Interval; DHA: Docosahexaenoic acid; EPA: Eicosapentaenoic; FFQ: Food Frequency Questionnaire; HR: Hazard Ratio; LCn-3PUFA: Long Chain omega-3 Poly-Unsaturated Fatty Acids; MBRN: Medical Birth Registry of Norway; MoBa: The Norwegian Mother and Child Cohort Study

Acknowledgment

We are grateful to all the participating families in Norway who take part in this on-going cohort study.

Funding

The Norwegian Mother and Child Cohort Study is supported by the Norwegian Ministry of Health and the Ministry of Education and Research, NIH/NIEHS (contract no N01-ES-75558), NIH/NINDS (grant no.1 UO1 NS 047537–01 and grant no.2 UO1 NS 047537-06A1). Payment of article-processing charges for this paper was covered by the Norwegian Institute of Public Health's institutional membership with BMC.

Authors' contributions

ALB and LE-Ö conducted the statistical analyses. ALB drafted the paper. MH, RM and VS were in charge of the coordination of the data file and analyses. BEB, HKK, JA, RMN, BJ and HMM contributed to the interpretation of the results. All authors were involved in the interpretation of the results and writing of the manuscript, and all approved the final version.

Competing interests

The authors declare that they have no competing interests.

Author details

[1]Department of Environmental Exposure and Epidemiology, Domain of Infection Control and Environmental Health, Norwegian Institute of Public Health, P.O. Box 4404Nydalen, NO-0403 Oslo, Norway. [2]Department of Obstetrics and Gynecology, Sahlgrenska University Hospital, Gothenburg, Sweden. [3]Unit for Nutrition Research, Landspitali University Hospital and University of Iceland, Reykjavik, Iceland. [4]Department of Genetics and Bioinformatics, Domain of Health Data and Digitalisation, Norwegian Institute of Public Health, Oslo, Norway. [5]Office of the Director-General, Norwegian Institute of Public Health, Oslo, Norway. [6]Department of Health and Social Sciences, Bergen University College, Bergen, Norway. [7]Department of Obstetrics and Gynecology, Sahlgrenska Academy, Gothenburg University, Gothenburg, Sweden.

References

1. Goldenberg RL, Culhane JF, Iams JD, Romero R. Epidemiology and causes of preterm birth. Lancet. 2008;371(9606):75–84.
2. Boyle JD, Boyle EM. Born just a few weeks early: does it matter? Arch Dis Child Fetal Neonatal Ed. 2013;98(1):F85–8.
3. Saigal S, Doyle LW. An overview of mortality and sequelae of preterm birth from infancy to adulthood. Lancet. 2008;371(9608):261–9.
4. Platt MJ. Outcomes in preterm infants. Public Health. 2014;128(5):399–403.
5. Chang HH, Larson J, Blencowe H, Spong CY, Howson CP, Cairns-Smith S, Lackritz EM, Lee SK, Mason E, Serazin AC, et al. Preventing preterm births: analysis of trends and potential reductions with interventions in 39 countries with very high human development index. Lancet. 2013; 381(9862):223–34.
6. Moster D, Lie RT, Markestad T. Long-term medical and social consequences of preterm birth. N Engl J Med. 2008;359(3):262–73.
7. Morken NH, Vogel I, Kallen K, Skjaerven R, Langhoff-Roos J, Kesmodel US, Jacobsson B. Reference population for international comparisons and time trend surveillance of preterm delivery proportions in three countries. BMC Womens Health. 2008;8:16.
8. Blencowe H, Cousens S, Oestergaard MZ, Chou D, Moller AB, Narwal R, Adler A, Vera GC, Rohde S, Say L, et al. National, regional, and worldwide estimates of preterm birth rates in the year 2010 with time trends since 1990 for selected countries: a systematic analysis and implications. Lancet. 2012;379(9832):2162–72.
9. Torloni MR, Betran AP, Daher S, Widmer M, Dolan SM, Menon R, Bergel E, Allen T, Merialdi M. Maternal BMI and preterm birth: a systematic review of the literature with meta-analysis. J Matern Fetal Neonatal Med. 2009;22(11): 957–70.
10. Khatibi A, Brantsaeter AL, Sengpiel V, Kacerovsky M, Magnus P, Morken NH, Myhre R, Gunnes N, Jacobsson B. Prepregnancy maternal body mass index and preterm delivery. Am J Obstet Gynecol. 2012;207(3):212–7.
11. Imhoff-Kunsch B, Briggs V, Goldenberg T, Ramakrishnan U. Effect of n-3 long-chain polyunsaturated fatty acid intake during pregnancy on maternal, infant, and child health outcomes: a systematic review. Paediatr Perinat Epidemiol. 2012;26 Suppl 1:91–107.
12. Larsen R, Eilertsen KE, Elvevoll EO. Health benefits of marine foods and ingredients. Biotechnol Adv. 2011;29(5):508–18.
13. Hosomi R, Yoshida M, Fukunaga K. Seafood consumption and components for health. Glob J Health Sci. 2012;4(3):72–86.
14. Lund EK. Health benefits of seafood; is it just the fatty acids? Food Chem. 2013;140(3):413–20.
15. Grandjean P, Bjerve KS, Weihe P, Steuerwald U. Birthweight in a fishing community: significance of essential fatty acids and marine food contaminants. Int J Epidemiol. 2001;30(6):1272–8.
16. Olsen SF, Østerdal ML, Salvig JD, Kesmodel U, Henriksen TB, Hedegaard M, Secher NJ. Duration of pregnancy in relation to seafood intake during early and mid pregnancy: prospective cohort. Eur J Epidemiol. 2006;21(10):749–58.
17. Guldner L, Monfort C, Rouget F, Garlantezec R, Cordier S. Maternal fish and shellfish intake and pregnancy outcomes: a prospective cohort study in Brittany, France. Environ Health. 2007;6:33.
18. Olsen SF, Secher NJ. Low consumption of seafood in early pregnancy as a risk factor for preterm delivery: prospective cohort study. BMJ. 2002; 324(7335):447.
19. Heppe DH, Steegers EA, Timmermans S, Breeijen H, Tiemeier H, Hofman A, Jaddoe VW. Maternal fish consumption, fetal growth and the risks of neonatal complications: the Generation R Study. Br J Nutr. 2011;105(6):938–49.
20. Oken E, Kleinman KP, Olsen SF, Rich-Edwards JW, Gillman MW. Associations of seafood and elongated n-3 fatty acid intake with fetal growth and length of gestation: results from a US pregnancy cohort. Am J Epidemiol. 2004; 160(8):774–83.
21. Mohanty AF, Siscovick DS, Williams MA, Thompson ML, Burbacher TM, Enquobahrie DA. Periconceptional seafood intake and pregnancy complications. Public Health Nutr. 2016;19(10):1795–803.
22. Yelland LN, Gajewski BJ, Colombo J, Gibson RA, Makrides M, Carlson SE. Predicting the effect of maternal docosahexaenoic acid (DHA) supplementation to reduce early preterm birth in Australia and the United States using results of within country randomized controlled trials. Prostaglandins Leukot Essent Fatty Acids. 2016;112:44–9.
23. Carlson SE, Colombo J, Gajewski BJ, Gustafson KM, Mundy D, Yeast J, Georgieff MK, Markley LA, Kerling EH, Shaddy DJ. DHA supplementation and pregnancy outcomes. Am J Clin Nutr. 2013;97(4):808–15.
24. Salvig JD, Lamont RF. Evidence regarding an effect of marine n-3 fatty acids on preterm birth: a systematic review and meta-analysis. Acta Obstet Gynecol Scand. 2011;90(8):825–38.
25. Makrides M, Gibson RA, McPhee AJ, Yelland L, Quinlivan J, Ryan P. Effect of DHA supplementation during pregnancy on maternal depression and neurodevelopment of young children: a randomized controlled trial. JAMA. 2010;304(15):1675–83.
26. Norwegian Health Authorities: Kostholdsråd for gravide/Dietary advice for pregnant women [in Norwegian]. Norwegian Food Safety Authority, Norwegian Directorate of Health, Norwegian Institute of Public Health. http://www.matportalen.no/rad_til_spesielle_grupper/tema/gravide/#tabs-1-2-anchor. Accessed Dec 2016.
27. Weichselbaum E, Coe S, Buttriss J, Stanner S. Fish in the diet: A review. Nutr Bull. 2013;38(2):128–77.
28. FAO/WHO. Report of the joint FAO/WHO Expert Consultation on the Risks and Benefits of Fish Consumption, vol. 978. Rome: Food and Agriculture Organization of the United Nations; Geneva, World Health Organization; 2011.
29. Knudsen VK, Hansen HS, Osterdal ML, Mikkelsen TB, Mu H, Olsen SF. Fish oil in various doses or flax oil in pregnancy and timing of spontaneous delivery: a randomised controlled trial. BJOG. 2006;113(5):536–43.
30. Szajewska H, Horvath A, Koletzko B. Effect of n-3 long-chain polyunsaturated fatty acid supplementation of women with low-risk pregnancies on pregnancy outcomes and growth measures at birth: a meta-analysis of randomized controlled trials. Am J Clin Nutr. 2006;83(6):1337–44.
31. Brantsaeter AL, Haugen M, Alexander J, Meltzer HM. Validity of a new food frequency questionnaire for pregnant women in the Norwegian Mother and Child Cohort Study (MoBa). Matern Child Nutr. 2008;4(1):28–43.
32. Meltzer HM, Brantsaeter AL, Ydersbond TA, Alexander J, Haugen M. Methodological challenges when monitoring the diet of pregnant women in a large study: experiences from the Norwegian Mother and Child Cohort Study (MoBa). Matern Child Nutr. 2008;4(1):14–27.
33. Brantsaeter AL, Haugen M, Thomassen Y, Ellingsen DG, Ydersbond TA, Hagve TA, Alexander J, Meltzer HM. Exploration of biomarkers for total fish intake in pregnant Norwegian women. Public Health Nutr. 2010;13(1):54–62.
34. Brantsaeter AL, Birgisdottir BE, Meltzer HM, Kvalem HE, Alexander J, Magnus P, Haugen M. Maternal seafood consumption and infant birth weight, length and head circumference in the Norwegian Mother and Child Cohort Study. Br J Nutr. 2012;107(3):436–44.
35. Magnus P, Irgens LM, Haug K, Nystad W, Skjaerven R, Stoltenberg C. Cohort profile: The Norwegian Mother and Child Cohort Study (MoBa). Int J Epidemiol. 2006;35(5):1146–50.
36. Irgens LM. The Medical Birth Registry of Norway. Epidemiological research and surveillance throughout 30 years. Acta Obstet Gynecol Scand. 2000; 79(6):435–9.
37. Norwegian Institute of Public Health: Questionnaire 1. English translation of the baseline questionnaire used in the Norwegian Mother and Child Cohort Study. https://www.fhi.no/globalassets/migrering/dokumenter/pdf/questionnaire—week-15-of-pregnancy-to-mother.pdf. Accessed Dec 2016.
38. Norwegian Institute of Public Health: Questionnaire 2, Your diet. English translation of the food Frequency Questionnaire used in the Norwegian Mother and Child Cohort Study. https://www.fhi.no/globalassets/migrering/dokumenter/pdf/questionnaire—week-22-of-pregnancy.pdf. Accessed Dec 2016.
39. Norwegian Institute of Public Health: The Norwegian Mother and Child Cohort Study, Revised PROTOCOL, End of Enrolment-Protocol II. https://www.fhi.no/globalassets/migrering/dokumenter/pdf/moba-protocol-2-end-of-enrolment-2010.pdf. Accessed Dec 2016.
40. Lauritsen J: FoodCalc. Data Program from the Project "Diet, Cancer and Health" at the Danish Cancer Society. http://www.ibt.ku.dk/jesper/foodcalc. Accessed Feb 2005.
41. Rimestad AH, Borgejordet A, Vesterhus KN, Sygnestveit K, Løken EB, Trygg K, Pollestad ML, Lund-Larsen K, Omholt-Jensen G, Nordbotten A. Den store matvaretabellen/The Norwegian Food Composition Table [in Norwegian]. Oslo: Norwegian Food Safety Authority; Norwegian Directorate of Health; University of Oslo, Department of Nutrition; 2001.
42. Brantsaeter AL, Haugen M, Hagve TA, Aksnes L, Rasmussen SE, Julshamn K, Alexander J, Meltzer HM. Self-Reported Dietary Supplement Use Is Confirmed by Biological Markers in the Norwegian Mother and Child Cohort Study (MoBa). Ann Nutr Metab. 2007;51(2):146–54.

43. Halldorsson TI, Meltzer HM, Thorsdottir I, Knudsen V, Olsen SF. Is high consumption of fatty fish during pregnancy a risk factor for fetal growth retardation? A study of 44,824 Danish pregnant women. Am J Epidemiol. 2007;166(6):687–96.

44. Symons MJ, Moore DT. Hazard rate ratio and prospective epidemiological studies. J Clin Epidemiol. 2002;55(9):893–9.

45. Khoury J, Henriksen T, Christophersen B, Tonstad S. Effect of a cholesterol-lowering diet on maternal, cord, and neonatal lipids, and pregnancy outcome: a randomized clinical trial. Am J ObstetGynecol. 2005;193(4):1292–301.

46. Haugen M, Meltzer HM, Brantsaeter AL, Mikkelsen T, Osterdal ML, Alexander J, Olsen SF, Bakketeig L. Mediterranean-type diet and risk of preterm birth among women in the Norwegian Mother and Child Cohort Study (MoBa): a prospective cohort study. Acta Obstet Gynecol Scand. 2008;87(3):319–24.

47. Englund-Ögge L, Brantsaeter AL, Sengpiel V, Haugen M, Birgisdottir BE, Myhre R, Meltzer HM, Jacobsson B. Maternal dietary patterns and preterm delivery: results from large prospective cohort study. BMJ. 2014;348:g1446.

48. Olsen SF, Hansen HS, Sorensen TI, Jensen B, Secher NJ, Sommer S, Knudsen LB. Intake of marine fat, rich in (n-3)-polyunsaturated fatty acids, may increase birthweight by prolonging gestation. Lancet. 1986;2(8503):367–9.

49. Olsen SF. Is supplementation with marine omega-3 fatty acids during pregnancy a useful tool in the prevention of preterm birth? Clin Obstet Gynecol. 2004;47(4):768–74.

50. Romero R, Espinoza J, Kusanovic JP, Gotsch F, Hassan S, Erez O, Chaiworapongsa T, Mazor M. The preterm parturition syndrome. BJOG. 2006;113 Suppl 3:17–42.

51. MacIntyre DA, Sykes L, Teoh TG, Bennett PR. Prevention of preterm labour via the modulation of inflammatory pathways. J Matern Fetal Neonatal Med. 2012;25 Suppl 1:17–20.

52. Klebanoff MA, Harper M, Lai Y, Thorp Jr J, Sorokin Y, Varner MW, Wapner RJ, Caritis SN, Iams JD, Carpenter MW, et al. Fish consumption, erythrocyte fatty acids, and preterm birth. Obstet Gynecol. 2011;117(5):1071–7.

53. Olsen SF, Osterdal ML, Salvig JD, Weber T, Tabor A, Secher NJ. Duration of pregnancy in relation to fish oil supplementation and habitual fish intake: a randomised clinical trial with fish oil. Eur J Clin Nutr. 2007;61(8):976–85.

54. Pot GK, Geelen A, Majsak-Newman G, Harvey LJ, Nagengast FM, Witteman BJ, van de Meeberg PC, Hart AR, Schaafsma G, Lund EK, et al. Increased consumption of fatty and lean fish reduces serum C-reactive protein concentrations but not inflammation markers in feces and in colonic biopsies. J Nutr. 2010;140(2):371–6.

55. Ramel A, Martinez JA, Kiely M, Bandarra NM, Thorsdottir I. Effects of weight loss and seafood consumption on inflammation parameters in young, overweight and obese European men and women during 8 weeks of energy restriction. Eur J Clin Nutr. 2010;64(9):987–93.

56. Maslowski KM, Mackay CR. Diet, gut microbiota and immune responses. Nat Immunol. 2011;12(1):5–9.

57. Urwin HJ, Miles EA, Noakes PS, Kremmyda LS, Vlachava M, Diaper ND, Godfrey KM, Calder PC, Vulevic J, Yaqoob P. Effect of salmon consumption during pregnancy on maternal and infant faecal microbiota, secretory IgA and calprotectin. Br J Nutr. 2013;111:1–12.

58. Stern AH, Korn LR. An approach for quantitatively balancing methylmercury risk and omega-3 benefit in fish consumption advisories. Environ Health Perspect. 2011;119(8):1043–6.

59. Mahaffey KR, Clickner RP, Bodurow CC. Blood organic mercury and dietary mercury intake: National Health and Nutrition Examination Survey, 1999 and 2000. Environ Health Perspect. 2004;112(5):562–70.

60. EFSA: European Food Safety Authority (EFSA). Opinion of the Scientific Panel on Contaminants in the Food Chain (CONTAM) on a Request from the European Parliament Related to the Safety Assessment of Wild and Farmed Fish. EFSA J. 2005;236:1–118.

61. Caspersen IH, Knutsen HK, Brantsaeter AL, Haugen M, Alexander J, Meltzer HM, Kvalem HE. Dietary exposure to dioxins and PCBs in a large cohort of pregnant women: Results from the Norwegian Mother and Child Cohort Study (MoBa). Environ Int. 2013;59C:398–407.

62. Ferguson KK, O'Neill MS, Meeker JD. Environmental contaminant exposures and preterm birth: a comprehensive review. J Toxicol Environ Health B Crit Rev. 2013;16(2):69–113.

63. Whitworth KW, Haug LS, Baird DD, Becher G, Hoppin JA, Skjaerven R, Thomsen C, Eggesbo M, Travlos G, Wilson R, et al. Perfluorinated compounds in relation to birth weight in the Norwegian Mother and Child Cohort Study. Am J Epidemiol. 2012;175(12):1209–16.

64. Papadopoulou E, Caspersen IH, Kvalem HE, Knutsen HK, Duarte-Salles T, Alexander J, Meltzer HM, Kogevinas M, Brantsaeter AL, Haugen M. Maternal dietary intake of dioxins and polychlorinated biphenyls and birth size in the Norwegian Mother and Child Cohort Study (MoBa). Environ Int. 2013;60C: 209–16.

65. Norwegian Scientific Committee for Food Safety. Benefit-risk assessment of fish and fish products in the Norwegian diet - an update. VKM Report 2014: 15: Norwegian Scientific Committee for Food Safety. 2014.

66. Nilsen RM, Suren P, Gunnes N, Alsaker ER, Bresnahan M, Hirtz D, Hornig M, Lie KK, Lipkin WI, Reichborn-Kjennerud T, et al. Analysis of self-selection bias in a population-based cohort study of autism spectrum disorders. Paediatr Perinat Epidemiol. 2013;27(6):553–63.

7

Specialist antenatal clinics for women at high risk of preterm birth: a systematic review of qualitative and quantitative research

Reem Malouf* and Maggie Redshaw

Abstract

Background: Preterm birth (PTB) is the leading cause of perinatal morbidity and mortality. Women with previous prenatal loss are at higher risk of preterm birth. A specialist antenatal clinic is considered as one approach to improve maternity and pregnancy outcomes.

Methods: A systematic review of quantitative, qualitative and mixed method studies conducted on women at high risk of preterm birth (PTB). The review primary outcomes were to report on the specialist antenatal clinics effect in preventing or reducing preterm birth, perinatal mortality and morbidity and women's perceptions and experiences of a specialist clinic whether compared or not compared with standard antenatal care. Other secondary maternal, infant and economic outcomes were also determined. A comprehensive search strategy was carried out in English within electronic databases as far back as 1980. The reviewers selected studies, assessed the quality, and extracted data independently. Results were summarized and tabulated.

Results: Eleven studies fully met the review inclusion criteria, ten were quantitative design studies and only one was a qualitative design study. No mixed method design study was included in the review. All were published after 1989, seven were conducted in the USA and four in the UK. Results from five good to low quality randomised controlled trials (RCTs), all conducted before 1990, did not illustrate the efficacy of the clinic in reducing preterm birth. Whereas results from more recent low quality cohort studies showed some positive neonatal outcomes. Themes from one good quality qualitative study reflected on the emotional and psychological need to reduce anxiety and stress of women referred to such a clinic. Women expressed their negative emotional responses at being labelled as high risk and positive responses to being assessed and treated in the clinic. Women also reported that their partners were struggling to cope emotionally.

Conclusions: Findings from this review were mixed. Evidence from cohort studies indicated a specialist clinic may be a means of predicting or preventing preterm birth. Testing this in a randomised controlled trial is desirable, though may be hard to achieve due to the growing focus of such clinics on managing women at high risk of preterm birth. Ongoing research has to recognize women's experiences and perceptions of such a clinic. Further clarification of the optimal referral route and a clear and standardized management and cost economic evaluation plan are also required. Fathers support and experience of PTB clinics should also be included in further research.

Keywords: High risk pregnancy, Preterm birth, Systematic review, Preterm birth clinic

* Correspondence: reem.malouf@npeu.ox.ac.uk
Policy Research Unit in Maternal Health and Care, National Perinatal
Epidemiology Unit, Nuffield Department of Population Health, University of
Oxford, Old Road Campus, Headington, Oxford OX3 7LF, UK

Background

An estimated 15 million babies are born prematurely (<37 weeks' gestation) each year and approximately one million die annually due to complications of prematurity [1]. The rate of preterm birth ranges from 5% in some European countries to 18% in some African countries [1]. In 2012, the national preterm birth rate in England and Wales was estimated to be 7% of all births [2]. Preterm birth remains the main cause of perinatal morbidity and mortality worldwide [3], it is the second leading cause of death in children under 5 years of age and the single most important direct cause of death in the first month of life [4]. The complications of preterm birth arise from immaturity in organ developments and survivors could suffer from long term disabilities. Therefore, a minor reduction in preterm births would lead to a substantial cost reduction [5]. Despite the improvement in neonatal care in recent decades and the marked impact on both mortality and morbidity, the incidence of preterm birth is still rising [6, 7]. A high proportion of preterm multiple gestations associated with assisted reproductive technologies is also an important contributor to the overall increase in preterm births. Singleton pregnancies after in-vitro fertilisation are also at increased risk of preterm birth [8].

The implications of preterm birth are not only associated with a significant neonatal hospital cost [9] but also with emotional and economic costs for the family and society [10]. Many pathways can lead to preterm birth (PTB) some resulting from pregnancy complications and others precipitated by concern for the health of the mother or the baby. However, spontaneous labour is responsible for 70–80% of preterm births and 20 to 30% occur as a result of intervention for maternal or foetal problems [11]. Factors contributing to an increased risk of spontaneous labour have been identified: prior preterm birth, Black ethnicity, advanced maternal age, lower and higher BMI, lower socioeconomic status, cervical injury or previous surgery and multiple pregnancy [12–14].

Various preventive options and tests are currently in use to prolong pregnancy such as progesterone supplementation, treating intra-uterine infection, surgical closure of the cervix with cerclage, improvement in maternal nutrition and lifestyle modification [15]. However, the complexity of managing these pregnancies led to the establishment of specialist preterm prevention clinics. Many hospitals have specialist gynaecology clinics, but relatively few have specifically preterm birth clinics, whose fundamental aim is to assist in avoiding preterm birth and reduce the associated perinatal mortality and morbidity [14]. The clinics focus on reducing preterm birth by providing a package of specialist care for high-risk women that could involve serial sonographic assessment, foetal fibronectin testing, vaginal PH testing and other management to prevent early labour. A Cochrane review [16] concluded that there was no clear evidence that specialized antenatal clinics reduce the preterm birth rate, reviewing only three randomised controlled trials from the USA. The three included studies were conducted in the 1980s, when many screening tests and ultrasounds, such as assessment of the cervix length and foetal fibronectin test that are currently in use in the clinic were not available. Moreover, the interventions across the studies were generally similar, offering only education about signs and symptoms of preterm birth in addition to more frequent antenatal visits to high risk women. The outcomes of interest across the studies were preterm birth rate and gestational age at delivery, with no reporting on maternal health and long term infant outcomes. Thus we believe it is necessary in our review to bring together evidence from primary quantitative and qualitative research to evaluate such clinics further.

Objectives

The review objective is to comprehensively assess the efficacy of specialist preterm clinics in preventing preterm birth and to report on the women's perceptions and experiences of accessing such services.

Methods

A review protocol was published at PROSPERO with a registration number CRD42015026976 and this is available at http://www.crd.york.ac.uk/PROSPERO/display_record.asp?ID=CRD42015026976.

In conducting this review, we followed the standard Preferred Reporting Items for Systematic Reviews and Meta-Analyses (PRISMA) checklist [17].

Types of study

Although randomised controlled trials (RCTs) provide the best evidence for estimating the effectiveness of any health interventions [18], this type of clinic is an accepted part of primary antenatal care in many settings and conducting RCTs may not be ethically possible. Evidence from both qualitative and quantitative research are therefore considered for inclusion in this review. All quantitative research methods, including randomised controlled trials, cohort studies, case-controlled studies, time series studies, cross-sectional and pre-post evaluation studies. Any observations and questionnaires which produce quantitative results were sought for inclusion. Qualitative research include range of designs: interviews, participant and non-participant observation, focus groups and documentary analyses.

Studies with mixed method designs were considered eligible for inclusion.

Types of participant
Studies conducted on women at high risk of preterm labour were eligible for inclusion in this review. Studies enrolling pregnant women with a singleton or multiple pregnancies were included.

Types of intervention
Specialist preterm prevention clinic: this could be called a specialist antenatal clinic, preterm birth prevention clinic, multi-disciplinary antenatal clinic and miscarriage follow-up clinic (this list is not exhaustive) compared or not compared with standard antenatal care. Studies involving other specialist antenatal clinics such as diabetes, hypertension and twins clinics were excluded.

Types of outcome measure
The primary outcomes relate to preterm birth defined as birth less than 37 completed weeks' gestation, very preterm birth (<34 weeks' gestation), moderate prematurity (32–33 weeks), severe prematurity (28–31 weeks) and extreme prematurity (<28 weeks), perinatal mortality and morbidity (neonatal intensive care admission, respiratory distress syndrome and disability in early life) and measures reflecting women's satisfaction and wellbeing. Other outcomes such as delivery mode, birth weight and cost associated with running the clinic (number or antenatal visits, hospital admission and length of maternal and neonatal hospital stay) were all considered.

Search and screening strategy
We developed a sensitive search strategy for five databases: MEDLINE, PsycINFO, Embase, Cinahl, and Cochrane. The strategy was designed to search the title and abstract fields or the thesaurus terms for pregnancy, antenatal, prenatal, prepartum, or preterm adjacent to following truncated words: project, program, service, clinic, meeting, or class. This set was then combined with the terms for high risk pregnancy such as hypertension, eclampsia, diabetes, HIV, epilepsy, previous preterm, or placenta praevia. We did not apply a qualitative search filter, and the "qualitative" term was introduced as the indexing system of databases only since 2003. We limited the search to English language references published from 1980 to March 2015. (See Appendix A for MEDLINE search report).

All retrieved references were imported into a referencing software program (ENDNOTE version 7). Two reviewers independently assessed the studies for inclusion in the review and any disagreement was resolved through discussion. Conference proceedings, reviews reference lists were also hand searched to identify additional studies.

Methodological quality assessments
The risk of bias of studies of a quantitative type were assessed by applying the Cochrane Effective Practice and Organization of Care group (EPOC) [19] criteria. The tool assesses the risk of bias for the following domains: sequence generation, allocation concealment, blinding, incomplete outcome data, selective reporting, baseline characteristics, baseline outcomes, protection against contamination and other bias. Each domain was given one of the following ratings: "yes", "no" or "unclear".

The Critical Appraisal Skills Programme (CASP) [20] for evaluating the risk of bias of studies of qualitative design was implemented. This tool has a checklist of ten questions covering the study objectives and rationale, study methods, study design, study value, recruitment strategies, method of data collection, information on ethical approval, researcher-participant relationship, reliability and validity method of analysing data and reporting of findings. Each domain was given "yes", "no" or "unclear".

The quality assessment was conducted independently by the two reviewers and any discrepancies in quality rating were resolved by discussion. For low risk of bias studies the low risk should be given to all domains in the risk of bias tool; for medium risk of bias studies at least 1 of the risk-of-bias criteria was not met, and a high risk of bias studies was assigned to studies with two or more risk-of-bias domains of the risk of bias tool. Unclear risk of bias was assigned for the studies when risk-of-bias criteria was poorly reported.

Data collection and analysis
Individual data extraction forms were designed for the quantitative and qualitative studies. The form for quantitative studies holds information about the study design, participants' characteristics, components of care provided in the clinics, outcome variables and reported results. For qualitative studies the study setting, study aims, ethics, participants' characteristics, and recruitment and sampling methods, methods used for data collection and analysis, reported themes and study conclusion were extracted.

Studies were summarized and grouped by their study designs and sub-grouped by their reported outcomes. A narrative synthesis only was implemented for data extracted from quantitative studies, as we identified heterogeneity and variation across the included studies. The heterogeneity arose from different study designs, variation in study inclusion criteria, intervention and reported outcomes. We originally planned to undertaken a meta-synthesis of data extracted from qualitative studies, however we only reported the common themes from one qualitative study found eligible for inclusion in this review.

All data were extracted and cross checked independently by the two reviewers.

Results

Results of database searching

The search strategy yielded 10,704 citations all generated from searching data bases electronically. Of these 6884 were duplications and 10,157 were unique study references. We identified 88 relevant references and full texts were retrieved and examined. Seventy-seven studies were excluded and 11 studies met the review inclusion criteria (See Fig. 1). One study was found via checking reference lists of the included studies [21]. The reference list of excluded publications with reasons is available on request from the authors.

Description of included studies

The review studies were organised by methodological design. Eleven studies met the review inclusion criteria, five were randomised controlled trials [21–25] and five were cohort studies [26–30]. Only one qualitative design study was included in this review [31].

Description of randomised studies

We included five randomised controlled trials [21–25] (Studies description is shown in Table 1). All were conducted in the USA from 1985 to 1990. One study was only available as an abstract [21]. Four studies were single centre studies [21, 22, 24, 25] and one [25] was a cluster randomised study involving eight clinics, five in the intervention group and three in the control.

Overall, 8986 women were involved and 5796 were categorised as being at high risk of preterm birth using the Creasy et al. [32] scoring system (low risk < 10 or high risk >10) in four studies [21–24], and one with a specifically designed risk assessment tool [25]. Similar entry criteria were utilized across the studies with women at less than 30–31 weeks gestational age at clinic first visit with no major congenital anomalies or disabling conditions included. Multiple pregnancy was an exclusion criteria in one study only [25]. The demographic characteristics and factors increasing the risk of preterm were not distinctly different, in the three studies [22, 24, 25] which were carried out in predominately Black or Hispanic women (See Table 1 for details). The intervention differed slightly between studies. In Iams and Johnson [21] and Muller-Heubach [23], women in the intervention group received a weekly visit to the clinic between 20 and 36 weeks gestation in which signs and symptoms of preterm labour were taught and the cervix was examined. Healthcare providers in Muller-Heubach [23] changed the study design by offering the intervention to all participants, and a historical control group

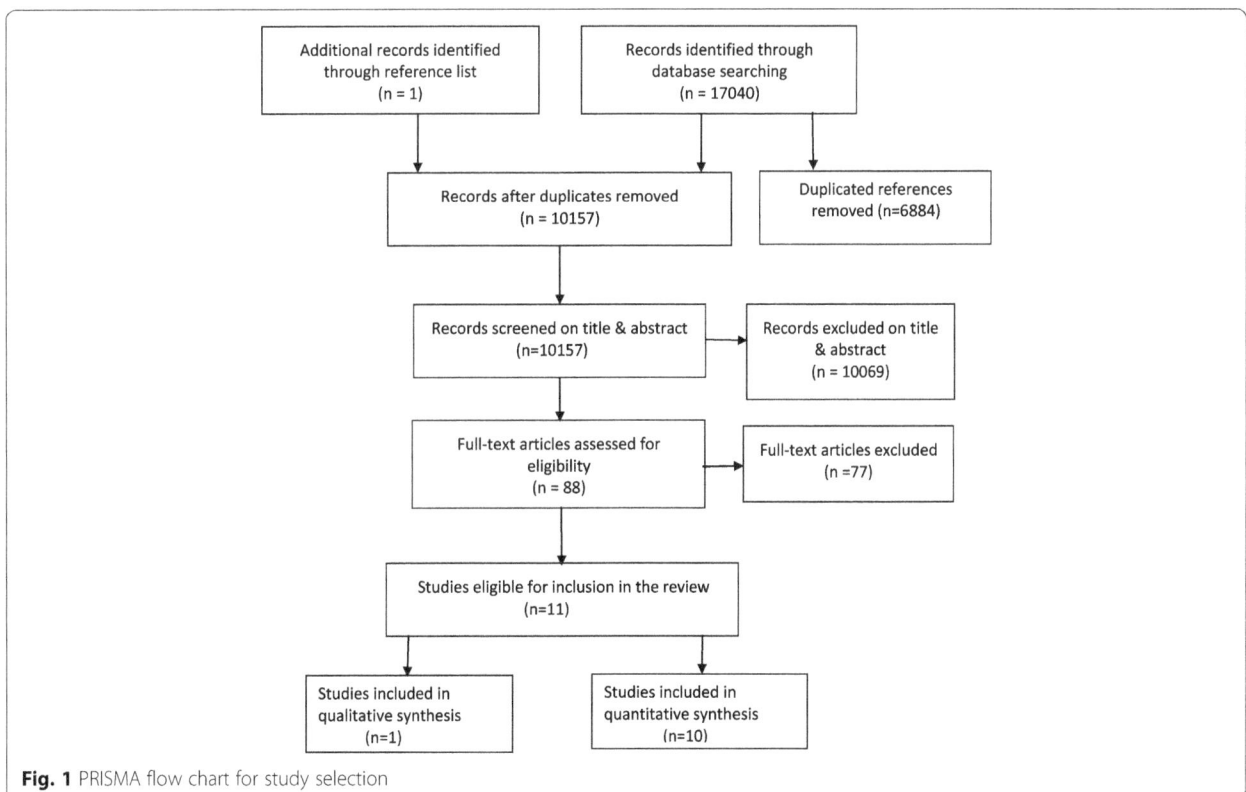

Fig. 1 PRISMA flow chart for study selection

Table 1 Characteristics of included quantitative studies

Study ID, design, country	Participants	Intervention	Outcomes	Results
Randomised controlled trials (RCTs)				
1. Iams and Johnson [21], single centre, study duration 1983 to 1986 (abstract only), USA	370 high-risk women based on Creasy scoring system were selected from 2829 women attending antenatal clinic. One hundred eighty-two women received routine antenatal care plus preterm birth prevention clinic the intervention and 188 women received routine antenatal care.	Preterm birth prevention clinic group received education about symptoms and signs of labour and the cervix examined at weekly visits between 20 and 36 weeks' gestation Control group received standard antenatal care.	1. Preterm labour (intervention vs control): 50/182 vs 40/188, $P = 0.17$ 2. Preterm birth < 37 weeks (intervention vs control): 24/50 (48%) vs 35/40 (87.5%), $P = 0.001$	No significant difference between the two groups with regards to the incidence of preterm labour. Significant difference between the two groups with regard to preterm birth among women who developed preterm labour.
2. Main et al. [22], single centre, study duration: 3.5 years, USA	367 black women at gestational age > 18 weeks were at high risk of preterm labour based on Creasy et al. [32] scoring criteria. Inclusion criteria: Black women with gestational age < 18 weeks were referred to the nurse specialist in the Preterm Labour Detection Clinic. Intervention group: $N = 178$, maternal age (yr) 23.9 ± 5.5, gravidity 3.7 ± 1.9, parity 1.4 ± 1.2, abortions ≤ 14 weeks 1.0 ± 1.0, abortion > 14 weeks 0.3 ± 0.7, women with previous preterm delivery 38%, gestational age at first visit (wk) 12.5 ± 3.7. Control group: $N = 198$, maternal age (yr) 24.1 ± 5.1, gravidity 3.8 ± 1.9, parity 1.6 ± 1.5, abortions ≤ 14 weeks 0.9 ± 1.1, abortion > 14 weeks 0.3 ± 0.7, women with previous preterm delivery 43%, gestational age at first visit (wk) 12.0 ± 3.3.	Attending a preterm labour detection clinic on a weekly or biweekly basis from 22 weeks' gestation and cervical assessment by 1 of 3 physicians at each visit. Also education provided by a nurse specialist regarding subtle signs of labour. High risk control: received usual prenatal care.	1. Preterm deliveries (intervention vs control): <28 weeks: 3% vs 3.9%, $p = 0.42$, 32 < 34 weeks: 6.6% vs 6.2%, $p = 0.51$, <36 weeks: 16.7% vs 13.4%, $p = 0.46$, <37 weeks: 23.2% vs 20.7%, $p = 0.32$. 2. Neonatal outcomes: 5-min Apgar <5 4.5% vs 6.1%, $p = 0.32$. Caesarean birth: 23.7% vs 21.2%, $p = 0.64$. NICU admission: 10.4% vs 16.4%, $p = 0.32$. Length of stay > 5 days: 21.4% vs 18.7%, $p = 0.33$. Stillborn: 4.8% vs 2.9%, $p = 0.53$. Neonatal deaths: 0% vs 0.7%, $p = 0.48$. 3. Cost/Hospital charges: Maternal charges: $5687 ± 4222 vs $5846 ± 4872, $p = 0.97$ Neonatal charges: $4958 ± 26,491 vs $4287 ± 24,247, $p = 0.83$. 4. Maternal hospital admission: Mean no. maternal hospital admissions: 1.7 ± 1.1 vs 1.3 ± 0.7, $p = 0.0001$, Women with one or more antepartum admissions: 44% vs 26%, $p = 0.001$.	No significant differences between the two high risk groups with respect to mean gestational age at delivery, birth weight or percentage delivering before term.

Table 1 Characteristics of included quantitative studies *(Continued)*

Study	Intervention	Results	Conclusion
3. Mueller-Heubach [23], study duration 3 years between September 1984 and August 1987, USA	5457 women were scored for risk of preterm birth using the Creasy scoring system 1980, and 18.1% were classified as high risk these were randomised into two groups. Exclusion criteria: Patients registered after 28 weeks' gestation.	The intervention group received weekly cervical examinations and teaching about signs and symptoms of preterm labour. Health care professionals received similar instructions. Historical control was used due to high contamination. The control group received the usual antenatal care.	Preterm birth rate (intervention vs control): 22.1% vs 20.8%, $p > 0.05$ Preterm birth in year one: 13.7%, in year two 9.3%, $p < 0.001$ and in year three 8.9%. Neonatal death (second and third year): 5/1755 vs 11/1203 the incidence: 2.8/1000 vs 9.1/1000.	There was no difference in preterm birth between the intervention and the control. There was a significant reduction in preterm birth rate in year 3 compared to year 1. There was a significant decrease in the neonatal death in the second and third year of the intervention compared with the control.
4. Goldenberg et al. [24], five centres, study duration 1982–1986 (singleton and multiple pregnancies), USA	1000 high risk women were randomized to intervention or control. Seventy percent were black and 35% were younger than 20 years and 4% were 35 years or older. 3.5% in the intervention had multiple pregnancy and 4.2% in the control. Inclusion criteria: women with an estimated date of delivery between 1 November, 1982 and April 1, 1986, at < 30 weeks gestational age, women were classified as high risk based on a score of 10 or more on the based on Creasy et al. [32] criteria.	The intervention group attended the clinic weekly and pelvic examination and education about preterm signs and symptoms. Primary care was provided by a specially trained nurse who saw the same woman. Women in the control group received usual prenatal care.	1. Pregnancy outcomes (intervention vs control): Spontaneous preterm labour: 26.9% vs 16.3% Spontaneous premature rupture of membranes (PROM) 6.3% vs 4.4% Preterm delivery incidence: 6.3% vs 2.5% Spontaneous delivery < 28 weeks: 2.7% vs 1.3%, $p > 0.05$ Spontaneous delivery < 36 weeks: 11.8% vs 10.5%, $p > 0.05$ Spontaneous delivery < 37 weeks: 15.9% vs 14.2%, $p > 0.05$ Birth weight 1500–2499 g: 37.7 ± 3.8 vs 38.1 ± 3.1, $p > 0.05$ Mean birth weight: 2892 ± 771 vs 2935 ± 679, $p > 0.05$ 2. Neonatal outcomes: Respiratory distress syndrome: 5.9% vs 3.8%, $p > 0.05$ Hyperbilirubinemia: 7.9% vs 9.4%, $p > 0.05$ Necrotizing enterocolitis: 0.6% vs 1.8%, $p > 0.05$ Patent ductus arteriosus: 2.4% vs 1.6%, $p > 0.05$ Interventricular haemorrhage: 1.8% vs0.4%, $p < 0.05$ Congenital anomaly: 6.75 vs 7.8%, $p > 0.05$	Preterm labour diagnosis and spontaneous preterm PROM diagnosis were higher in the intervention group, but the difference was not significant. No significant difference between the groups on most the neonatal outcomes.

Table 1 Characteristics of included quantitative studies *(Continued)*

Study	Population	Intervention	Results	Conclusion
5. Hobel et al. [25], multicentre study, 5 clinics in the intervention and three in the control, recruitment lasted from 1983 to 1986, USA	1774 high-risk women in the intervention clinics and 880 in the control clinics. Women were predominantly Hispanics. Inclusion criteria: Had a gestational age of <31 week, no disabling condition, and were English or Spanish speaking. Exclusion criteria: major congenital anomaly, multiple births, pregnancies with missing charts of cost information.	Intervention group received preterm birth prevention education plus increased antenatal visits to the clinic and selected prophylactic interventions. Visits were scheduled at 2 weeks intervals, 3 educational classes about preterm birth prevention, nutritional and psychosocial screening and offered treatment when it was needed. The control clinics offered visits at 4 weeks intervals up to 30 weeks 'gestation, then every 2 weeks from 30 to 35 weeks' gestation, then weekly until delivery.	1. Number of clinic visits(intervention vs control): 6.4 ± 3.4 vs.9 $\pm$ 2.5, $p < 0.05$ 2. Preterm rate: 7.4% vs 9.1%, $p = 0.063$ 3. Birth weight <2500gm: 5.8% vs 6.4%, $p = 0.15$ 4. Gestatioanl age: 39.8 ± 2.3 vs 39.9 ± 2.5, $p = 0.38$ 4. Inpatient costs per New born: <37 weeks: ($n = 95$, $17,206 \pm 3995$ vs $n = 55$, $31,129 \pm 8572$) ≥37 weeks: ($n = 70$, 2025 ± 273 vs $n = 70$, 2763 ± 628) 5. Average new born inpatient cost:$3146 vs $5342 Sepsis: 0.8% vs 0.8%, $p > 0.5$ Hypoglycaemia:2.3% vs 4%, $p > 0.5$ Need for resuscitation: 8.2% vs 8%, $p > 0.05$ NECU: 27.4% vs 26.6%, $p > 0.05$ Time on ventilator: <12 h:93.5 vs 97.4, $P < 0.05$; >12 h: 6.5% vs 2.4%, $p < 0.05$ Babies days in hospital: ≤7: 89% vs 91.8%, $p > 0.5$; >7 11% vs 8.2%, $p > 0.05$	No significant difference between the two groups with regards to the incidence of preterm birth, low birth weight and gestational age. High risk prevention clinics had an average cost savings of $2196 for new born care ($p = 0.2$).

Cohort studies

Study	Population	Intervention	Results	Conclusion
1. Herron et al. [26], prospective-cohort, single centre, between July 1, 1978 and June 30, 1979, USA.	Patients were screened based on the Creasy criteria 1980 and divided into two groups: 176 (15.2%) women assigned to the high risk group and 974 (84.8%) to the low-risk group.	For the high risk group: The intervention involved: the first visit to the clinic included education regarding the signs and symptoms of preterm labour and training the participants in self-detection of painless contractions. Weekly antenatal visit to the clinic, if the symptoms of painless labour occurs then patients were monitored for 1–2 h. Reporting to the clinic immediately if one of the preterm signs and symptoms occurred. AT the weekly visit the pelvic examination was performed by the same physician. If preterm	1.Preterm labour(comparing high risk group to low risk): 30/176 (17.5%) vs 24/974 (2.5%), $p < 0.05$, 2. Preterm delivery (comparing high risk group to low risk group): 7/176 (4%) vs 9/974 (0.9%), $p > 0.05$. 3. Men gestational age at delivery (comparing high to low group):	A significant decrease in preterm birth with the clinic.

Table 1 Characteristics of included quantitative studies (Continued)

Study	Participants	Intervention/clinic description	Outcomes	Conclusions
		labour occurred then patients admitted to hospital and tocolytic therapy was given. Staff training and education to prompt response to patients' complaints, of any preterm signs and symptoms, early admission to patients having a mild increase uterine activity, aggressive therapeutic approach in patients with documented preterm labour, awareness of long term side effects of the tocolysis.	33.7 ± 2.6 vs 33.3 ± 3.6 weeks 4. Preterm birth ≤ 36 weeks at year 1 after introducing the clinic: 2.4% compared with 6.75% before the clinic.	
2. Manuck et al. [27], Retrospective cohort, multi-centre study from 17 hospitals, participants' enrolment from 2008 to 2010, USA.	Inclusion criteria: Single pregnancy, previous PTB <35 weeks. Exclusion criteria: Women who delivered preterm babies <37 weeks due to medical or foetal complications, eg, preeclampsia, foetal growth restriction. Women excluded from the study analysis if they had a history of incompetent cervix (painless cervical dilation <24 week's gestation). Total number of patients: 223 PTB clinic group: $n = 70$ Maternal age 28.5 years, white 83.1%, smoking 3.4%, married 86.4%, primary obstetrics provider is perinatalogist 18.6%; number of PTB <37 weeks 1.7 (mean) Usual care group: $n = 153$ Maternal age 28.8% years, white 88.8%, smoking 9.8%, married 83%, primary obstetrics provider is perinatalogist 11.8%; number of PTB <37 weeks 1.6 (mean)	The recurrent PTB prevention clinic includes three visits (10–18 weeks, 19–24 weeks, and 28–32 weeks): Detailed obstetric history and personal recurrence risk assessment: at visit 1 (10–18 weeks) Screen for BV and treat if positive with oral metronidazole at all three visits. Urinalysis : at all three visits Urine culture: at all visits (symptoms positive or urinalysis is positive). Transvaginal cervical length: at all visits. Cervical length <2.5 cm is abnormal. Offer 17 alpha hyroxyprogesterone caproate: at visit one for all patients, patients who declined were offered the treatment again at week 24 if cervical shortening is noted. Usual care group: Managed by their primary obstetrician without being referred to the clinic.	Primary outcome (PTB clinic vs usual care): 1. PTB < 37 weeks,%: 48.6% vs 63.4%, $p=0.02$ 2. PTB < 37 weeks,%: 5.7% vs 13.7%, $p=0.08$ 3. Delivery GA, mean wk: 36.1 vs 34.9, $p = 0.02$ Secondary outcomes: 1. Neonatal morbidity, %: 5.7 vs 16.3, $p = 0.03$ 2. NICU admission, %: 44.3 vs 41.2, $p = 0.66$ 3. Mean inpatient maternal cost: $6929 vs $7706, $p = 0.48$ 4. Mean inpatient neonatal cost: $11,818 vs $15,662, $p = 0.05$	28% reduction in the risk of recurrent PTB <37 weeks and >1 week of pregnancy prolongation and reduced the rate of major neonatal morbidity with the intervention.
3. Karkhanis et al. [28], retrospective-cohort from November 2007 to January 2009, Birmingham-UK (abstract)	180 high risk women, mean age 29.85 years (18-41), mean BMI = 27.52 kg/m2, $N = 158$ with previous preterm labour or mid trimester loss.	All patients in the preterm prevention clinic underwent serial transvaginal scan monitoring and infection screening between 16 and 28 weeks. 40 women underwent cervical cerclage and progesterone 35 women received progesterone only	1. Term delivery > 37 weeks: $n = 123/180$ 2. Term delivery >37 weeks after one preterm delivery (PTD): 79% 3. Term delivery > 37 weeks after 2 PTD:71% 4. Term delivery >37 weeks after 3 PTD:60% 5. NICU admission: $n = 36$ babies 6. Infant mortality: $n = 7$	The preterm prevention clinic reduced prematurity rate.
4. Burul et al. [29], retrospective-cohort, clinic cases from January 2005 to December 2008, London-UK (abstract).	210 cerclage cases: 85 cases before the establish of the clinic and 125 afterwards	Cervical cerclage	1. Elective cervical cerclage 44% before the clinic vs 88% after establishing the clinic	

Table 1 Characteristics of included quantitative studies (*Continued*)

5. Cohen et al. [30], audit of two London preterm surveillance clinics between January 2013 and May 2014, UK (abstract).	509 pregnancies reviewed; mean age 33.6 years (18–49 years), BMI 24.4 (range 17–48), 59% White and 15% Afro-Caribbean. Reasons for referral to the clinics: Previous cervical treatment (50%) Previous preterm birth before 34 weeks 926%), mid trimester miscarriage (MTL) (17%) Uterine anomalies (2%) Multiple pregnancy (3%)	Clinic interventions: Cervical shortening found in 44% Progesterone supplementations 25% Cervical cerclage 27%
	2. GA at delivery 28 + 2/ 40 before the PTBC compared with 35 + 2/40 with the clinic care	Preterm delivery: <28 weeks 0.7% delivered <34 weeks 4% delivered <37 weeks 11% derived
		Early referral to the clinics for better monitoring.

was thus established. Women were also seen weekly or biweekly starting at 22 weeks' gestation and offered a comprehensive education in Main et al. [22]. Whereas, in Hobel et al. [25], women attending five clinics received the intervention, and in three the control. High risk women in the intervention cluster received three educational classes on preterm birth prevention and visits to the clinic scheduled every 2 weeks. In a nested study, women were also randomised to one of the four following interventions: protocols of bed rest, psychosocial support, Provera (progesterone) or placebo, or no additional intervention. Additionally, nutritional screening, psychosocial support and crisis intervention were offered to participants from both groups. In all studies the women in the control groups were assigned to receive the usual antenatal care. Ultimately, all five studies had similar primary outcomes of preterm labour and gestational age at delivery.

Description of cohort studies

Five cohort studies [26–30] were included in this review (Table 1 is a summary of the study characteristics). Three studies were conducted in the UK [28–30] and two in the USA [26, 27]. Herron et al. [26] was a prospective cohort single centre study where participants were assigned one of two group, high and low risk, based on the Creasy et al. [32] criteria [30]. Participants were then instructed on how to identify early signs of preterm labour and to be followed weekly in a specialist clinic, in addition to their usual antenatal care. If preterm labour occurred, women were admitted to hospital for further treatment. In Manuck [27], 223 women were identified from a clinic data base retrospectively. Women were included if they had at least one PTB < 35 weeks' gestation and one subsequent singleton pregnancy carried to at least 20 weeks gestation. Three clinic visits were scheduled at 10–18 weeks, 19–24 weeks and 28–32 weeks gestation. Screening for bacterial vaginosis (BV), urine culture and transvaginal ultrasound for cervix length were performed at each visit. Hydroxyprogesterone was also offered to all women. The study primary outcome was recurrent PTB < 35 weeks' gestation.

The three most recent UK studies were published only as abstracts [28–30] and involved a retrospective case-note analysis of patients registered at the clinics. In Burul [29] the focus of the study was to collect data on cervical cerclage and pregnancy outcomes. A total 210 cerclage cases were identified at the PTB clinic, 85 cases before the PTB clinic was established (January 2005–December 2012) and 120 cases since January 2005–December 2012.

Karkhanis et al. [28] reviewed the clinic notes of 180 women from November 2007 to November 2009. All women underwent serial transvaginal scans and infection screening between 16 and 28 weeks. Forty women underwent cervical cerclage and 35 received progesterone.

An audit of two London preterm surveillance clinics between January 2013 and May 2014, described by Cohen et al. [30] aimed to assess the outcomes of 509 high risk pregnancies, among which 27% of women underwent cervical cerclage and 25% received progesterone.

Description of qualitative studies

One qualitative study [31] conducted in a single centre in the North West of England was included in this review (Table 2 is a summary of the study characteristics). Data were collected by a mixture of focus groups and one to one interviews. Fourteen Women with high risk pregnancies and at risk of preterm birth who were referred to a specialist antenatal clinic for their antenatal care were interviewed. Three focus groups ($n = 4$), ($n = 2$), ($n = 4$) and 4 individual interviews were conducted. Interviews took place in the clinic or the women's homes. Data on gravidity, parity, current treatment and demographic data were collected prior to interview. Women were encouraged to discuss their views of high risk pregnancy and their individual care and their management which could include activity restriction, inpatient admission, antibiotics, aspirin and progesterone treatment. Data were analysed thematically.

Quality assessment of quantitative research

The quality of studies included in this review was mixed, varying from good to low. Two of the included five randomised trials [24, 25] were considered good quality; the other two RCTs [22, 23] were low quality and one RCT [21] was published as an abstract and information to assess the study quality were missing. All four cohort studies were considered low quality (See Table 3 for details).

For the risk of bias assessment in the randomised studies, the allocation concealment technique was described in the three studies [22, 24, 25]. Hobel et al. [25] was a cluster randomisation study with eight clinics allocated to intervention and control using the blocked technique. A quasi-randomisation method was used in Main et al. [22] whereas, in Iams et al. [21] and Mueller-Heubach [23], little was available on study methodology and randomisation allocation was reported with no further information. For this type of intervention blinding of women and health care professionals is difficult as both would be aware of the

Table 2 Characteristics of included qualitative study

Study ID, country	O'Brien et al. [31], UK
Study Aims	High risk pregnant women's views on attending a specialised antenatal clinic.
Ethics	Study was reviewed by the hospital's Research & development committee and gained ethical approval from local research ethics committee.
Participants	Women who had a previous preterm birth, experience antenatal care for the current pregnancy was provided in preterm clinic and English speaking. Women were excluded if they had a known foetal malformation.
Recruitment	Specialist preterm clinic.
Sampling method	Women were identified for inclusion in the study through obstetrician referral.
Participants characteristics	37 women were interested in participating in the study and 14 were interviewed. Age range 23–44 years; 13 were white and one Black Caribbean. Gestational age an interview range (14–32 weeks).
Data quality rating	Two independent researchers analysed the data.
Data collection	Three focus groups and face to face interviews.
Data analysis	Interpretative approach (thematic coding method) was used.
Data extracts	Data transcribed anonymously, coding and categories and themes were developed by two researchers.
Themes	1. Balancing the risks: Women were aware of their risk, but viewed positively due to the extra care ("I would prefer to know and I would see it as a positive thing because you would expect that they would monitor you closely and if necessary give you medication or obviously try and lower the risk somehow to have a successful pregnancy"). 2. Threat of preterm labour: All women felt paranoid about potential signs or symptoms of PTB "Just get through this bit. 3) Personal coping buy developing strategies to survive the pregnancy however, women tried not to focus on their pregnancy avoiding bonding with the baby and were reluctant to look too far to the future. a) Recognizing that something does not feel right: Ignoring the warning signs of PTL with previous pregnancies, however, the PTB was realised they were feeling guilty and not ignoring their intuition again: ("When I look back, leading up to actually having her there were some little signs. And I was very much ignoring them because I was thinking I was being paranoid and silly… the promise that we made to ourselves and particularly to myself was that I am just not going to take any risks….. I don't care if anyone thinks I 'm paranoid, you know, or nuts, whatever, as long as I eventually have a healthy baby"). Some women struggled with the health professional to have their concerns taken seriously. Some felt worse after interactions with health professionals in the clinic. c) Need regular reassurance from health professionals were not always sensitive to women's worries about the risk of PTL, felt better with the routine reassurance of the clinic screening and scanning.

frequent visits to the clinics. A cluster randomisation method at the clinic level would be the preferable approach to reduce bias associated with contamination between the intervention and control groups. In three RCTs [22, 24, 25] women were not aware of their intervention status. In both Main et al. [22] and Goldenberg [24] health care professionals were not aware of the intervention status. In Mueller-Heubach [23], a high contamination occurred between the intervention and the control, resulting in the use of historical controls. The numbers of participants lost to follow-up for most outcomes were not reported clearly in most studies [22, 24, 25].

All five cohort studies were rated at high risk of bias. Three studies were published as abstracts and information on their methodology was absent. Only one study was a prospective cohort [26] and involved a good sample size ($n = 179$) in the high risk group and ($n = 974$) in the control. Both were selected from the same clinic. The follow-up rate was sufficient, with only three women missing from year 2 results. The second fully-published paper Manuck et al. [27] was a retrospective cohort study and participants were selected from the same clinic with no baseline difference with regards to maternal age, gravidity, parity and the number of previous preterm births. Potential confounding variables were measured and adjusted for in this study (progesterone prophylactic use, history of spontaneous PTB <28 weeks, maternal smoking, male foetus, a short cervix or carrying of private health insurance). In all cohort studies there is no information about whether outcomes were assessed blindly. The risk of bias from allocation to interventions was high and risk of contamination bias was low across included cohort studies.

Quality of evidence of qualitative study

Based on the CASP 2013 criteria O'Brien et al. [31], was a good quality study as reflected in the adequate formulation of the study aims and the appropriate use of qualitative methods (See details in Table 4). The characteristics and the recruitment criteria of the study sample were appropriately specified. Validity of data collection was also established with two different methods for gathering data, focus groups and face to face interviews. Additionally, the reliability of data analysis was established as coding and thematic analysis were conducted by two researchers independently.

Effects of the interventions from quantitative research

The following primary outcomes were addressed across the included studies:

Table 3 Risk of bias of quantitative studies based on the EPOC tool

Study/year	Selection bias	Allocation to intervention	Performance bias	Baseline differences in characteristics	Baseline differences in outcomes	Contamination	Attrition bias	Selective reporting	Other bias
Randomized controlled trials (RCTs)									
1. Hobel et al. [25]	Low: Cluster randomization with a restricted block	Low: cluster randomization.	Low: women were not aware of their intervention status nor the clinics teams	Low: participants were comparable with respect to age, marital status, gravidity, parity and preterm birth rate	Low: no difference between the groups with regards to high risk preterm problems at baseline	Low: intervention was provided on a clinic-basis rather than patients	Unclear: the number of women who left the study was not reported	Low	low
2. Main et al. [22]	High: a random numbers table was used for the first 479 participants then the second sample of464 women was divided into groups by birthday date	High: women's' date of birth was used to allocate women to intervention or control	Low: In the control group neither the doctors nor the women were made aware they were at high risk of preterm birth.	Low: no differences between groups with respect to maternal age, gravidity, parity, previous preterm deliveries, and gestational age at first visit	High: More women with previous preterm birth were assigned to the intervention.	High: 8 women from the control group transferred to the clinic	High: insufficient reporting on the rate of attrition.	Unclear	Low
3. Iams and Johnson [21]	Unclear	Unclear	Unclear	Unclear	Unclear	Unclear	Unclear	Unclear	Unclear
4. Goldenberg et al. [24]	Low: randomization by a randomization officer	Unclear: allocation to intervention or control method was not reported	Low: nobody was aware of the intervention status	Low: No significant difference between high-risk control group and high-risk intervention with regard to number of birth, race, age and parity	Low: no differences of previous preterm birth and multiple pregnancies between the two groups	low	Unclear: the number of missing women was not reported	Low	Low
5. Mueller-Heubach [23]	Low: participants were selected to intervention and controlled randomly	Unclear: method of allocation to intervention or control was not reported	High: nurses were aware of the intervention status of the participants	Low	Low	High: a historical control was used in the analysis	Unclear	low	low
Cohort studies									
1. Herron et al. [26]	High	High	High	Low	Unclear	Low	Low	Low	Low
2. Manuck et al. [27]	High	High	High	Low	Low	Low	Low	Low	Low
3. Karkhanis et al. [28] (abstract)	High	High	High	Unclear	Unclear	Low	Unclear	Unclear	Unclear
4. Burul [29] (abstract)	High	High	High	unclear	Unclear	Low	Unclear	Unclear	Unclear
5. Cohen et al. [30] (abstract)	High	High	High	Unclear	Unclear	Low	Unclear	Unclear	Unclear

Table 4 Risk of bias qualitative studies using the CASP tool for qualitative studies

Study ID	O'Brien et al. [31]
Study objective	Yes, understanding the women's experiences of attending and being referred to the specialist antenatal clinic.
Appropriate method	Yes, qualitative methodology is appropriate to seek women's experience of the clinic.
Study design	Yes, through focus groups and in depth face to face interviews.
Recruitment strategy	Yes, women were enrolled from a specialist clinic which is a major referral centre in the North West England.
Data collection	Yes, data collected through focus groups and face to face interview. All were recorded and transcribed and data saturation was discussed.
Researcher-participant relationship	Unclear, no information was given.
Ethical approval	Yes, study reviewed by Hospital's Research and development Committee.
Data analysis	Yes, data was analysed by two independent researchers using the constant comparative method.
Study findings	Yes, three themes were explicitly defined and the credibility of the findings was also clearly discussed.
Study values	Yes, researchers identify a new area for further research.

Preterm birth: (birth < 37 weeks' gestation):
Results from all RCTs [21–25] showed no significant difference between the intervention and the control groups in preterm delivery (7.4% vs 9.1%, $p = 0.063$; 23.2% vs 20.7%, $p = 0.32$; 22.1% vs 20.8%, $p > 0.05$; 15.9% vs 14.2%, $P > 0.05$; and 22.1% vs 20.8%, $P > 0.05$?) respectively. In contrast, results from cohort studies showed a reduction of preterm birth incidence after the clinic was introduced. A 28% reduction in the risk of preterm birth in comparison to data from women receiving usual care was reported in Herron et al. [26]. In Karkhanis et al. [28], the prematurity rate was reduced and the term delivery > 37 weeks' figures were reported for women with one (74%), two (42%) and three (41%) previous preterm deliveries.
Very preterm birth (birth before 34 weeks' gestation) and extremely preterm birth (birth <28 weeks' gestation):
Data from two RCTs [21, 24] contributed to both outcomes. There was no significant differences between the number of women attending the specialist clinic and delivering very or extremely preterm babies compared to those receiving usual care.
Gestational age at birth:
Results from one study [25] showed no significant differences between women attending the specialist

clinic mean gestation 39.8 (2.3) and women receiving usual care 39.9 (2.3) weeks, $p = 0.32$. The median gestational age at delivery increased from 28 + 2/40 to 35 + 2/40, $P = 0.6$, in the cohort study reported by Burul et al. [29].
Stillbirth:
One RCT [22], reported no significant difference between the women in the two groups, with seven deaths reported in the intervention group compared with six in the control.

Secondary outcomes
For neonatal outcomes such as birth weight, admission to neonatal intensive care and length of hospital stay, there were no significant differences between women receiving the intervention in comparison to women in the control groups. The only significant difference was more women were treated with tocolytics in the intervention group ($p = 0.3$) in Main et al. [22].

The cerclage rate per 1000 women delivered fell from 6 to 5 as reported by Burul et al. [29], and the gestational age at cerclage placement fell after introducing the clinic (17 + 0/40, 13 + 2–23 + 3 to 15 + 2/40, 12 + 2–23 + 4 weeks, $P > 0.05$). The proportion of rescue cerclage also fell (26% to 12%, $P > 0.05$), whereas the proportion of elective cerclage doubled significantly (44 to 88%).

Cost effective outcomes
Three included studies [22, 25, 27] calculated maternal and neonatal cost-effectiveness associated with care in the clinic. In Ross et al. [33], a cost effectiveness evaluation for Hobel et al [25], data on costs were only available for a subgroup of women and cost were collected for prenatal care, maternal inpatient costs for preterm labour, delivery and postpartum care, and newborn inpatient care cost. The results indicated a net savings of $1768 for every high risk mother-infant pair. The estimated outpatient cost per patient was significantly higher for women attending preterm clinic in Main et al. [22]. Both inpatient maternal and neonatal care costs were higher among women receiving routine care in Manuck et al. [27] as the outpatient cost was not available.

Findings from qualitative research
In O'Brien et al. [31], women's response to high preterm risk pregnancy was a mixture of being reassured by the treatments and frequent clinic appointments and feeling anxious and emotionally drained. Therefore, women in this study developed coping strategies during their pregnancy and the following three main themes were emerged: balancing the risks associated with the threat of preterm birth, developing personal coping strategies to survive the pregnancy (focusing on the present and

not looking too far into the future) and developing a family coping strategy.

Women also acknowledged that their physical and emotional needs were considered and addressed in the clinic, however their partners who were struggling to cope emotionally were ignored.

Discussion

Summary of main findings

A strength of this review arises from searching for evidence from both quantitative and qualitative research studies although those included were predominantly of a quantitative design. This is because our aim was initially to enhance the integrity of review findings, reflecting on women's perspectives in addition to clinical outcomes.

The review findings were mixed. Evidence from randomised controlled studies suggested that there was no differences between usual care and care provided at a specialist preterm clinic. In contrast, evidence from cohort studies emphasized that a specialist clinic for managing high risk women is associated with a reduction in preterm birth and lower rates of adverse neonatal outcomes. Moreover, results from individual studies sometimes produced mixed results. In Goldenberg et al. [24] results were not in favour of the clinic and some outcome measures such as foetal and neonatal mortality were slightly worse in the intervention group than in the control. This was explained by the poor compliance with the individual clinic visits. The included RCTs in this review were conducted in late 1980s and 1990s before the usage of cerclage or other new management to prevent preterm birth and before the availability of new screening tests such as the foetal fibronectin screening test (fFN). The intervention itself in these old studies was only by increasing the frequency of antenatal visit to weekly or biweekly and educating the pregnant women about preterm labour signs and symptoms.

The included studies referred to specialist clinics which were established to prevent the onset of preterm labour and facilitate its early identification and treatment. Although these clinics shared a similar goal, the studies varied in their primary outcome focus, target populations, study designs, and specific intervention components. Another common component of the clinic was the initial screening for women at risk, which in the earliest included studies involved using the Creasy et al. [32] scoring system to identify high risk women. However, more recent studies have relied on specific screening tests such as measuring cervical length and fibronectin testing to identify this group of women. In general women are most likely to

be referred if they have had a previous preterm birth, late miscarriage, multiple pregnancy or cervical surgery [14, 34].

A particular limitation of the available quantitative studies is the absence of data collection relating to women's mental health and wellbeing in the context of specialist preterm clinic care in addition to the lack of women's experiences of care. In the single included qualitative study on women's views, some themes reflected psychological issues, namely their anxieties and a need for continuous reassurance and support. The experiences of women accessing this clinic was only addressed in the one qualitative study included in this review [31], women felt relieved by being labelled as "high risk" of preterm birth and by being referred to the clinic, which had offered them a sense of reassurance and frequent clinical assessments. However, only a small number of participants from a single centre who could speak English were interviewed. The views of women from ethnic minority backgrounds were not heard. Other qualitative studies of women who experienced preterm labour, unrelated to the use of a specialist preterm birth clinic, for example MacKinnon and McIntyre [35] have explored women's fear about preterm birth, guilt, feelings of being judged and their sense of personal responsibility in preventing labour. Both parents may be involved in clinic attendance, however no studies of fathers' experience and support in relation to PTB clinics were found.

Another limitation in this review is the lack of accurate economic costing of the clinics with only three studies reporting on relative cost outcomes and using various measure. Results from two studies suggested a cost saving effect of the clinic when compared with standard care, including only inpatient maternal and neonatal care in the economic model. However, the outpatients care cost was higher in the clinic as suggested by the third study.

We conclude that the current literature suggests some benefit of specialist clinics aimed at preventing preterm labour and delivery, but methodological weakness across these studies indicate caution as the most positive reported outcomes are from retrospective cohort studies. While effective intervention may be possible, some risk factors for preterm birth cannot be changed, for example greater maternal age and a previous history of preterm birth. However, the way in which antenatal care is delivered for this population in terms service organisation and care clearly can be changed. First of all the current screening for the risk of preterm birth has changed and the usage of foetal fibronectin testing (fFN) and cervical ultrasound will identify quite a different risk group to those included in earlier studies where the risk of preterm birth was based on the woman scoic-demographics and a previous history of preterm birth. Additionally, other models of antenatal care to prevent and reduce preterm birth such as midwife led continuity of care has been proposed, this is a comprehensive and specialized antenatal clinic-based care or a shared antenatal midwife-obstetric model of care. Alternative antenatal care models are systematically studied and it has been found to be effective in reducing preterm birth for all pregnant women when compared to standard care [36]. Therefore, in arguing for a population health strategy in preventing preterm birth Heaman et al. [37] emphasized that a comprehensive model in preventing preterm birth should be based on targeting the social and economic environment, the physical environment, personal health practices and individual capacity and coping skills, in addition to healthcare services. Thus while maternity services may include such specialist clinics, it must be held in mind that other factors may be more powerfully influencing preterm birth rates and outcomes.

Review limitations

The lack of meta-analysis to identify the efficacy of such a clinic in reducing preterm birth is one of the major limitations of this review. We are aware of the result of a meta-analysis of the preterm birth outcome in the Cochrane review [16] illustrating that there is no significant difference between a specialist clinic and standard care for high risk women. As stressed earlier, this was a result of combining three old studies only. However, the most recent data on clinic efficacy were collected from four cohort studies and combining data from different study design is not feasible.

Another limitation was the absence of any measurement of the women's well-being in the included studies.

Review agreement and disagreements with other reviews

We are not totally with agreement with the conclusion of the 2011 Cochrane review [16], as positive outcomes about the clinic were suggested by more recent cohort studies. The Cochrane review stated that specialist clinics for preterm birth prevention are not effective in preventing preterm labour. As mentioned previously, this was a result of combining results data of three RCTs conducted before 1994, two of which are included in this review [21, 22].

Another and more recent systematic review with meta-analysis [36], looked at the existing models of antenatal care and their effectiveness in reducing preterm birth. Fifteen randomized controlled trials were included and the risk of preterm birth was significantly lower among pregnant women receiving alternative antenatal care compared to women receiving standard care. In Fernandez et al. [37] review, studies including women with low or high risk of pregnancy complications and or preterm birth were eligible for inclusion. The review investigated various antenatal care models such as midwife-led model of care, preterm prevention programmes, clinic-based specialised care and standalone intervention. The overall risk of preterm birth was reduced by 16% by implementing alternative care model. However, subgroup meta-analysis including specialist antenatal care studies showed no significant difference when compared with standard antenatal care on reducing preterm birth. These results were derived from combining data from six randomised controlled trials, three of these are included in this review [21, 22, 25].

Implications of research

There are numerous papers in the literature dealing with interventions to prevent preterm birth, however there is still a gap to identify which interventions are most effective in improving preterm birth maternal and perinatal outcomes [38]. Specialist preterm birth clinics provide a complex package of care and thus, with an agreed standard protocol and guidelines on screening criteria, diagnostic tests and a treatment plan for women attending the clinic. Future studies should include a standardized reporting of the intervention and the relevant outcomes as well as establishing a standardized economic model. More research in screening tests to predict preterm birth is also needed. A well-designed cluster randomisation study would be therefore the preferred design to establish the efficacy of such an intervention, but this approach might be hard to achieve as such clinics are currently a well-established means of providing antenatal care for high risk women in many settings. However, given the heterogeneity of clinics and variations in practice [14, 39], such a study has not yet been undertaken. Women's well-being, mental health and satisfaction and experience of care provided and that of their partners should be included in the design of future studies. Fathers support and experience of PTB is also in need of further research.

Conclusion

There is no evidence yet, either in support of or to refute the effect of a preterm prevention clinic in reducing preterm birth. However, this kind of specialist clinic serves the purpose of offering coordinated and individualized antenatal care to women at high risk of preterm labour. Further clarification is necessary on the optimal referral route and a clear and standardized management plan for this service.

Appendix A

Table 5 Medline Search results in March 2015

1	((specialist or specialised or specialized) adj3 clinic?).ti,ab.	2620
2	((specialist or specialised or specialized) adj3 (class or classes)).ti,ab.	124
3	((specialist or specialised or specialized) adj3 meeting?).ti,ab.	60
4	((specialist or specialised or specialized) adj3 service?).ti,ab.	3588
5	1 or 2 or 3 or 4	6279
6	(pregnan* or antenatal or ante-natal or antepartum or ante-partum or prenatal or pre-natal or prepartum or pre-partum or preterm or pre-term).ti,ab,hw.	798,714
7	5 and 6	294
8	((miscarriage? or high risk pregnan* or pregnancy complication? or complicated pregnanc* or pre-eclampsia or eclampsia or gestational diabet* or gestational hyper-tens* or pregnancy induced hypertens*) adj3 clinic?).ti,ab.	108
9	((miscarriage? or high risk pregnan* or pregnancy complication? or complicated pregnanc* or pre-eclampsia or eclampsia or gestational diabet* or gestational hyper-tens* or pregnancy induced hypertens*) adj3 service?).ti,ab.	29
10	7 or 8 or 9	425
11	Prenatal Care/og [Organization & Administration]	1081
12	Prenatal Care/and (ambulatory care facilities/or outpatient clinics, hospital/)	282
13	Pregnancy/and (ambulatory care facilities/or outpatient clinics, hospital/)	1067
14	((antenatal or ante-natal or antepartum or ante-partum or prenatal or pre-natal or prepartum or pre-partum or pre-term or pre-term) adj3 clinic?).ti,ab.	4113
15	((antenatal or ante-natal or antepartum or ante-partum or prenatal or pre-natal or prepartum or pre-partum or pre-term or pre-term) adj3 (class or classes)).ti,ab.	395
16	((antenatal or ante-natal or antepartum or ante-partum or prenatal or pre-natal or prepartum or pre-partum or pre-term or pre-term) adj3 meeting?).ti,ab.	17
17	((antenatal or ante-natal or antepartum or ante-partum or prenatal or pre-natal or prepartum or pre-partum or pre-term or pre-term) adj3 service?).ti,ab.	1134
18	((antenatal or ante-natal or antepartum or ante-partum or prenatal or pre-natal or prepartum or pre-partum or pre-term or pre-term) and clinic?).ti.	565
19	((antenatal or ante-natal or antepartum or ante-partum or prenatal or pre-natal or prepartum or pre-partum or pre-term or pre-term) and service?).ti.	300
20	11 or 12 or 13 or 14 or 15 or 16 or 17 or 18 or 19	7461
21	*Pregnancy, High-Risk/	1611
22	*Abortion, Habitual/	3894
23	((recur* or history or habitual) adj3 (miscarriage* or abortion?)).ti,ab.	4898
24	*Hypertension/or *Hypertension, Pregnancy-Induced/	133,497
25	*eclampsia/or *hellp syndrome/or *pre-eclampsia/	19,170
26	(hypertens* or high blood pressure or eclampsia or pre-eclampsia or preeclampsia).ti.	160,268

Table 5 Medline Search results in March 2015 *(Continued)*

27	*Diabetes Mellitus, Type 1/or *Diabetes, Gestational/	51,216
28	(diabet* and (gestational or pregnan*)).ti.	8126
29	Placenta Previa/	2183
30	(placenta previa or placenta praevia).ti,ab.	2165
31	Pregnancy Complications/	70,144
32	((high risk* or complicat*) and pregnan*).ti.	6659
33	*HIV Infections/or *HIV Seropositivity/or exp *HIV/	161,063
34	(hiv or hiv1 or hiv2 or human immunodeficiency virus).ti.	162,191
35	exp *Sexually Transmitted Diseases/	226,680
36	21 or 22 or 23 or 24 or 25 or 26 or 27 or 28 or 29 or 30 or 31 or 32 or 33 or 34 or 35	609,992
37	20 and 36	2328

* is a truncation symbol and was used to retrieve terms with a common root within MEDLINE search

Abbreviations
CASP: Critical Appraisal Skills Programme; EPOC: Cochrane Effective Practice and Organization of Care group (EPOC); PRISMA: Preferred Reporting Items for Systematic Reviews and Meta-Analyses; PTB: Preterm birth; RCTs: Randomised Controlled Trials

Acknowledgements
We would like to thank Eli Harriss from the Bodleian Health Care Libraries for her assistance with searching the literature.

Funding
This paper reports on an independent study which was funded by the Policy Research Programme in the Department of Health. The views expressed are not necessarily those of the Department.

Authors' contributions
RM and MR wrote the protocol, assessed potentially relevant articles for inclusion/exclusion and conducted the methodological quality reviews. RM tabulated the extracted data and wrote the first draft of the paper. MR commented, was involved in interpretation of the findings and edited the manuscript. Both authors agreed the final version of the manuscript.

Competing interests
The authors declare that they have no competing interests.

References
1. Wold Health Organization (WHO). Preterm birth. 2015. http://www.who.int/mediacentre/factsheets/fs363/en/. Accessed 22 Sept 2015.
2. Office of National Statistics (ONS). Birth characteristics in England and Wales. 2014. http://www.ons.gov.uk/ons/rel/vsob1/birth-characteristics-in-england-and-wales/2014/stb-birth-characteristics-2014.html. Accessed 22 Sept 2015.
3. Blencowe H, Vos T, Lee AC, et al. Estimates of neonatal morbidities and disabilities at regional and global levels for 2010: introduction, methods overview, and relevant findings from the Global Burden of Disease study. Pediatr Res. 2013;74 Suppl 1:4–16. doi:10.1038/pr.2013.203.
4. Liu L, Johnson HL, Cousens S, Perin J, Scott S, Lawn JE, Rudan I, Campbell H,

Cibulskis R, Li M, Mathers C, Black RE. Child Health Epidemiology Reference Group of WHO and UNICEF: Global, regional, and national causes of child mortality: an updated systematic analysis for 2010 with time trends since 2000. Lancet. 2012;379(9832):2151–61. doi:10.1016/S0140-6736(12)60560-1. Epub 2012 May 11.

5. Raju TN. Epidemiology of late preterm (near-term) births. Clin Perinatol. 2006;33:751–63.

6. Blencowe H, Cousens S, Oestergaard MZ, Chou D, Moller AB, Narwal R, Adler A, Vera Garcia C, Rohde S, Say L, Lawn JE. National, regional, and worldwide estimates of preterm birth rates in the year 2010 with time trends since 1990 for selected countries: a systematic analysis and implications. Lancet. 2012;379(9832):2162–72. doi:10.1016/S0140-6736(12)60820-4.

7. Webb DA, Coyne JC, Goldenberg RL, Hogan VK, Elo I, Bloch JR, Mathew L, Bennett IM, Dennis EF, Culhane JF. Recruitment and retention of women in a large randomized control trial to reduce repeat preterm births: the Philadelphia Collaborative Preterm Prevention Project. BMC Med Res Methodol. 2010;10:88.

8. Jackson RA, Gibson KA, Wu YW, Croughan MS. Perinatal outcomes in singletons following in vitro fertilization: a meta-analysis. Obstet Gynecol. 2004;103(3):551–63.

9. Gilbert WM, Nesbitt TS, Danielsen B. The cost of prematurity: quantification by gestational age and birth weight. Obstet Gynecol. 2003;102:488–92.

10. Petrou S. Economic consequences of preterm birth and low birthweight. BJOG. 2003;110 Suppl 20:17–23.

11. Slattery MM, Morrison JJ. Preterm delivery. Lancet. 2002;360(9344):1489–97.

12. Kugler JP, Connell FA, Henley CE. Lack of difference in neonatal mortality between blacks and whites served by the same medical care system. J Fam Pract. 1990;30:281–7.

13. Alexander GR, Baruffi G, Mor JM, Kieffer EC, Hulsey TC. Multiethnic variations in the pregnancy outcomes of military dependents. Am J Public Health. 1993;83:1721–5.

14. Lamont RF. Setting up a preterm prevention clinic: a practical guide. BJOG. 2006;113 Suppl 3:86–92.

15. Newnham JP, Dickinson JE, Hart RJ, Pennell CE, Arrese CA, Keelan JA. Strategies to Prevent Preterm Birth. Front Immunol. 2014;5:584. doi:10.3389/fimmu.2014.00584.

16. Whitworth M, Quenby S, Cockerill RO, Dowswell T. Specialised antenatal clinics for women with a pregnancy at high risk of preterm birth (excluding multiple pregnancy) to improve maternal and infant outcomes. Cochrane Database Syst Rev. 2011. doi:10.1002/14651858.CD006760.pub2.

17. Moher D, Liberati A, Tetzlaff J, Altman DG, The PRISMA Group. Preferred Reporting Items for Systematic Reviews and Meta-Analyses: The PRISMA Statement. PLoS Med. 2009;6(6):e1000097. doi:10.1371/journal.pmed1000097.

18. Higgins JPT, Green S (editors). Cochrane Handbook for Systematic Reviews of Interventions Version 5.0.0 [updated March 2011]. The Cochrane Collaboration. 2011. http://handbook.cochrane.org/. Accessed 27 Jan 2017.

19. Effective Practice and Organisation of Care (EPOC): Suggested risk of bias criteria for EPOC reviews. EPOC Resources for review authors. Oslo: Norwegian Knowledge Centre for the Health Services. 2015. http://epoc.cochrane.org/epoc-specific-resources-review-authors. Accessed 8 Jan 2015.

20. Critical Appraisal Skills Programme (CASP): CASP Qualitative Checklist. http://www.casp-uk.net/#!casp-tools-checklists/c18f8. Accessed 10 Jan 2015.

21. Iams JD, Johnson FF. Effect of a preterm birth prevention program on the diagnosis and treatment of preterm labor in high risk patients. In: Proceedings of 9th Annual Meeting of the Society of Perinatal Obstetricians. New Orleans, Louisiana, USA; Feb 1-4. Am J Obstet Gynecol. 1989;161:387.

22. Main DM, Richardson DK, Hadley CB, Gabbe SG. Controlled trial of a preterm labor detection program: efficacy and costs. Obstet Gynecol. 1989;74:873–7.

23. Mueller-Heubach E, Reddick D, Barnett B, Bente R. Preterm birth prevention: evaluation of a prospective controlled randomized trial. Am J Obstet Gynecol. 1989;160:1172–8.

24. Goldenberg RL, Davis RO, Copper RL, Corliss DK, Andrews JB, Carpenter AH. The Alabama Preterm Birth Prevention Project. Obstet Gynecol. 1990;75:933–9.

25. Hobel CJ, Ross MG, Bemis RL, Bragonier JR, Nessim S, Sandhu M, et al. The West Los Angeles preterm birth prevention project: I. program impact on high-risk women. Am J Obstet Gynecol. 1994;170:54 62.

26. Herron MA, Katz M, Creasy RK. Evaluation of a preterm birth prevention program: preliminary report. Obstet Gynecol. 1982;59(4):452–6.

27. Manuck TA, Henry E, Gibson J, Varner MW, Porter FT, Jackson GM, Esplin MS. Pregnancy outcomes in a recurrent preterm birth prevention clinic. Am J Obstet Gynecol. 2011;204:320.e1–6.

28. Karkhanis P, Patni S, Gargeswari S. Performance of the preterm prevention clinic at heart of England NHS trust. Int J Gynaecol Obstet. 2012;119(Suppl 1):S386.

29. Burul G, James CP, Forya F, Casagrandi D, Burul G, James CP, Forya F, Casagrandi D. Does specialist antenatal care for women at risk of preterm birth affect patient selection, rate and outcomes of cervical cerclage? Arch Dis Fetal Neonatal Ed. 2014;99 Suppl 1:A1–A180.

30. Cohen A, Kindinger L, Clifford K, Bennett P, Teoh TG. Who is most at risk: a preterm surveillance clinic audit. BJOG. 2014;121:16.

31. O'Brien ET, Quenby S, Lavender T. Women's views of high risk pregnancy under threat of preterm birth. Sex Reprod Healthc. 2010;1(3):79–84.

32. Creasy PK, Gummer BA, Liggins GC. System predicting spontaneous preterm birth. Obstet Gynecol. 1980;55:692–5.

33. Ross MG, Sandhu M, Bemis R, Nessim S, Bragonier JR, Hobel C. The West Los Angeles preterm birth prevention project: II. cost-effectiveness analysis of high-risk pregnancy interventions. Obstet Gynecol. 1994;83:506–11.

34. Esplin MS, O'Brien E, Fraser A, Kerber RA, Clark E, Simonsen SE, et al. Estimating recurrence of spontaneous preterm delivery. Obstet Gynecol. 2008;112(3):516–23.

35. MacKinnon K, McIntyre M. From Braxton Hicks to preterm labour: The constitution of risk in pregnancy. Can J Nurs Res. 2006;38(2):56–72.

36. Heaman M, Sprague A, Stewart P. Reducing the preterm birth rate: a population health strategy. J Obstet Gynecol Neonatal Nurs. 2001;30(1):20–9.

37. Fernandez Turienzo C, Sandall J, Peacock JL. Models of ntenatal care to reduce and prevent preterm birth: a systematic review and meta-analysis. BMJ Open. 2016;6:e009044. doi:10.1136/bmjopen-2015-009044.

38. James Lind Alliance Priority setting partnership (JLA). Preterm Birth Top 10. 2017. http://www.jla.nihr.ac.uk/priority-setting-partnerships/preterm-birth/top-10-priorities/. Accessed 27 Jan 2017.

39. Sharp AN, Alfirevic Z. Provision and practice of specialist preterm labour clinics: a UK survey of practice. BJOG. 2014;121(4):417–21.

Morbidity and mortality among very preterm singletons following fertility treatment in Australia and New Zealand, a population cohort study

Alex Y Wang[1]*, Abrar A. Chughtai[2], Kei Lui[3] and Elizabeth A. Sullivan[1]

Abstract

Background: Due to high rates of multiple birth and preterm birth following fertility treatment, the rates of mortality and morbidity among births following fertility treatment were higher than those conceived spontaneously. However, it is unclear whether the rates of adverse neonatal outcomes remain higher for very preterm (<32 weeks gestational age) singletons born after fertility treatment. This study aims to compare adverse neonatal outcomes among very preterm singletons born after fertility treatment including assisted reproductive technology (ART) hyper-ovulation (HO) and artificial insemination (AI) to those following spontaneous conception.

Methods: The population cohort study included 24069 liveborn very preterm singletons who were admitted to Neonatal Intensive Care Unit (NICU) in Australia and New Zealand from 2000 to 2010. The in-hospital neonatal mortality and morbidity among 21753 liveborn very preterm singletons were compared by maternal mode of conceptions: spontaneous conception, HO, ART and AI. Univariate and multivariate binary logistic regression analysis was used to examine the association between mode of conception and various outcome factors. Odds ratio (OR) and adjusted odds ratio (AOR) and 95% confidence interval (CI) were calculated.

Results: The rate of small for gestational age was significantly higher in HO group (AOR 1.52, 95% CI 1.02–2.67) and AI group (AOR 2.98, 95% CI 1.53–5.81) than spontaneous group. The rate of birth defect was significantly higher in ART group (AOR 1.71, 95% CI 1.36–2.16) and AI group (AOR 3.01, 95% CI 1.47–6.19) compared to spontaneous group. Singletons following ART had 43% increased odds of necrotizing enterocolitis (AOR 1.43, 95% CI 1.04–1.97) and 71% increased odds of major surgery (AOR 1.71, 95% CI 1.37–2.13) compared to singletons conceived spontaneously. Other birth and NICU outcomes were not different among the comparison groups.

Conclusions: Compared to the spontaneous conception group, risk of congenital abnormality significantly increases after ART and AI; the risk of morbidities increases after ART, HO and AI. Preconception planning should include comprehensive information about the benefits and risks of fertility treatment on the neonatal outcomes.

Keywords: Preterm birth, Very preterm birth, Assisted reproductive technology, Hyper-ovulation, Artificial insemination

---

* Correspondence: alex.wang@uts.edu.au
[1]Faculty of Health, University of Technology Sydney, PO Box 123, Broadway, NSW 2007, Australia
Full list of author information is available at the end of the article

Background

The latest report of Australia's mothers and babies shows that 25113 of the 301810 babies (8.3%) born in Australia in 2012 were preterm (<37 weeks gestational age), the most common cause of death among infants [1]. Worldwide, around 14.9 million babies were born preterm in 2010 (11.1% of total birth in the same year). Of these, about 5% were extreme preterm (<28 weeks), 11% were very preterm (28–31 weeks gestational age) and 84% moderate to late preterm (32–36 weeks gestational age) [2]. In comparison, of preterm births in Australia in 2012, 11% were extreme preterm, 9% were very preterm and 80% were moderate to late preterm [1]. Evidence shows that extreme preterm and very preterm births are at increased risk of severe morbidity and mortality compared to moderate preterm births (32–36 weeks) and term births (>36 weeks) [3].

With the advanced care in neonatal intensive care units (NICU), the survival of very preterm babies has been improved in recent years, especially in developed countries. The 2012 annual report by the Australian and New Zealand Neonatal Network (ANZNN) shows that the survival rate before NICU discharge was 70% for births of 24 weeks gestational age and 98% for births of 31 weeks gestational age [4]. The ANZNN data also shows that the NICU survival rates varied by plurality, with significantly higher survival rates for singletons than for multiples.

The literature suggests that multiple birth is the most significant risk factor of preterm birth and subsequent adverse neonatal outcome [5]. Preterm birth occurred in 60.8% of twins and in 94.8% of higher order multiple births compared to 6.9% of singletons [1]. The neonatal death rates of twins (10.9 per 1,000 live births) and higher order multiples (28.7 per 1,000 live births) were significantly higher than that of singletons (2.1 per 1,000 live births) [1]. Given the higher rate of multiple pregnancy following assisted reproductive technology (ART), births following ART were at increased risk of preterm birth and subsequent adverse neonatal outcomes. Previous studies also reported increased morbidity and mortality among births following ART compared to those following spontaneous conception [6, 7]. However, it is unclear whether increased risk of subsequent adverse neonatal outcomes among very preterm singletons is related to ART treatment itself or more attributable to the underlying subfertility [8]. The study using a population cohort approach aims to compare adverse neonatal outcomes among very preterm singletons born after fertility treatment including ART, hyper-ovulation (HO) and artificial insemination (AI) to those born following spontaneous conceptions. We hypothesized that very preterm singletons following fertility treatment have increased risk of morbidity and mortality.

Methods

Data

This study used data and definitions from the ANZNN data collection. The ANZNN is collected annually from all NICUs in Australia and New Zealand. Liveborn babies included in ANZNN are either born at less than 32 weeks gestation, or weighed less than 1,500 g at birth, or those who received assisted ventilation or major surgery (surgery that involved opening a body cavity). A research dataset including all liveborn singletons ($N = 24,069$) of <32 weeks gestation born between 2000 and 2010 was supplied from ANZNN for this study. Of these, 17696 (73.5%) were with birthweight < 1500 g, 9854 (40.9%) required assisted ventilation and 1946 (8.1%) had major surgery.

Main outcome measures

The primary outcomes are morbidity and mortality before NICU discharge. Outcome measures were categorised into conditions at birth and NICU complications. Conditions at birth include small for gestational age (SGA, <10th percentile for the gestation), 5 min APGAR score (less than 7 was categorised as moderate/severe depressed), extreme low birth weight (extreme LBW; <1000 g), intubation during resuscitation and presence of congenital abnormalities (defined as structural abnormalities including deformations that are present at birth and diagnosed prior to separation from care). SGA for non-ART singletons were estimated from already published birthweight for gestational age percentile charts [9, 10]. SGA for ART singletons was estimated using published birthweight percentiles by gestational age for ART births [11]. NICU complications include hyaline membrane disease, necrotizing enterocolitis (NEC), intraventricular haemorrhage, retinopathy of prematurity, major surgery and death.

Comparison group

Conditions at birth and NICU complications were compared among liveborn singletons by four modes of conceptions flagged the ANZNN database: spontaneous conception (no fertility treatment used for this pregnancy), HO (any hormone therapy used to stimulate ovulation), ART (any method of in-vitro handling oocyte or embryos including in-vitro fertilisation, gamete intra-fallopian transfer, zygote intra fallopian transfer) and AI. ANZNN data collection does not have detailed information about the ART fertilisation procedures, fresh or frozen embryos, and the number of embryo transferred and stage of embryo development (blastocyst or cleavage stage). Other study factors include maternal age, ethnicity, gestational age and maternal complications, including pregnancy inducted hypertension in pregnancy (A systolic blood pressure > 140 mmHg and/or diastolic blood pressure > 90 mmHg, or a rise in systolic blood pressure > 25 mmHg and/or a rise in diastolic blood pressure > 15 mmHg from a reading before conception or in 1st trimester; confirmed by 2 readings 6 h apart), antepartum haemorrhage (Significant haemorrhage in the time from 20 weeks gestation to the end of second stage of labour) and premature rupture of membranes (Confirmed spontaneous rupture of membranes occurring prior to the onset of labour and before 37 weeks gestation).

Statistical analysis

Demographics characteristics (maternal age, aboriginal status, gestational age, previous preterm birth and previous perinatal death) and other maternal conditions (premature rupture of membranes, pregnancy inducted hypertension, antepartum haemorrhage and antenatal steroid) were compared among mode of conception and differences in the means and proportions were tested. Analysis of variance was used for continuous variables and Chi-square test was used for categorical variables. Univariate and multivariate binary logistic regression analysis was used to examine the association between mode of conception and various outcome factors. Odds ratio (OR) and adjusted odds ratio (AOR) (adjusted for maternal age, gestational age, ethnicity, previous pre term, previous prenatal death, maternal hypertension, antepartum haemorrhage, PROM and antenatal steroid) and 95% CI were calculated. The level of significance was set at 0.05, and 95% CIs were used to minimize the risk of chance findings. Statistical Package for Social Sciences (SPSS, Inc., Chicago, IL, USA Version 21) was used for data analysis.

Results

The information on mode of conception was available for 21,753 (90.4%) singletons. Among these, 94.4% (20,530/21,753) of singletons were born following spontaneous conception, 4.4% (953/21,753) after ART, 1% (216/21,753) after HO, 0.2% (54/21,753) after AI. Figure 1 presents the distribution of gestational age by the mode of conceptions. The proportion of extreme preterm was 26.1% in AI group, compared to 30.6% in ART group, 33.7% in HO group and 32.9% in spontaneous conception group.

The average age of mother following ART (34.6 ± 4.7 years), AI (33.3 ± 4.7 years) and HO (30.2 ± 4.9 years) was significantly higher compared to those who conceived spontaneously (28.9 ± 6.3 years) ($p < 0.01$). Similarly, the mean gestational age was significantly different among four groups ($p = 0.01$) (Table 1). Compared to the spontaneously conceived singletons, mothers of ART singletons had higher proportions of pregnancy inducted hypertension and use of antenatal steroids ($p < 0.01$).

Figure 2 shows the number of singletons admitted to NICU by the mode of conceptions over the period of 10 years. NICU admissions for the singletons conceived spontaneously and after ART treatment increased by 11.7% and 48.8% respectively from 2001–10.

The rates of adverse birth outcomes were higher in HO, ART and AI singletons, compared to the spontaneous conception. In the univariate analysis, HO was associated with SGA, and extreme LBW; ART was associated with extreme LBW, intubation during resuscitation and major malformation; and AI was associated with SGA and congenital abnormalities (Table 2). Compared to very preterm singletons conceived spontaneously, the odds of SGA was about 3 times higher for those after AI (AOR 2.98, 95% CI

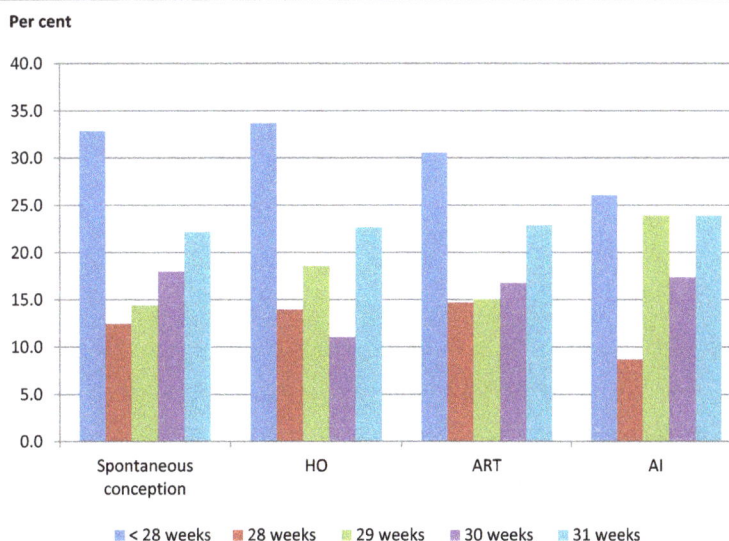

Fig. 1 Distribution of gestational age of very preterm and extreme preterm singletons by mode of conceptions

Table 1 Demographics of very preterm singletons by mode of conceptions

	Spontaneous (20,530)		HO (216)		ART (953)		AI (54)		P value[a]
	#	%	#	%	#	%	#	%	
Maternal age (years) Mean ± SD	28.87	±6.3	30.36	±4.9	34.64	±4.7	33.33	±4.7	<0.05[b]
Gestational age (weeks) Mean ± SD	28.44	±2.5	28.12	2.4±	28.25	2.3±	28.19	2.3±	0.01
Aboriginal status									
Yes	1274	6.2	4	1.9	10	1.0	0	0.0	<0.05
no	17079	83.2	186	86.1	830	87.1	52	96.3	
Not stated	2177	10.6	26	12	113	11.9	2	3.7	
Previous preterm birth									
Yes	3928	19.1	24	11.1	78	8.2	7	13.0	<0.05
No	16506	80.4	192	88.9	874	91.7	47	87.0	
Not stated	96	0.5	0	0.0	1	0.1	0	0.0	
Previous perinatal death									
Yes	1239	6.0	11	5.1	38	4.0	5	9.3	<0.05
No	19218	93.6	205	94.9	915	96.0	49	90.7	
Not stated	73	0.4	0	0.0	0	0.0	0	0.0	
Premature rupture of membranes									
Yes	5243	25.5	44	20.4	246	25.8	10	18.5	0.301
No	15256	74.3	171	79.2	704	73.9	44	81.5	
Not stated	31	0.2	1	0.5	3	0.3	0	0.0	
Pregnancy inducted hypertension									
Yes	3619	17.6	58	26.9	199	20.9	20	37.0	<0.05
No	16895	82.3	157	72.7	752	78.9	34	63.0	
Not stated	16	0.1	1	0.5	2	0.2	0	0.0	
Antepartum haemorrhage									
Yes	5028	24.5	47	21.8	262	27.5	13	24.1	0.063
No	15488	75.4	168	77.8	689	72.3	41	75.9	
Not stated	14	0.1	1	0.5	2	0.2	0	0.0	
Antenatal steroid									
None	2724	13.3	17	7.9	76	8	3.0	5.6	<0.05
Incomplete	5514	26.9	56	25.9	234	24.6	13	24.1	
Complete	9377	45.7	111	51.4	468	49.1	33	61.1	
More than 7 days	2548	12.4	31	14.4	156	16.4	5	9.3	
Not stated	367	1.8	1	0.5	19	2.0	0	0.0	
Gender of baby									
Male	11279	54.9	122	56.5	517	54.2	33	61.1	0.98
Female	9233	45.0	94	43.5	436	45.8	21	38.9	
Ambiguous	2	0.0	0	0.0	0	0.0	0	0.0	
Not stated	16	0.1	0	0.0	0	0.0	0	0.0	

[a] chi square test.
[b] Analysis of variance

1.53–5.81) and 1.5 times higher for those after HO (AOR 1.52, 95% CI 1.02–2.67). Similarly, the odds of major abnormalities was 3 times (AOR 3.01, 95% CI 1.47–6.19) higher for AI singletons and 1.7 times (AOR 1.71, 95% CI 1.36–2.16) higher for ART singletons than spontaneous singletons. Other birth outcomes were not significantly different between spontaneous conception group and the three fertility treatment groups.

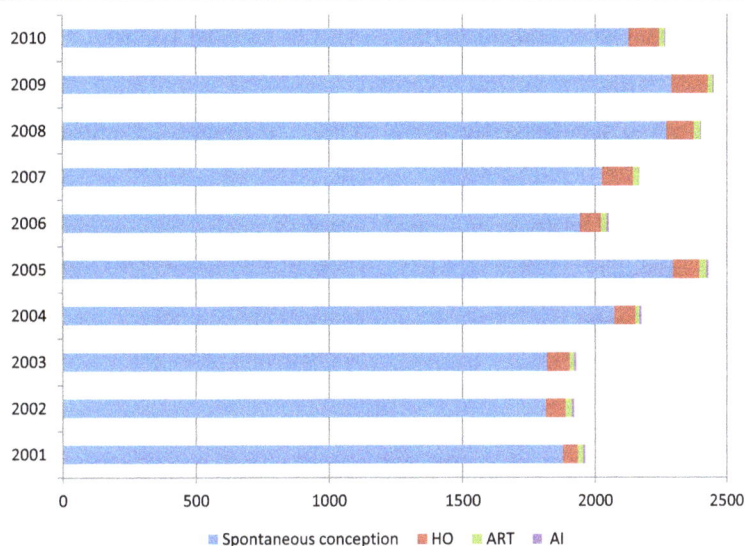

Fig. 2 Number of very preterm and extreme preterm singletons by mode of conceptions 2001–2010

Table 2 Birth conditions of very preterm singletons by mode of conceptions

	Number	Percent	OR (95% CI)	AOR (95% CI)[a]
Small for gestational age				
Spontaneous conception	1833	8.9	Ref	Ref
HO	35	16.2	**1.97 (1.37–2.84)**	**1.52 (1.02–2.67)**
ART	102	10.7	1.22 (0.99–1.51)	1.09 (0.87–1.38)
AI	16	29.6	**4.29 (2.39–7.71)**	**2.98 (1.53–5.81)**
5 min APGAR (Mod/ severe depressed)				
Spontaneous conception	3659	18.0	Ref	Ref
HO	35	16.2	0.88 (0.61–1.27)	0.78 (0.52–1.18)
ART	176	18.6	1.04 (0.88–1.23)	1.02 (0.85–1.24)
AI	10	18.5	1.04 (0.52–2.06)	1.07 (0.52–2.22)
Extreme Low birth weight (<1000 g)				
Spontaneous conception	6676	32.5	Ref	Ref
HO	88	40.7	**1.43 (1.09–1.87)**	1.13 (0.72–1.79)
ART	351	36.8	**1.21 (1.06–1.38)**	1.11 (0.88–1.40)
AI	22	40.7	1.43 (0.83–2.46)	1.01 (0.43–2.42)
Intubation during resuscitation				
Spontaneous conception	8405	41.0	Ref	Ref
HO	101	46.8	1.26 (0.97–1.65)	1.16 (0.84–1.60)
ART	440	46.3	**1.24 (1.09–1.41)**	1.11 (0.94–1.30)
AI	22	40.7	0.97 (0.57–1.70)	0.87 (0.46–1.64)
Congenital abnormalities				
Spontaneous conception	1197	6.0	Ref	Ref
HO	10	4.9	0.80 (0.42–1.51)	0.80 (0.42–1.52)
ART	93	10.1	**1.75 (1.40–2.19)**	**1.71 (1.36–2.16)**
AI	9	16.7	**3.12 (1.52–6.40)**	**3.01 (1.47–6.19)**

[a] Adjusted for maternal age, gestational age, ethnicity, previous pre term, previous prenatal death, maternal hypertension, antepartum haemorrhage, premature rupture of membranes and antenatal steroid
Significant results are in bold

The multivariate analysis shows that very preterm singletons born after ART have 43% higher odds of having NEC (AOR 1.43, 95% CI 1.04–1.97) and 71% higher odds of having major surgery (AOR 1.71, 95% CI 1.37–2.13) compared to those conceived spontaneously. Data stratification shows that major surgery was closely related to congenital abnormalities. Major surgery was reported in 33% and 11% of ART singletons with and without congenital abnormalities respectively (p value <0.05). Other NICU outcomes were not significantly different spontaneous conception group and the three fertility treatment groups (Table 3).

Discussion

This bi-national population study showed that the rates of some adverse neonatal outcomes are significantly increased among the very preterm singletons following fertility treatment. Compared to the spontaneous conception group, ART and AI groups had 1.7 times and 3.0 times increased odds of major malformation. Very preterm singletons following HO and AI had 1.5 times and 3.0 times increased odds of SGA than spontaneous conception group. ART is associated with 43% and 71% higher odds of NEC and major surgery compared to spontaneous conception group.

Table 3 NICU outcomes of very preterm singletons by mode of conceptions

	Number	Percent	OR (95% CI)	AOR (95% CI)[a]
Hyaline membrane disease				
Spontaneous conception	14574	71.9	Ref	Ref
HO	154	72.0	1.00 (0.74–1.36)	0.87 (0.62–1.21)
ART	724	76.9	**1.30 (1.11–1.52)**	1.18 (0.99–1.40)
AI	38	72.1	0.93 (0.52–1.67)	0.75 (0.41–1.42)
Necrotizing enterocolitis				
Spontaneous conception	817	4.0	Ref	Ref
HO	3	1.4	0.34 (0.11–1.04)	0.33 (0.10–1.05)
ART	49	5.2	1.30 (0.97–1.75)	**1.43 (1.04–1.97)**
AI	2	3.7	0.92 (0.22–3.80)	0.85 (0.20–3.60)
Intra ventricular haemorrhage				
Spontaneous conception	4327	23.1	Ref	Ref
HO	53	26.0	1.17 (0.85–1.60)	1.23 (0.86–1.75)
ART	229	25.6	1.14 (0.98–1.33)	1.20 (1.00–1.43)
AI	12	23.1	0.99 (0.52–1.90)	1.21 (0.61–2.40)
Retinopathy of prematurity				
Spontaneous conception	3896	26.6	Ref	Ref
HO	49	31.6	1.27 (0.91–1.79)	1.04 (0.70–1.52)
ART	187	27.2	1.03 (0.87–1.22)	1.00 (0.82–1.24)
AI and other	10	23.3	0.83 (0.41–1.70)	0.99 (0.44–2.17)
Major surgery				
Spontaneous conception	1642	8.1	Ref	Ref
HO	23	10.7	1.37 (0.89–2.11)	1.27 (0.79–2.02)
ART	122	12.9	**1.70 (1.39–2.06)**	**1.71 (1.37–2.13)**
AI	6	11.1	1.43 (0.61–2.34)	1.00 (0.389–2.60)
Deaths				
Spontaneous conception	1852	9.0	Ref	Ref
HO	20	9.3	1.02 (0.65–1.63)	0.67 (0.38–1.18)
ART	98	10.3	1.15 (0.93–1.43)	1.11 (0.86–1.42)
AI	9	16.7	2.01 (0.98–4.13)	2.10 (0.93–4.76)

[a] Adjusted for maternal age, gestational age, ethnicity, previous pre term, previous prenatal death, maternal hypertension, antepartum haemorrhage, premature rupture of membranes and antenatal steroid
Significant results are in bold

The literature shows that fertility treatments including ART, AI, HO and use of Clomiphene are associated with increased risk of adverse pregnancy and perinatal outcomes [12]. Very preterm and preterm birth are such adverse perinatal outcomes associated fertility treatment, and are leading causes of other morbidity and mortality [13, 14]. We selected very preterm singletons as our study population which reduced the confounding and interaction effects between the fertility treatment and adverse perinatal outcomes due to multiple pregnancies and prematurity. Agreed with the literature, our findings suggested that very preterm singletons following ART and other fertility treatment are at increased risk of fetal and neonatal outcomes [15–18].

A number of studies reported higher incidence of low birthweight among births following fertility treatment than spontaneous births [6, 19–22]. Since our study population was limited to very preterm singletons, the low birthweight is not a measure relevant to our study population. Instead, we used SGA to measure birthweight outcomes. Babies are SGA if their weights are below the 10th percentile for their gestational ages. Although the majority babies born SGA catch up in growth at 2 years old, SGA babies are at increased risk of morbidity and mortality [7]. Apart from genetic reasons, SGA is related to fetal, maternal and placental conditions. Subfertility, one of the maternal conditions is associated with increased risk of SGA [23]. Since all couples who access ART treatment have some level of subfertility, they are more likely to have a SGA baby [17]. Zhu and colleagues also reported a high rate of SGA in sub-fertile women regardless of ART treatment [23]. Even for very preterm singletons, those born to mothers following fertility treatment, an indicator of subfertility, have a higher rate of SGA than those following spontaneous conceptions.

Congenital anomaly is the one of the leading causes of neonatal death among the preterm babies [24]. Many studies have reported an increased rate of congenital anomalies among births following fertility treatment compared to spontaneous births [18, 25, 26], with the prevalence of congenital anomalies ranges from 4–9% among ART births according to various studies [12, 17, 27], and 4–6% in general population [28, 29]. Even though our rates are comparable with other published studies, it should be interpreted with cautions as we only included very preterm births in this study. Increase risk of congenital abnormality may be due to generally increased risk of congenital amorality in ART group or due to shift of gestational duration toward lower values among a normal rate of congenital amorality. Moreover, congenital anomalies may be on the casual pathway to low birth weight or preterm birth [30, 31].

Presence of congenital abnormalities is one of the major causes of surgery and other adverse neonatal outcomes in the neonatal period [32]. The most common reasons for major surgery in our study include vascular system (418 cases), skeletal system (151 cases), gastrointestinal (146 cases), genital tract (136 cases) and respiratory (105 cases). The higher rate of major surgery among ART singletons in our study is likely due to associated congenital abnormalities. Rates of major surgery were significantly in ART singletons with congenital abnormalities, compared to ART singletons without congenital abnormalities (p value <0.05). Similarly we need to assume that a chain of event might happen and in most cases birth conditions are related to the common NICU outcomes including NEC, intraventricular haemorrhage, hyaline membrane disease and retinopathy of prematurity among the very preterm babies [24]. Although the rates of all conditions were high in the ART group, only NEC was significantly associated with the ART in this study.

Necrotizing Enterocolitis is one of the most common severe diseases among preterm births, with high morbidity and mortality. Yee and colleagues suggested that the mortality for NEC can be up to 50% and 20–40% cases may need surgical treatment [33]. The rates of NEC in our study were 5.2% among ART and 4.0% among spontaneous conceived very preterm singletons. These are within the range between 3% and 15% reported by other studies [34]. The increase rate of NEC and very preterm ART singletons in our study remains unclean as the cause necrotizing enterocolitis is incompletely understood. Neu and Walker suggested that the cause of NEC is multifactorial, but it is preventable by withholding enteral feedings, using enteral antibiotics, feeding with expressed breast milk, and administering probiotic agents [35].

Death rates in ART treatment groups were high in our study, compared to the spontaneous conception group, however the difference was not statistically significant. In a previous NICU study in Australia, low mortality was observed in the ART twins and triplets compare to spontaneously conceived twins and triplets and authors attributed it "protective effect" to the "dichorionic pregnancies" and specialized care offered to the ART mothers [20]. Another study reported low rate of death among the babies born after the ART treatment and authors attributed it to the single embryo transfer practices and comparison of ART healthy babies with sick non ART babies [24]. However both these studies included multiple pregnancies in the analysis and there is ample of evidence suggests that ART singletons have high mortality compared to non-ART singletons [21].

Survival rates of the very preterm babies have been improved in the last few decades due to increase use of ventilator support, steroids and surfactants [36, 37]. However the outcome is still poor among the babies born after the fertility treatment. It is not clear whether this is due to complication of treatment such as congenital abnormalities or due to maternal conditions such as pregnancy induced hypertension. These babies are at risk of long term neurological and behavioural complications which are not well studied [38]. The outcome in the very preterm singletons also may be different as it is associated with the gestational age. Among the preterm babies, the mortality is generally very high among the those born at 23 weeks (84%) compared to those born at 28 week (13%) [39]. The potential risk of very preterm birth and subsequent neonatal morbidity and mortality should be explained to the women undergoing ART treatment.

There are some limitations of this study, which are important while interpreting the results. In the ANZNN database four categories are mentioned under the flag "Assisted conception": spontaneous conception, HO, ART and AI. It is possible that some HO and AI singletons were misreported into spontaneous conception group given the small number of HO and AI singletons were identified in this study. However, we are unable to track the assisted conception from other records. Similarly we are unable to track the pregnancies characterises including gestational sacs and fetal hearts. It is suggested that singletons born as a result of vanish twins/triples have increased risk of adverse perinatal outcomes those born with initial one gestational sac/fetal heart (Wang et al. 2009). This is especially relavent to HO and ART singletons where multiple gestational sacs pregnancies are prevalent [12, 14].

ART included complex procedures such as oocyte collection, ICSI procedure, cleavage stage transfer, frozen embryo transfer, and number of embryos transferred. Detailed information on types of cycle, ART procedures, and embryo transfers which may be associated with adverse maternal and fetal outcomes is not available in the database [40, 41]. For example high rate of congenital abnormalities are reported after the ICSI procedure [12] and cleavage stage transfer [42]. Perinatal outcomes are usually favourable following frozen embryo transfers than fresh embryo transfers [13, 43]. Similarly, double embryo transfer is related to multiple birth [44] and multiple births had higher chances of congenital abnormalities than the singletons [45]. Compared to the single embryo transfers, 1.5 fold increase in fetal death has been reported for births following double embryo transfers [14].

Another limitation of this study was restricting analysis to only extreme preterm and very (<32 weeks) births, which limits the study generalisation to all preterm births. ANZNN data collection includes births of gestational age < 32 weeks in Australia and New Zealand, however the evidence suggests that the rate of preterm in the developed countries are mainly increased for the moderate preterm birth (32–36 weeks gestation) [46]. As ANZNN only includes babies of birth weight <1,500 g, many LBW babies may not be admitted to NICU and were not included from the study. Comparison between babies of birth weight <1,500 g and those of birth weight 1500–2499 g is important since the later have less complications compared to very preterm babies. Another limitation of this study is that we are unable to identify women who have a history of subfertility but conceived spontaneously. These women were included in the spontaneous conception group although they were inherently different from women without history of infertility [47, 48]. Previous studies also show that maternal and childhood complications are more common in subfertile women compared to fertile women [49–51]. This indicates that some biological factors may play a role however there is limited evidence.

Our multivariate analysis was adjusted for maternal age, gestational age, ethnicity, previous pre term, previous prenatal death, maternal hypertension, antepartum haemorrhage, PROM and antenatal steroid. The residual confounding may exist as we were unable to adjust factors such as maternal smoking, BMI, location and size of NICU, method of delivery and parental social-economic status. Moreover, increase risk of congenital abnormality and other morbidities after fertility treatments in NICU setting may not be generalised to the all babies born after fertility treatment. We only examined morbidity and mortality among cases admitted to NICUs. Fetal deaths and terminations due to prenatally diagnosed congenital abnormality are not included. Finally the comparison was made between spontaneous conceived singletons and those following ART, HO and AI. We did not make comparison across fertility treatment groups due to small sample size in HO and AI groups. Further studies need be conducted by directly comparing outcomes in sub-fertile/infertile women conceived with or without fertility treatment and type of fertility treatment [52, 53].

Conclusions

Very preterm (<32 weeks gestational age) singletons following HO, ART and AI had higher rates of some neonatal morbidity than spontaneous singletons. Compared to the spontaneous conception group, risk of birth defects significantly increases after ART and AI; the risk of morbidities increases after ART, HO and AI. Preconception planning should include comprehensive information about the benefits and risks of fertility treatment on the neonatal outcomes.

Abbreviations

AI: Artificial insemination; ANZNN: Australian and New Zealand Neonatal Network; AOR: Adjusted odds ratio; ART: Assisted reproductive technology; CI: Confidence interval; HO: Hyper-ovulation; LBW: Low birth weight; NICU: Neonatal Intensive Care Unit; OR: Odds ratio; SGA: Small for gestational age

Acknowledgement

We acknowledge the Advisory Council Members of ANZNN: Ross Haslam* Chair of the Executive Committee; Flinders Medical Centre, SA: Peter Marshall. Gosford University Hospital, QLD: Peter Schmidt. Gosford District Hospital, NSW: Adam Buckmaster*. John Hunter Hospital, NSW: Paul Craven, Koert de Waal*. King Edward Memorial and Princess Margaret Hospitals, WA: Karen Simmer, Andy Gill*, Jane Pillow*. Liverpool Hospital, NSW: Jacqueline Stack. Mater Mothers' Hospital, QLD: Lucy Cooke. Mercy Hospital for Women, VIC: Dan Casalaz, Jim Holberton*. Monash Medical Centre, VIC: Charles Barfield,. Nepean Hospital, NSW: Lyn Downe Vijay Shingde. Newborn Emergency Transport Service (VIC): Michael Stewart. NSW Newborn and Pregnancy Services Network: Barbara Bajuk*. NSW Newborn & Paediatric Emergency Transport Service: Andrew Berry. Royal Children's Hospital, VIC: Rod Hunt. Royal Darwin Hospital, NT: Charles Kilburn. Royal Hobart Hospital, Tasmania: Tony De Paoli. Royal Hospital for Women, NSW: Kei Lui*. Royal North Shore Hospital, NSW: Mary Paradisis. Royal Prince Alfred Hospital, NSW: Ingrid Rieger, Shelley Reid*. Royal Brisbane and Women's Hospital, QLD: David Cartwright, Pieter Koorts. Royal Women's Hospital, VIC: Carl Kuschel, Lex Doyle. Sydney Children's Hospital, NSW: Andrew Numa. The Canberra Hospital, ACT: Hazel Carlisle. The Children's Hospital at Westmead, NSW: Nadia Badawi, Robert Halliday. The Townsville Hospital, QLD: Guan Koh*. Western Australia Neonatal Transport Service: Steven Resnick. Westmead Hospital, NSW: Melissa Luig. Women's & Children's Hospital, SA: Chad Andersen. National Perinatal Epidemiology and Statistics Unit, University of New South Wales: Georgina Chambers*. New Zealand: Christchurch Women's Hospital: Adrienne Lynn, Brian Darlow. Dunedin Hospital: Roland Broadbent*. Middlemore Hospital: Lindsay Mildenhall. Auckland City Hospital: Malcolm Battin. North Shore and Waitakere Hospitals: Jutta van den Boom*. Waikato Hospital: David Bourchier, Lee Carpenter*. Wellington Women's Hospital: Vaughan Richardson. Singapore: KK Women's and Children's Hospital, Singapore: Victor Samuel Rajadurai*.
* denotes the ANZNN Executive Committee.

Funding

There is no specific funding related to this research.

Authors' contributions

AW designed the study, prepared the data, drafted the manuscript, and approved the final manuscript as submitted. AC prepared the data, carried out the initial analyses, drafted the manuscript and approved the final manuscript as submitted. KL reviewed and revised the manuscript, and approved the final manuscript as submitted. ES conceptualised and designated the study, reviewed and revised the manuscript, and approved the final manuscript as submitted.

Competing interests

The authors declare that they have no competing interests.

Author details

[1]Faculty of Health, University of Technology Sydney, PO Box 123, Broadway, NSW 2007, Australia. [2]School of Public Health and Community Medicine, University of New South Wales, Sydney, NSW 2031, Australia. [3]School of Women's and Children's Health, University of New South Wales, Sydney, NSW 2031, Australia.

References

1. Hilder LZZ, Parker M, Jahan S, Chambers GM. 014. Australia's mothers and babies 2012. Perinatal statistics series no. 30. Cat. no. PER 69. Canberra: AIHW; 2014.
2. Blencowe H, Cousens S, Oestergaard MZ, Chou D, Moller AB, Narwal R, et al. National, regional, and worldwide estimates of preterm birth rates in the year 2010 with time trends since 1990 for selected countries: a systematic analysis and implications. Lancet. 2012;379(9832):2162–72.
3. Kramer MS, Demissie K, Yang H, Platt RW, Sauve R, Liston R. The contribution of mild and moderate preterm birth to infant mortality. Fetal and Infant Health Study Group of the Canadian Perinatal Surveillance System. JAMA. 2000;284(7):843–9.
4. Chow SSW. Report of the Australian and New Zealand Neonatal Network 2012. Sydney: ANZNN; 2014.
5. Beck S, Wojdyla D, Say L, Betran AP, Merialdi M, Requejo JH, et al. The worldwide incidence of preterm births: a systematic review of maternal mortality and morbidity. Bulletin World Health Organization. 2010;88:31–8.
6. Nyirati I, Orvos H, Bártfai G, Kovács L. Iatrogenic multiple pregnancy: Higher risk than a spontaneous one? J Reprod Med. 1997;42(11):695–8.
7. Battaglia FC, Lubchenco LO. A practical classification of newborn infants by weight and gestational age. J Pediatr. 1967;71(2):159–63.
8. Thomson F, Shanbhag S, Templeton A, Bhattacharya S. Obstetric outcome in women with subfertility. Bjog. 2005;112(5):632–7.
9. Dobbins TA, Sullivan EA, Roberts CL, Simpson JM. Australian national birthweight percentiles by sex and gestational age, 1998–2007. Med J Aust. 2012;197(5):291.
10. Roberts C, Lancaster P. National birthweight percentiles by gestational age for twins born in Australia. J Paediatr Child Health. 1999;35(3):278–82.
11. Li Z, Wang YA, Ledger W, Sullivan EA. Birthweight percentiles by gestational age for births following assisted reproductive technology in Australia and New Zealand, 2002–2010. Hum Reprod. 2014;29(8):1787–800.
12. Davies MJ, Moore VM, Willson KJ, Van Essen P, Priest K, Scott H, et al. Reproductive technologies and the risk of birth defects. N Engl J Med. 2012;366(19):1803–13.
13. Wang YA, Sullivan EA, Black D, Dean J, Bryant J, Chapman M. Preterm birth and low birth weight after assisted reproductive technology-related pregnancy in Australia between 1996 and 2000. Fertil Steril. 2005;83(6):1650–8.
14. Wang YA, Sullivan EA, Healy DL, Black DA. Perinatal outcomes after assisted reproductive technology treatment in Australia and New Zealand: single versus double embryo transfer. Med J Aust. 2009;190(5):234–7.
15. Hansen M, Bower C, Milne E, Klerk N, Kurinczuk J. Assisted reproductive technologies and birth outcomes: overview of recent systematic reviews. Reprod Fertil Dev. 2005;17(3):329–33.
16. Koivurova S, Hartikainen A-L, Gissler M, Hemminki E, Sovio U, Järvelin M-R. Neonatal outcome and congenital malformations in children born after in-vitro fertilization. Hum Reprod. 2002;17(5):1391–8.
17. Bower C, Hansen M. Assisted reproductive technologies and birth outcomes: overview of recent systematic reviews. Reprod Fertil Dev. 2005; 17(3):329–33.
18. Halliday JL, Ukoumunne OC, Baker HW, Breheny S, Jaques AM, Garrett C, et al. Increased risk of blastogenesis birth defects, arising in the first 4 weeks of pregnancy, after assisted reproductive technologies. Hum Reprod. 2010; 25(1):59–65. doi:10.1093/humrep/dep364.
19. Pandian Z, Bhattacharya S, Templeton A. Review of unexplained infertility and obstetric outcome: a 10 year review. Hum Reprod. 2001;16(12):2593–7.
20. Garg P, Abdel-Latif ME, Bolisetty S, Bajuk B, Vincent T, Lui K. Perinatal characteristics and outcome of preterm singleton, twin and triplet infants in NSW and the ACT, Australia (1994–2005). Arch Dis Child Fetal Neonatal Ed. 2010;95(1):10.
21. Helmerhorst FM, Perquin DA, Donker D, Keirse MJ. Perinatal outcome of singletons and twins after assisted conception: a systematic review of controlled studies. BMJ. 2004;328(7434):261.
22. Jackson RA, Gibson KA, Wu YW, Croughan MS. Perinatal outcomes in singletons following in vitro fertilization: a meta-analysis. Obstet Gynecol. 2004;103(3):551–63.
23. Zhu JL, Obel C, Bech BH, Olsen J, Basso O. Infertility, infertility treatment and fetal growth restriction. Obstet Gynecol. 2007;110(6):1326.
24. Feng Y, Abdel-Latif ME, Bajuk B, Lui K, Oei JL. Causes of death in infants admitted to Australian neonatal intensive care units between 1995 and 2006. Acta Paediatr. 2013;102(1):1.
25. Kallen B, Finnstrom O, Nygren KG, Olausson PO. In vitro fertilization (IVF) in

Sweden: infant outcome after different IVF fertilization methods. Fertil Steril. 2005;84(3):611–7.

26. Hansen M, Bower C, Milne E, de Klerk N, Kurinczuk JJ. Assisted reproductive technologies and the risk of birth defects–a systematic review. Hum Reprod. 2005;20(2):328–38.

27. Kallen B, Finnstrom O, Nygren KG, Olausson PO. In vitro fertilization (IVF) in Sweden: risk for congenital malformations after different IVF methods. Birth Defects Research. 2005;73(3):162–9.

28. Gibson CS vEP, Scott H, Baghurst P, Chan A, Scheil W. Annual Report of the South Australian Birth Defects Register, incorporating the 2007 Annual Report of Prenatal Diagnosis in South Australia. Adelaide: SA Birth Defects Register, Children, Youth and Women's Health Service; 2007.

29. Bower C, Rudy E, Callaghan A, Quick J, Cosgrove P. Report of the Birth Defects Registry of Western Australia 1980–2009. 2010.

30. Honein MA, Kirby RS, Meyer RE, Xing J, Skerrette NI, Yuskiv N, et al. The association between major birth defects and preterm birth. Matern Child Health J. 2009;13(2):164–75.

31. Mili F, Edmonds LD, Khoury MJ, McClearn AB. Prevalence of birth defects among low-birth-weight infants: a population study. Am J Dis Child. 1991; 145(11):1313–8.

32. Van den Berg BJ, Yerushalmy J. The relationship of the rate of intrauterine growth of infants of low birth weight to mortality, morbidity, and congenital anomalies. J Pediatr. 1966;69(4):531–45.

33. Yee WH, Soraisham AS, Shah VS, Aziz K, Yoon W, Lee SK. Incidence and timing of presentation of necrotizing enterocolitis in preterm infants. Pediatrics. 2012;129(2):e298–304.

34. Wolf EJ, Vintzileos AM, Rosenkrantz TS, Rodis JF, Lettieri L, Mallozzi A. A comparison of pre-discharge survival and morbidity in singleton and twin very low birth weight infants. Obstet Gynecol. 1992;80(3 Pt 1):436–9.

35. Neu J, Walker WA. Necrotizing enterocolitis. N Engl J Med. 2011;364(3):255–64.

36. Blickstein I, Shinwell ES, Lusky A, Reichman B. Plurality-dependent risk of respiratory distress syndrome among very-low-birth-weight infants and antepartum corticosteroid treatment. Am J Obstet Gynecol. 2005;192(2): 360–4.

37. Saigal S, Doyle LW. An overview of mortality and sequelae of preterm birth from infancy to adulthood. Lancet. 2008;371(9608):261–9.

38. Msall ME, Park JJ. The spectrum of behavioral outcomes after extreme prematurity: regulatory, attention, social, and adaptive dimensions. Semin Perinatol. 2008;32(1):42–50.

39. Synnes AR, Ling EW, Whitfield MF, Mackinnon M, Lopes L, Wong G, et al. Perinatal outcomes of a large cohort of extremely low gestational age infants (twenty-three to twenty-eight completed weeks of gestation). J Pediatr. 1994;125(6):952–60.

40. Wang JX, Norman RJ, Kristiansson P. The effect of various infertility treatments on the risk of preterm birth. Hum Reprod. 2002;17(4):945–9.

41. Shih W, Rushford DD, Bourne H, Garrett C, McBain JC, Healy DL, et al. Factors affecting low birthweight after assisted reproduction technology: difference between transfer of fresh and cryopreserved embryos suggests an adverse effect of oocyte collection. Hum Reprod. 2008;23(7):1644–53.

42. Wang YA, Kovacs G, Sullivan EA. Transfer of a selected single blastocyst optimizes the chance of a healthy term baby: a retrospective population based study in Australia 2004–2007. Hum Reprod. 2010;25(8):1996–2005.

43. Maheshwari A, Bhattacharya S. Elective frozen replacement cycles for all: ready for prime time? Hum Reprod. 2013;28(1):6–9.

44. Kjellberg AT, Carlsson P, Bergh C. Randomized single versus double embryo transfer: obstetric and paediatric outcome and a cost-effectiveness analysis. Hum Reprod. 2006;21(1):210–6.

45. Wennerholm U-B, Bergh C, Hamberger L, Lundin K, Nilsson L, Wikland M, et al. Incidence of congenital malformations in children born after ICSI. Hum Reprod. 1999;15(4):944–8.

46. Martin JA, Hamilton BE, Sutton PD, Ventura SJ, Menacker F, Munson ML. Births: final data for 2003. Natl Vital Stat Rep. 2005;54(2):1–116.

47. Lisonkova S, Janssen PA, Sheps SB, Lee SK, Dahlgren L. The effect of maternal age on adverse birth outcomes: does parity matter? J Obstet Gynaecol Can. 2010;32(6):541–8.

48. Fretts RC. Etiology and prevention of stillbirth. Am J Obstet Gynecol. 2005; 193(6):1923–35.

49. Tandberg A, Bjorge T, Nygard O, Bordahl PE, Skjaerven R. Trends in incidence and mortality for triplets in Norway 1967–2006: the influence of assisted reproductive technologies. Bjog. 2010;117(6):667–75.

50. Pelkonen S, Koivunen R, Gissler M, Nuojua-Huttunen S, Suikkari AM, Hyden-Granskog C, et al. Perinatal outcome of children born after frozen and fresh embryo transfer: the Finnish cohort study 1995–2006. Hum Reprod. 2010; 25(4):914–23.

51. Schieve LA, Cohen B, Nannini A, Ferre C, Reynolds MA, Zhang Z, et al. A population-based study of maternal and perinatal outcomes associated with assisted reproductive technology in Massachusetts. Matern Child Health J. 2007;11(6):517–25.

52. Basso O, Olsen J. Subfecundity and neonatal mortality: longitudinal study within the Danish national birth cohort. BMJ. 2005;330(7488):393–4.

53. Barnhart KT. Assisted reproductive technologies and perinatal morbidity: interrogating the association. Fertil Steril. 2013;99(2):299–302.

Congenital tuberculosis in an extremely preterm infant conceived after in vitro fertilization

Veronica Samedi[1], Stephen K. Field[2], Essa Al Awad[1], Gregory Ratcliffe[3] and Kamran Yusuf[1,4,3]*

Abstract

Background: Congenital tuberculosis is a rare manifestation of tuberculosis. The diagnosis is often delayed, especially in preterm neonates because of the non-specific clinical presentation and the lack of awareness of maternal disease prior to pregnancy.

Case Presentation: We report a case of congenital tuberculosis in an infant born at 24 weeks of gestation to a mother who presented with uncontrolled seizures during preterm labor. Maternal diagnosis was initially made by placental pathology, and later confirmed by isolation of Mycobacterium tuberculosis in urine, gastric aspirates and sputum. Full screening was performed on the newborn infant, and both mother and infant were successfully treated for tuberculosis with a four drug regimen.

Conclusion: Pregnancy can exacerbate latent tuberculosis and women originating from endemic areas are especially susceptible. The best way to prevent congenital tuberculosis is to have a high index of suspicion and identify and treat tuberculosis in pregnant women.

Keywords: Tuberculosis, Congenital, Placenta, Preterm neonate, Maternal, Case Report

Background

Despite advances in therapeutics and diagnostic techniques, tuberculosis (TB) continues to be a major infectious cause of morbidity and mortality worldwide. According to the World Health Organization, in 2015 there were 10.4 million new cases of TB worldwide of which 3.5 million were women and 1 million children [1]. TB continues to be amongst the top ten causes of death worldwide [1]. Although, over 95% of TB deaths occurs in low - and middle-income countries, the disease prevalence is increasing in developed countries due to migration from endemic areas [2]. While the burden of TB among pregnant women is equal to or greater than in the general population, many cases remain undiagnosed because of low threshold of suspicion and similarity of TB symptoms with physiological symptoms of pregnancy [3]. Even in high risk countries of Asia and Africa where severity of TB in pregnant women is confounded by HIV infection and malnutrition, screening for TB in preterm or term neonates born to mothers with confirmed or suspected TB infection remains inconsistent at best [4].

The burden of TB in children is not well established but is thought to account for 11% of all TB cases [2]. In 2014, 5% of the 1568 reported cases of TB in Canada were in children 14 years or younger with 2.9% in infants less than a year old [5]. Although data is limited, the prevalence of vertically transmitted TB from infected mothers to their off-springs can be as high as 16% [4]. Congenital TB can occur by hematogenous placental transmission of the organism from the mother to the fetus and also by ingestion of infected amniotic fluid or by direct contact with the organism during birth [6]. Although congenital TB is rare with about 350 cases reported in the literature, the numbers may be much higher as some cases could be missed as the diagnosis of congenital TB is challenging with some cases not diagnosed and others not reported [7, 8]. Initially based on

* Correspondence: kyusuf@ucalgary.ca
[1]Department of Pediatrics, Section of Neonatology, Cumming School of Medicine, University of Calgary, Calgary, AB, Canada
[4]Rm 273, Heritage Medical Research Building 3330 Hospital Drive NW, Calgary, AB T2N 4N1, Canada
Full list of author information is available at the end of the article

autopsy findings, the criteria for diagnosis of congenital TB were revised in 1994 by Cantwell. These include the presence of tuberculous lesions in the infant with at least one of the following: lesions in the first week of life, a primary hepatic complex or caseating granulomas, tuberculous infection of the placenta or endometrium and exclusion of post-natal transmission of TB by screening contacts [8–10].

Genital TB, a major cause of infertility in women from endemic countries or belonging to high-risk ethnic groups, is also a risk factor for congenital TB especially I with increasing access to assisted reproductive technology including in vitro fertilization (IVF) [11–14]. We report a case of congenital TB in a 24-week gestation infant whose mother had genital TB and who was conceived by in vitro fertilization (IVF). To the best of our knowledge, only five cases of congenital TB following IVF have been described and of the 350 reported cases, very few have reported adequate pathological evaluation of the placenta.

Case Report

A 37-year-old South Asian woman with no significant past medical history except for infertility and thalassemia minor underwent IVF for the first time. Infertility workup before IVF detected no abnormalities of the uterus or tubal lesions but endometrial biopsies were not performed. She had regular prenatal follow up, and used folic acid and prenatal vitamins. With the exception of intermittent vaginal bleeding noted since 10 weeks of pregnancy, her pregnancy was uneventful until 20 weeks of gestational age (GA) when she had spontaneous rupture of membranes. Fetal ultrasound (US) showed severe oligohydramnios. Repeat US at 23 weeks showed absence of the septum pellucidum and right talipes equino varus in the fetus. At 24 weeks GA, the mother presented with generalized seizures, went into precipitous labour delivering a male infant by spontaneous vaginal delivery with a birthweight of 590 g and APGAR scores of 4, 6, and 6 at 1, 5 and 10 min respectively.

Resuscitation of the infant in the case room included intubation, intermittent positive pressure ventilation with up to 100% oxygen and surfactant administration. High Frequency Oscillatory Ventilation (HFOV) was started in the case room due to the high oxygen requirements and absent chest movement.

The mother was admitted to the Intensive Care Unit with continuous seizure activity for a diagnostic workup. Diagnosis of TB was made by placental pathology on day three post-delivery that showed necrotizing granulomatous deciduitis and sub-chorionitis with acid-fast bacilli (AFB) apparent on Ziehl-Neelsen staining (Fig. 1a, b). The findings were suggestive of placental involvement from chronic endometrial infection rather than recently acquired or

haematogenous infection. The parents denied any family history of TB or contact with a known tuberculous patient. Anti-tuberculosus treatment was started while awaiting confirmation of the diagnosis. The diagnosis was confirmed by a positive Polymerase Chain Reaction (PCR) on placental tissue for Mycobacterium Tuberculosis and culture of the organism from sputum and urine after 15 and 17 days of incubation respectively. Her chest X ray was suggestive of military TB and CT scan of the chest confirmed the pulmonary involvement. An abdomen ultrasound was reported to be normal. Her brain magnetic resonance imaging (MRI) showed multiple small ring-enhancing cerebral and cerebellar lesions, consistent with an atypical infection such as TB (Fig. 2).

Immediately after the diagnosis of maternal TB and due to the complicated respiratory course of the infant (HFOV in case room, repeated doses of surfactant, presentation with Persistent Pulmonary Hypertension of Newborn (PPHN) within 24 h of life that required nitric oxide (iNO)), the infant was fully screened for TB.

Given the florid miliary and placental TB in the mother and the infant's critical condition, he was started empirically on anti-tuberculous treatment on day 3 of life. Mycobacterial culture of blood, cerebro-spinal fluid (CSF), endotracheal aspirates, gastric aspirates, urine and stool were, however, negative. Since confirming the diagnosis of congenital TB is difficult and the associated high mortality and morbidity, it was decided to continue anti-tuberculous treatment. The infant was started on isoniazid (10 mg/kg/d), rifampin (20 mg/kg/d), pyrazinamide (30 mg/kg/d), and ethambutol (20 mg/kg/d) for 2 months with a plan for isoniazid and rifampin for a further 4 months. His course in NICU was complicated by severe respiratory insufficiency, radiological evidence of pulmonary interstitial emphysema and early signs of chronic lung disease (CLD).

The baby remained on HFOV for 25 days and required iNO support for 29 days. A course of dexamethasone was required to facilitate extubation to Continuous Positive Airway Pressure.

At 42 weeks of corrected GA the infant's growth is appropriate, he has CLD requiring oxygen via nasal cannula and a brain MRI was reported to be normal. His eye examination and liver function tests are normal. The mother continues her anti-TB treatment and is doing well.

Discussion and conclusions

Our case report highlights the need to raise awareness about the possibility of latent genital tuberculosis in an infertile woman and initiating timely anti-tuberculous therapy in newborns. Genital TB is a common cause of infertility in women from areas where TB is prevalent [12]. However, with increasing global migration, genital TB is being

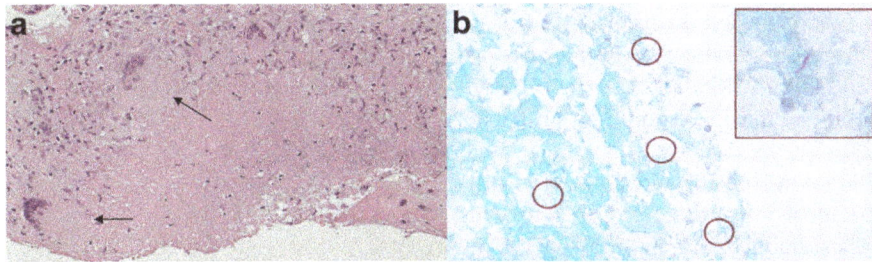

Fig. 1 a Maternal surface of the placenta showing necrotizing granulomatous deciduitis. **b** Ziehl-Neelsen stain showing acid fast bacilli

increasingly recognized in developed countries [2]. Although congenital TB due to maternal genitourinary TB is uncommon, the increasing availability of assisted reproductive technologies, especially IVF, has the potential to increase the prevalence of congenital TB [13, 15, 16]. Currently, IVF is one of the commonest treatment for infertility, and the number of babies conceived through IVF is increasing [14]. Presently, many women whose infertility was caused by genital TB choose IVF as an option to conceive [13, 16]. In developed countries, immigrants for endemic areas, such as the mother of our patient and HIV infected mothers in resource limited countries would be at high risk for TB. Screening for latent TB during pregnancy can, however, be problematic. The tuberculin skin test can be false positive in mothers who have received BCG vaccine and be false negative in mothers with HIV. Some investigators do not recommend chest X-ray in pregnancy and the

AFB smear has a low sensitivity. AFB culture is time consuming and may not be easily available everywhere. The interferon-gamma release assays (IGRA) test is recommended by some investigators as the results are not affected by BCG vaccination or HIV status [17]. Thus, a high level of clinical suspicion has to be maintained in high risk populations with a thorough assessment including a detailed clinical history at the time of prenatal visits [3, 17]. Importantly, pregnant women with TB who are treated appropriately do not have increased levels of maternal or neonatal complications [17].

The infant in our case did not meet all of Cantwell's criteria as we were unable to isolate mycobacterium tuberculosis from any of the biological samples. The diagnosis of congenital TB can, however, be challenging. Diagnostic tests for TB have extremely poor sensitivity in newborns and some investigators suggest that the

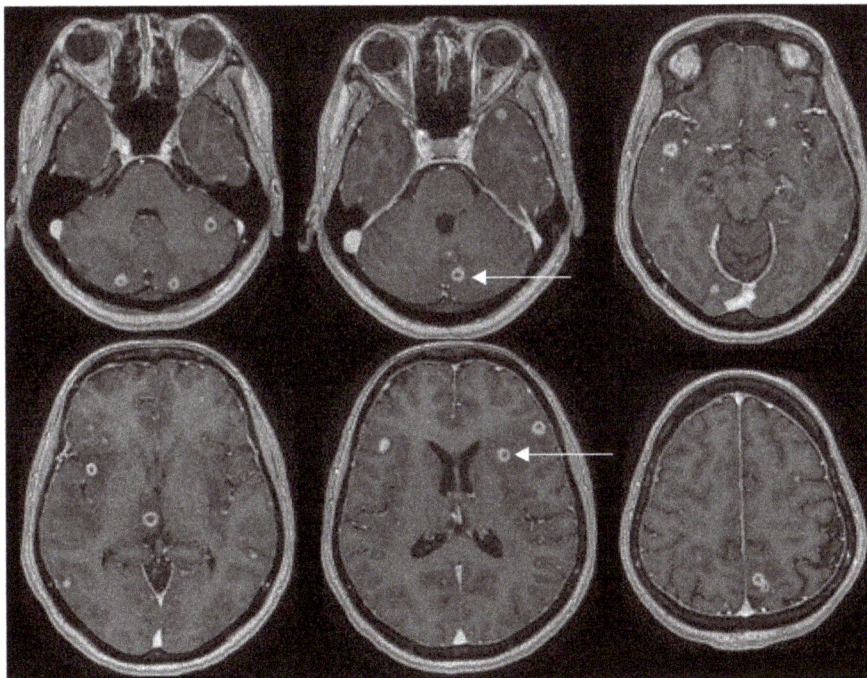

Fig. 2 Maternal MRI showing small ring-enhancing lesions in both cerebral and cerebellar hemispheres

diagnosis of congenital TB should be based on clinical criteria [9, 10]. The tuberculin test is universally negative in newborns and the IGRA is also usually negative as the T lymphocytes in newborns do not have the capacity to generate interferon-gamma in response to antigenic stimulation [7, 9, 11]. The clinical symptoms associated with congenital TB are non- specific and similar to those in viral or other bacterial infections [2, 6, 9]. Furthermore, radiological chest findings may be non-specific [2, 6, 11]. Mycobacterial smears and PCR detection can be negative in 30% of cases [7, 9]. However, a number of clinical features placed this infant at extremely high risk of having TB. The greatest risk of transmission to the fetus is miliary or bacillemic TB in the mother at the time of or just prior to delivery, like our case. Endometrial and placental granulomas were present and AFB were demonstrated in the placenta. The infant's chest x-ray also deteriorated rapidly although it was difficult to ascertain whether this was due to prematurity or TB. The neutrophil count was low (1.2×10^9/L) which has been suggested as a bad prognostic sign in congenital TB [11]. Importantly, mortality of untreated disease is 100% [9, 11]. Given these concerns, the infant was empirically treated for TB. Amongst the five cases of congenital TB following IVF reported by Flibotte, the organism could not be isolated from one infant [13]. Stuart et al. have reported a case after IVF where the organism was not detected in CSF, blood or gastric aspirate by PCR or culture but was present in a lymph node biopsy [15].

In summary, pregnancy can exacerbate latent TB infection. Women from high TB prevalence areas are especially at risk and those with genital TB may transmit the disease to the fetus. The diagnosis of congenital TB can be difficult as diagnostic tests are insensitive and the clinical signs and symptoms non-specific. The best way to prevent congenital TB is to maintain a high index of suspicion in women from high prevalence areas and to identify and treat TB in pregnancy. Multicentre trials to establish diagnostic tests including molecular tests such as PCR, with better sensitivity and specificity for TB are needed, especially in pregnancy and neonates.

Acknowledgement
We thank Dr. Kyle Kurek from the Department of Pathology and Laboratory Medicine, Cumming School of Medicine, University of Calgary, Alberta, Canada for providing the placental pathology images.

Funding
There was no funding from any source for this case report.

Author's contributions
VS: Acquired data, drafted the first version of the paper. EA-A: Drafted the paper and revised it critically for important intellectual content. SKF: Made substantial contributions to analysis, or interpretation of data and critically appraised the paper. GR: Interpreted and provided the MRI images, critically appraised the paper. KY: Substantial contributions to the conception or design of the paper, contributions to the acquisition, analysis, or interpretation of data for the paper, critically revised the paper, and finalized the manuscript. All authors approved the version to be published.

Competing interests
The authors declare no conflict of interest, financial or otherwise.

Author details
[1]Department of Pediatrics, Section of Neonatology, Cumming School of Medicine, University of Calgary, Calgary, AB, Canada. [2]Department of Medicine, Section of Respiratory Medicine, Cumming School of Medicine, University of Calgary, Calgary, AB, Canada. [3]Department of Radiology, Section of Neuroradiology, Cumming School of Medicine, University of Calgary, Calgary, AB, Canada. [4]Rm 273, Heritage Medical Research Building 3330 Hospital Drive NW, Calgary, AB T2N 4N1, Canada.

References
1. WHO. Global Tuberculosis Report. 2016. Retrieved from http://www.hoint/tb/publications/global_report/gtbr2016_executive_summarypdf?ua=1. Accessed 16 Jan 2017.
2. Perez-Velez CM, Marais BJ. Tuberculosis in children. N Engl J Med. 2012; 367(4):348–61.
3. Bates M, Ahmed Y, Kapata N, Maeurer M, Mwaba P, Zumla A. Perspectives on tuberculosis in pregnancy. Int J Infect Dis. 2015;32:124–7.
4. Pillay T, Sturm AW, Khan M, Adhikari M, Moodley J, Connolly C, Moodley D, Padayatchi N, Ramjee A, Coovadia HM, et al. Vertical transmission of mycobacterium tuberculosis in KwaZulu natal: impact of HIV-1 co-infection. Int J Tuberculosis Lung Dis. 2004;8(1):59–69.
5. Kitai I, Morris S, Kordy F, Lam R. Diagnosis and management of pediatric tuberculosis in Canada. CMAJ. 2017;9(189):E11–16.
6. Skevaki CL, Kafetzis DA. Tuberculosis in neonates and infants: epidemiology, pathogenesis, clinical manifestations, diagnosis, and management issues. Paediatr Drugs. 2005;7(4):219–34.
7. Schaaf HS, Collins A, Bekker A, Davies PD. Tuberculosis at extremes of age. Respirology. 2010;15(5):747–63.
8. Di Comite A, Esposito S, Villani A, Stronati M, Grp IPTS. How to manage neonatal tuberculosis. J Perinatol. 2016;36(2):80–5.
9. Smith KC. Congenital tuberculosis: a rare manifestation of a common infection. Curr Opin Infect Dis. 2002;15(3):269–74.
10. Cantwell MF, Shehab ZM, Costello AM, Sands L, Green WF, Ewing Jr EP, Valway SE, Onorato IM. Brief report: congenital tuberculosis. N Engl J Med. 1994;330(15):1051–4.
11. Peng WS, Yang J, Liu EM. Analysis of 170 cases of congenital TB reported in the literature between 1946 and 2009. Pediatr Pulmonol. 2011;46(12):1215–24.
12. Tripathy SN, Tripathy SN. Infertility and pregnancy outcome in female genital tuberculosis. Int J Gynaecol Obstet. 2002;76(2):159–63.
13. Flibotte JJ, Lee GE, Buser GL, Feja KN, Kreiswirth BN, McSherry GD, Nolan SM, Tolan Jr RW, Zhang H. Infertility, in vitro fertilization and congenital tuberculosis. J Perinatol. 2013;33(7):565–8.
14. CDC: Centres for Disease Control and Prevention. Reproductive Health. Assissted Reproductive Technology. National Summary and Fertility Clinic Reports. 2014. http://www.cdcgov/art/reports/. Accessed 16 Jan 2017.
15. Stuart RL, Lewis A, Ramsden CA, Doherty RR. Congenital tuberculosis after in-vitro fertilisation. Med J Aust. 2009;191(1):41–2.
16. Doudier B, Mosnier E, Rovery C, Uters M, D'Ercole C, Brouqui P. Congenital tuberculosis after in vitro fertilization. Pediatr Infect Dis J. 2008;27(3):277–8.
17. Nguyen HT, Pandolfini C, Chiodini P, Bonati M. Tuberculosis care for pregnant women: a systematic review. BMC Infect Dis. 2014;14:617.

The prevalence and risk factors of preterm small-for-gestational-age infants: a population-based retrospective cohort study in rural Chinese population

Shi Chen[1†], Rong Zhu[2,9†], Huijuan Zhu[1], Hongbo Yang[1], Fengying Gong[1], Linjie Wang[1], Yu Jiang[3], Bill Q. Lian[4], Chengsheng Yan[5], Jianqiang Li[6], Qing Wang[7], Shi-kun Zhang[8] and Hui Pan[1*]

Abstract

Background: Preterm birth and small for gestational age (SGA) are strong indicators of neonatal adverse outcomes. With the growing importance of preterm SGA infants, we aim to evaluate the prevalence and risk factors for preterm SGA in China.

Method: We analyzed the data of parents and infants from a population-based cohort research of the free National Pre-pregnancy Checkups Project (NPCP) in rural China. Only singleton live births that occurred between 24 weeks +0 days and 36 weeks +6 days of pregnancy were included in this study. SGA was defined as birth weight less than the 10th percentile of the reference birth-weight-for-gestational-age population. A multiple logistic regression model was built using the statistically significant variables from the 371 variables in the questionnaire.

Results: A total of 11,474 singleton, preterm, live-birth infants were included. Of the total infants, 317 (2.77%) were preterm SGA infants. A higher risk of preterm SGA infants was observed among mothers who were on oral contraceptives (OR: 8.162, 95% CI: 1.622–41.072), mothers who had syphilis (OR: 12.800, 95% CI: 1.250–131.041), and mothers with a high eosinophil percentage (OR: 13.292, 95% CI: 1.282–135.796). Maternal intake of folic acid at least 3 months before pregnancy (OR: 0.284, 95% CI:0.124–0.654) and paternal intake of egg and meat (OR: 0.097,95% CI:0.030–0.315) were protective factors. Compared with North China, the incidence of preterm SGA infants was higher in South China.

Conclusion: Preterm SGA infants were associated with both maternal and paternal factors.

Keywords: Preterm delivery, Small for gestational age, Folic acid supplementation, Oral contraceptive

Background

Gestational age and birth weight are two of the most important factors for evaluating the prognosis of infants. Small for gestational age (SGA) infants may show a decrease in their growth due to intrauterine growth restriction. Limitations in fetal growth affect the development of the cardiovascular system or other organs, which can have life-long effects on an individual [1]. Preterm birth is a significant causative factor of infant and child morbidity and mortality. Preterm birth complications are estimated to be the second most common cause of death in children under 5 years old [2]. In addition to its contribution to mortality, preterm birth has lifelong effects, and increased risk of neurodevelopmental disorders and chronic diseases in adulthood [3]. There is a growing consensus on the differentiation of preterm SGA from term SGA infants from both the clinical and research perspectives [4]. In particular, preterm SGA infants have

* Correspondence: panhui20111111@163.com

†Equal contributors

[1]Department of Endocrinology, Key Laboratory of Endocrinology of Ministry of Health, Chinese Academy of Medical Sciences & Peking Union Medical College, Peking Union Medical College Hospital, No.1, Shuaifuyuan Road, Beijing, Dongcheng district 100730, China

Full list of author information is available at the end of the article

a 10–40 times greater risk of dying in the first month of life than term appropriate for gestational age (AGA) infants [5]. Further, preterm SGA infants have a relatively low body fat percentage and would experience a postnatal catchup growth. Many epidemiological studies have demonstrated that the catch-up growth is associated with cardiovascular diseases, obesity, hypertension, type-2 diabetes, and metabolic syndrome in later life [6]. Few studies have evaluated the risk factors of preterm SGA infants [7, 8]. The purpose of present study is to identify the risk factors of preterm small-for-gestational age infants. The knowledge gained from this study will be crucial in prevention and treatment of preterm SGA.

Methods
Subjects
A population-based retrospective cohort study was performed on 248,501 couples and their children who were part of the free National Pre-pregnancy Checkups Project (NPCP) in 220 pilot counties in 30 provinces in China between January 2010 and December 2012. The project was implemented by the Chinese National Health and Family Planning Commission and Ministry of Finance with aim of preventing birth defects in China, it is the largest pregnancy retrospective cohort study of the preconception stage in China. It covered all volunteer couples who planned to conceive within the next 6 months. The clinical data were collected during the preconception medical examination. Information on socioeconomic background, reproductive history and history of illness, lifestyle, and dietary habits was carefully collected through face-to-face

interviews by qualified nurses. Physical examinations and biochemical studies were also carried out by medical staff at the same time [9].

SGA was defined by a 1995 WHO expert committee as infants with body weight below the 10th percentile of a birth-weight-for-gestational-age, using the gender-specific reference population with the local growth standards of Li Zhu et al. [10] Zhu's neonatal growth standards were derived from birth weight data obtained from a nationwide neonatology network of 161,420 live births in China from 2011 to 2014. Preterm SGA infants in our study were defined as infants born small for gestational age between 24 weeks + 0 days and 36 weeks +6 days of gestation.

The inclusion and exclusion criteria are shown in Fig. 1. A couple and their children was considered as a single subject. We included a total of 11,474 subjects.

Design and setting
Data collection
A structured questionnaire was constructed by well-trained investigators; the questionnaire included 371 variables from the National Free Preconception Health Examination Project [9, 11]. As the adverse effect of preterm large-for-gestational age (LGA) infants is controversial [12, 13], we compared preterm SGA infants with preterm non-SGA infants including the preterm AGA and LGA infants. We divided China into North and South region by the Qinling Mountain-Huaihe River Line and we compared the prevalence of preterm SGA infants in both regions. We also assessed the risk factors of preterm SGA infants.

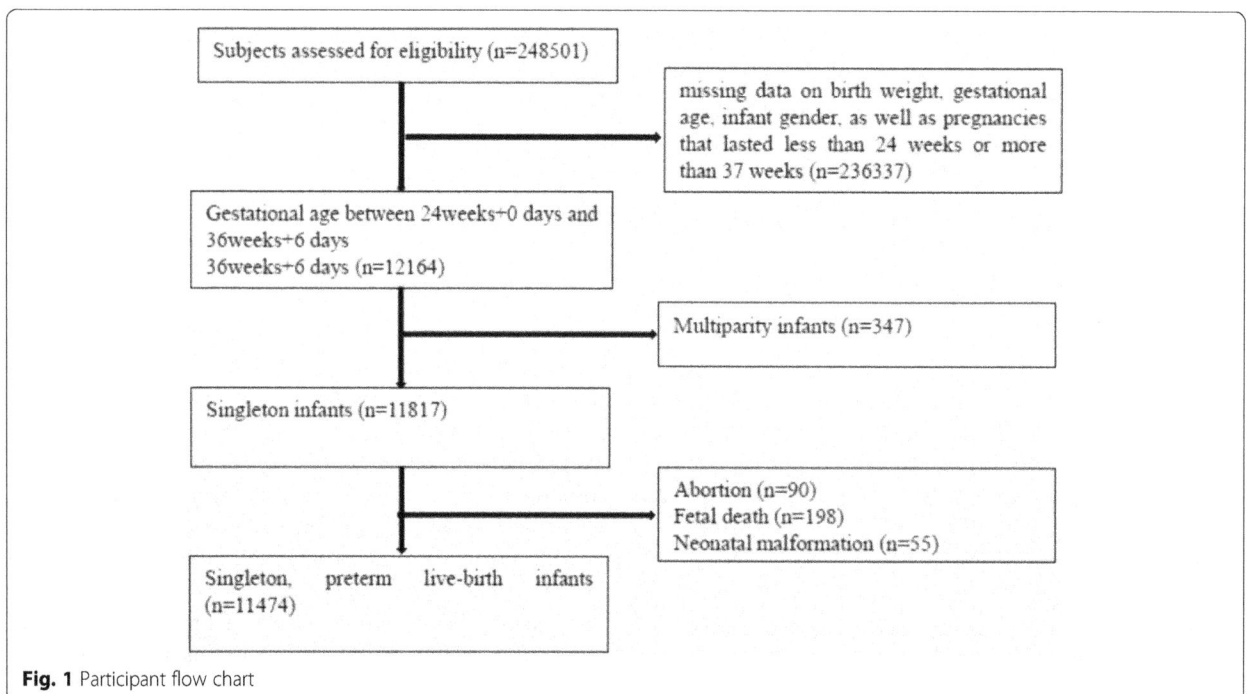

Fig. 1 Participant flow chart

Selection of risk factors

The questionnaire involves 19 aspects including baseline characters of couples, physical examination, laboratory examination family history of couples etc. We chose the variables with a high data integrity over 80%. Among these variables, 38 variables were statistically significant exposures in univariate analysis including education level of the parents, maternal preconception intake of narcotics and paternal second-hand smoking, maternal intake of eggs and meat, the beginning time of maternal intake of folic acid, paternal intake of eggs and meat and paternal intake of vegetables, tense maternal and paternal relationship with relatives and co-workers, paternal exposure to heavy metals, organic solutes and vibrations, maternal syphilis and Candida infection, maternal drug use, pet exposure and influenza virus infection during pregnancy, maternal medical history of diabetes mellitus (DM), maternal medical history of hepatitis B, maternal oral contraceptive use, maternal family history of neonatal death, paternal hepatitis B vaccination and paternal family history of DM, maternal height (meter), maternal weight (kilogram), maternal BMI (kg/m2), maternal red blood cell count (109/L), maternal eosinophil percentage, maternal blood glucose level (mmol/L) and paternal height. It also included the presence of maternal HBe antibodies, maternal rubella virus IgG antibodies, maternal CMV IgG antibodies, maternal toxoplasma IgG antibodies, paternal HBs antibodies. The folic acid supplementation, the preconception habits and socio-economic status of the parents were based on self-report. The location was classified as North or South region of China by the Qinling Mountain-Huaihe River Line.

Statistical analysis

All risk factor variables were first examined by univariate analysis to assess the importance of each of them on preterm SGA. We used chi-square test for analysis of categorical variables, and the Mann-Whitney U test for analysis of continuous variables with a skewed distribution as all of continuous variables were of skewed distribution in this cohorts examined by Kolmogorov-Smirnov test. The continuous skewed variables were expressed in the form of mid-values (25th percentile, 75th percentile). When a variable was found to be significant at the 0.1 level, it was entered into the multivariate model. Stepwise logistic regression was used to examine the correlation between risk factors and preterm SGA. In logistic regression, $p < 0.05$ was considered statistical significance. The results were presented using the OR and 95% CI values. The analyses were performed with SPSS (version 19.0; SPSS Inc., Chicago, IL, USA).

Results

Baseline characteristics of SGA and non-SGA

A total of 248,501 infants were recruited in our database, of which 12,164 were preterm infants (5.63%). The preterm neonatal mortality was 1.69% in our study. The mean weight of 11,474 preterm singleton live-birth infants was 3104.87 ± 636.03 g, 6307 infants of them were male (54.97%). Among them, 317 (2.77%) were preterm singleton live-birth SGA infants. The mean weight of them was 1778.26 ± 438.58 g, 189 of them were male (59.62%). 11,157 of them were preterm singleton live-birth non-SGA infants, the mean weight was 3141.73 ± 595.51 g, 6118 of them were male (54.84%).

Univariate analysis

The following tables show the risk factors in preterm SGA deliveries. Table 1 indicates that maternal intake of narcotics lead to a higher risk of preterm SGA. Nutrition status is also described in Table 1. Parents who did not consume enough vegetables, eggs or meat were more likely to deliver preterm SGA infants, which reflects the paternal level of essential vitamin and proteins. Starting time of maternal folic acid supplement is described in Table 1. Mothers who used folic acid at least 3 months before last menstrual period (LMP) had a lower risk of giving birth to preterm SGA infants. We also noticed that a total of 3701 women (32.6%) in our study did not take folic acid before or after their pregnancy, even though it is routinely recommended by their health care providers.

Paternal exposure to heavy metals, organic solutes and vibrations were associated with a higher incidence of preterm SGA. Parental infections were also identified as important risk factors. Syphilis, Candida infection, rubella virus infection, CMV infection, toxoplasma infection were associated with higher rate of preterm SGA. Hepatitis B is common in China. Positive maternal HBe antibodies is associated with higher prevalence of preterm SGA. Moreover, maternal family history of hepatitis B was associated with higher rate in preterm SGA infants while paternal hepatitis B vaccination was associated with lower rate in preterm SGA infants.

Mothers who were taking medications, came into contact with pets or had influenza virus infection were more likely to have preterm SGA infants. With regard to the medical history of the parents, maternal family history of neonatal death were associated with a higher rate of preterm SGA.

The Qinling Mountain-Huaihe River Line is an important demarcation line of climate, hydrology, and topography in China [14]. The North China has a lower rate of preterm SGA rate (1.61% vs. 3.32%). The mean birth weight of preterm live-birth was 3188.58 ± 650.67 g in North China and 3061.78 ± 636.03 g in South China.

Table 1 The univariate analysis of risk factors of preterm SGA infants (categorical variables)

Risk factors	Number of SGA	Number of Non-SGA	P value
Maternal Education years			
0	2	27	0.000
0–6	19	444	
6–9	181	7743	
9–12	71	1713	
12–16	38	966	
> 16	1	6	
Paternal Education years			
0	1	13	0.008
0–6	13	337	
6–9	189	7464	
9–12	70	1922	
12–16	33	1066	
> 16	0	10	
Maternal intake of narcotics			
Yes	4	29	0.012
No	208	10,782	
Paternal second-hand smoking			
Regular	13	358	0.091
Occasional	90	3732	
No	191	6089	
Maternal intake of eggs and meat			
No	9	155	0.045
Yes	292	10,675	
Maternal intake of vegetable			
No	10	94	0.000
Yes	290	10,737	
Maternal intake of folic acid from at least 3 months before LMP			
Yes	73	3448	0.003
No	241	7584	
Paternal intake of eggs or meat			
No	8	125	0.003
Yes	286	10,073	
Paternal intake of vegetables			
No	5	81	0.094
Yes	289	10,104	
Maternal tense relationship with relatives and co-workers			
No	272	10,098	0.000
Low	29	597	
Moderate	0	143	
High	2	3	

Table 1 The univariate analysis of risk factors of preterm SGA infants (categorical variables) *(Continued)*

Paternal tense relationship with relatives and co-workers			
No	261	9403	0.075
Low	2	627	
Moderate	4	162	
High	0	5	
Paternal exposure to heavy metals			
Yes	4	28	0.011
No	313	11,489	
Paternal exposure to organic solutes			
Yes	5	528	0.006
No	312	10,989	
Paternal exposure to vibrations			
Yes	4	54	0.076
No	313	11,463	
Maternal syphilis infection			
Yes	4	29	
No	293	10,656	
Maternal Candida infection			
Yes	2	80	0.003
No	269	10,138	
Maternal HBe antibodies			
Positive	31	770	0.024
Negative	255	9855	
Maternal rubella virus IgG antibodies			
Positive	136	4114	0.022
Negative	153	6355	
Maternal CMV IgG antibodies			
Positive	79	2312	0.068
Negative	204	8022	
Maternal toxoplasma IgG antibodies			
Positive	9	148	0.052
Negative	273	10,190	
Paternal HBs antibodies			
Positive	83	2555	0.077
Negative	198	7413	
Maternal medication us after LMP			
Yes	20	274	0.000
No	294	10,758	
Maternal pet exposure after LMP			
Yes	11	171	0.018
No	305	10,942	

Table 1 The univariate analysis of risk factors of preterm SGA infants (categorical variables) *(Continued)*

Maternal influenza virus infection after LMP			
Yes	9	92	0.002
No	305	11,021	
Maternal medical history of hepatitis B			
Yes	4	51	0.076
No	299	10,811	
Maternal oral contraceptive use			
Yes	4	56	
No	300	10,732	
Maternal family history of neonatal death			
Yes	2	4	0.010
No	300	10,846	
Paternal hepatitis B vaccination			
Yes	66	2980.017	
No	230	7273	
Paternal family history of DM			
Yes	4	47	0.055
No	292	10,716	
Location			
North	60	3671	0.000
South	257	7486	

As expected, the parental weight, height and BMI were associated with preterm SGA as shown in Table 2. The median values were used for risk factors that showed skewed distribution. The maternal weight, height, BMI and paternal height were significantly lower and the maternal eosinophil ratio was higher in preterm SGA group.

Multivariable analysis
Table 3 shows the results of multiple logistic regression of preterm SGA. Higher risks of preterm SGA infants were observed among women who took oral contraceptives (OR: 8.162, 95% CI: 1.622–41.072), women

with higher eosinophil percentage (OR: 1.067, 95% CI: 1.010–1.127) and women with syphilis infection (OR: 13.292, 95% CI: 1.282–135.796). Frequent intake of meat and egg of father (OR: 0.097, 95% CI: 0.030–0.315) was found to be a protective factor for infants. Comparing with women who did not use folic acid or started using folic acid after 3 months before LMP, intake of folic acid from 3 months before LMP (OR: 0.284, 95% CI:0.124–0.654) was also a protective factor for preterm SGA infants. It is well accepted that maternal BMI before LMP is related to the rate of preterm and SGA. So we put the maternal BMI before LMP (OR: 0.945, 95% CI: 0.828–1.709) in the regression model although it was not statistically significant. Moreover, the confidence intervals are wide for some of the factors in the logistic model may due to the small sample size of preterm SGA.

Discussion
Birth weight and gestational age are considered as strong predictors of short-term and long-term prognosis of infants. Given the growing attention paid to preterm SGA infants, our study attempted to determine the incidence of the preterm SGA infants and the risk factors associated with delivering preterm SGA infants.

A major strength of this study is its large sample size and the large number of variables analyzed. To the best of our knowledge, this is the most extensive multi-center study in China to evaluate the risk factors associated with preterm SGA infants. The large number of variables allows us to analyze more risk factors than previous studies on preterm SGA infants. The effect of paternal factors on preterm SGA infants, for example, the maternal eosinophil percentage has rarely been reported before.

This database has several unique features. Compared with earlier study, the mortality rate of preterm infants in our study (5.63%) was lower than the average rate reported for eastern Asia (7.2% (5.4–9.0)) [15]. With economic growth and improvements in perinatal care, the neonatal mortality rate has decreased by 59.3% from 2000 to 2010 in China [16], which could be due to lower rate of preterm SGA. With regard to the low prevalence

Table 2 The univariate analysis of risk factors of preterm SGA infants (continuous variables)

Risk factors	SGA Median(quartile)	Non-SGA Median(quartile)	P value
Maternal age	24.00 (22.00–27.00)	24.00 (22.00–27.50)	0.571
Maternal height (meter)	159.00 (156.00–161.00)	160.00 (156.00–162.00)	0.081
Maternal weight (kilogram)	52.00 (48.00–56.00)	52.00 (49.00–57.00)	0.027
Maternal BMI before LMP (kg/m2)	20.32 (18.89–22.31)	20.70 (19.38–22.38)	0.063
Maternal red blood cell count (10^9/L)	4.22 (3.90–4.51)	4.13 (3.80–4.48)	0.005
Maternal eosinophil percentage	2.00 (0.73–3.48)	1.10 (0.10–2.50)	0.017
Maternal blood glucose level (mmol/L)	4.90 (4.39–5.50)	4.82 (4.30–5.30)	0.018
Paternal height (meter)	170.00 (168.00–173.25)	171.00 (169.00–175.00)	0.031

Table 3 Multiple logistic regression of preterm SGA infants

Risk factors	B	P value	OR	95% C.I. for OR	
				Lower	Upper
Maternal intake of folic acid from at least 3 months before LMP	−1.257	0.003	0.284	0.124	0.654
Maternal oral Contraceptive use	2.100	0.011	8.162	1.622	41.072
Maternal eosinophil percentage	0.064	0.021	1.067	1.010	1.127
Maternal syphilis infection	2.580	0.030	13.191	1.281	135.796
Paternal intake of egg and meat	−2.336	0.000	0.097	0.030	0.315
Maternal BMI before LMP	−0.056	0.403	0.945	0.828	1.709
Constant	1.357	0.401	3.886		

of preterm SGA infants in the North China, it could be explained by the significant difference in body weight and height between the Northern and Southern Han Chinese. It also fit the Bergmann's rule as body mass increases with colder climate [17, 18]. The greater weight and height of parents in the North could explain the lower incidence of preterm SGA in North China.

In our study, we discovered a gender-based difference in the incidence of preterm SGA infants in China; 59.62% of preterm SGA infants were male. It has been reported that boys are more likely to be born before term in a different of populations [19]. A possible explanation is that in preterm infants, the growth-promoting effect of androgen is not obvious. Moreover, the male preterm infants were more likely to meet the preterm SGA criteria, as the weight standard for males is higher than that for females.

Folic acid

Insufficient periconceptional folic acid intake is associated with a number of birth defects that may also be related to genetic and environmental factors before conception or during early pregnancy [20]. Recent study has shown that supplementation of folic acid could protect against preterm birth. This study also suggests that the duration of folic acid supplementation may be as important as the dose. The risk of spontaneous preterm birth was inversely related to the duration of folic acid supplementation, and was lowest in women who reported using folic acid supplementation for more than a year prior to conception [21]. However, it is controversial whether folic acid supplementation influence the incidence of low birth weight or SGA [21–23]. In our study, taking folic acid supplementation more than 3 months before LMP was associated with a significant reduction in incidence of preterm SGA. As mentioned before, 32.6% of the women in this study did not take

folic acid before or during pregnancy, even it is routinely recommended. Considering the large percentage of subjects were from rural areas with relatively poor nutrition status, we think that health care providers in these areas, in particular, should emphasize on folic acid supplementation before pregnancy.

Oral contraceptive

Oral contraceptives use is one of the most popular reversible methods of contraception. However, the adverse effects of oral contraceptives on fetal development are unclear. Previous studies have reported the association of oral contraceptive use and preterm birth and low birth weight [24, 25]. It should be noted that oral contraceptive use is rare in China compared to developed countries; only 1.31% of women who delivered preterm SGA infants and 0.47% of women who delivered preterm non-SGA infants used oral contraceptives. In contrast, it was reported that oral contraceptive account for 79% of all contraception in America for the same period [26]. Nonetheless, we observed that the use of oral contraceptives was associated with preterm SGA infants. A possible explanation is that increased levels of estrogen at the time of blastocyst implantation may contribute to an increased risk of preterm birth, which has been shown in women undergoing fresh embryo-based transfer for in vitro fertilization [27, 28]. It is undeniable that oral contraceptives have many advantages in birth control and regulating the menstrual cycle, but physicians should be aware of its potential side effects of delivering preterm SGA infants.

Maternal eosinophil percentage

Eosinophils have been shown to be a significant cellular infiltrate of the placenta and uterus, including the infiltration and degranulation of eosinophils in the cervix of pregnant humans [29]. The roles of eosinophils in preterm delivery or SGA remains unknown. Elevation of the eosinophil level is associated with chronic inflammation or enhanced immune reactions, which may associate with preterm SGA infants. As the eosinophil percentage is not routinely determined in pregnancy, further research needs to be conducted to explore the relationship between the eosinophil percentage and pregnancy.

Infection of syphilis

Despite being easily detectable and treatable during pregnancy, syphilis remains an important cause of adverse pregnancy outcomes [30]. Syphilis in pregnancy may lead to severely adverse pregnancy outcome such as abortion, prematurity, neonatal death and congenital syphilis in the newborn [31]. In China, the incidence of congenital syphilis has increased at an alarming rate of 71.9% per year from 0.01 to 19.68 cases per 100,000 live births from 1997 to 2005 [32]. A study released in 2013 indicated that total incidence of maternal syphilis in China was estimated as 0.30% (95% CI: 0.28–0.32) [32]. In our study, the incidence of maternal syphilis was 1.35% in women who delivered preterm SGA infants, which was much higher than the incidence in women who delivered preterm non-SGA infants (0.271%). Unless testing and treatment of syphilis during pregnancy are made universally available, over half of the pregnancies in women with syphilis will have adverse outcome [33]. Primary prevention and prenatal care are needed to be addressed to reduce the incidence of syphilis associated preterm SGA infants.

Nutrition status of father

Our study showed that diet containing egg and meat of the father, which reflected the paternal nutritional status, particularly protein intake, was significantly associated with lower incidence of preterm SGA infants. Animal studies have demonstrated that all stages of gamete maturation and preimplantation embryo development are influenced directly by parental nutrition and hormonal status [34]. Moreover, an animal model showed that the diet during the preconception period and pregnancy of the males and females differentially affects embryonic growth and fatty acid content [35]. Also, there is an animal study showed that paternal nutrition can influence the amount of seminiferous tissue, spermatogenic capacity and spermatogenic efficiency [36]. However, our understanding of the influence of paternal nutritional status on human offspring is still limited.

Limitation

The primary limitation of our study is that several risk factors such as the beginning time of maternal folic acid intake, the paternal intake of egg and meat, and the use of oral contraceptive were based on self-report of the parents. More quantitative variables are needed in our questionnaire. With the large number of subjects, it is difficult to assure the completeness of data. This study identified several factors that are associated with preterm SGA, due to diverse culture and social economic status of these subjects, some confounding factors might be overlooked.

Conclusion

Our results show that preterm SGA infants were associated with both maternal and paternal factors. Maternal use of oral contraceptives, maternal syphilis infection, maternal higher eosinophil percentage, maternal folic acid intake less than 3 months before pregnancy and paternal low protein diet were associated with preterm SGA.

Abbreviations
AGA: Appropriate for gestational age; DM: Diabetes mellitus; LGA: Large for gestational age; LMP: Last menstrual period; SGA: Small for gestational age

Acknowledgments
We thank all the participants in this research and all the medical staffs in the 220 counties for their hard work in NFPC. We also gratefully thank the valuable support of Xu Ma (National Research Institute for Family Planning, No. 12, Dahuisi Road, Haidian District, Beijing 100081, China), QiaoMei WANG, HaiPing SHEN and YiPING ZHANG (National health and family planning commission of the people's republic of China).

Funding
This study was supported by the "Five-twelfth" National Science and Technology Support Program (No.2012BAI41B08, No.2013BAI12B01) and the National Natural Science Foundation (No.41401469), People's Republic of China.

Authors' contributions
SC data analysis and drafting of manuscript. RZ data analysis and drafting of manuscript. HZ paper review and analysis of data. HY acquisition and interpretation of data and paper review. FG study design and drafting of manuscript. LW technical support, acquisition of data and paper review. YJ acquisition and interpretation of data and drafting of manuscript. BQL data analysis and paper review. CY acquisition and interpretation of data and drafting of manuscript. JL acquisition of data, technical support and paper review. QW acquisition of data, technical support and paper review. SZ study design and paper review. HP paper review and study supervision. All authors read and approved the final manuscript.

Competing interests
The authors declare that they have no competing interests.

Author details
[1]Department of Endocrinology, Key Laboratory of Endocrinology of Ministry of Health, Chinese Academy of Medical Sciences & Peking Union Medical College, Peking Union Medical College Hospital, No.1, Shuaifuyuan Road, Beijing, Dongcheng district 100730, China. [2]Intern of medicine, PUMCH, Beijing 100730, China. [3]School of public health, PUMC, Beijing 100730, China. [4]University of Massachusetts Medical Center, 55 Lake Ave., North Worcester, MA 01655, USA. [5]Hebei Center for women and children's health, Shijiazhuang 050031, China. [6]School of Software Engineering, Beijing University of Technology, Beijing 100124, China. [7]Tsinghua National Laboratory for Info. Science and Technology, Tsinghua University, Beijing 100084, China. [8]Research association for women and children's health, Beijing 100081, China. [9]Department of Gynaecology and Obsterics, Peking University First Hospital, Beijing 100034, China.

References
1. Sochet AA, Ayers M, Quezada E, et al. The importance of small for gestational age in the risk assessment of infants with critical congenital heart disease. Cardiol Young. 2013;23:896–904.
2. Liu L, Johnson HL, Cousens S, Perin J, et al. Global, regional, and national causes of child mortality: an updated systematic analysis for 2010 with time trends since 2000. Lancet. 2012;379:2151–61.

3. Mwaniki MK, Atieno M, Lawn JE, Newton CR. Long-term neurodevelopmental outcomes after intrauterine and neonatal insults: a systematic review. Lancet. 2012;379:445–52.

4. Crispi F, Llurba E, Dominguez C, Martin-Gallan P, Cabero L, Gratacos E. Predictive value of angiogenic factors and uterine artery Doppler for early-versus late-onset pre-eclampsia and intrauterine growth restriction. Ultrasound Obstet Gynecol. 2008;31:303–9.

5. Katz J, Lee ACC, Kozuki N, et al. Mortality risk in preterm and small-for-gestational-age infants in low-income and middle-income countries: a pooled country analysis. Lancet. 2013;382:417–25.

6. Okada T, Takahashi S, Nagano N, Yoshikawa K, Usukura Y, Hosono S. Early postnatal alteration of body composition in preterm and small-for-gestational-age infants: implications of catch-up fat. Pediatr Res. 2015;77:136–42.

7. Ota E, Ganchimeg T, Morisaki N, et al. Risk factors and adverse Perinatal outcomes among term and preterm infants born small-for-gestational-age: secondary analyses of the WHO multi-country survey on maternal and newborn health. PLoS One. 2014;9:e105155.

8. Zeitlin JA, Ancel PY, Saurel-Cubizolles MJ, Papiernik E. Are risk factors the same for small for gestational age versus other preterm births? Am J Obstet Gynecol. 2001;185:208–15.

9. Wang Y, Cao Z, Peng Z, et al. Folic acid supplementation, preconception body mass index, and preterm delivery: findings from the preconception cohort data in a Chinese rural population. BMC Pregnancy Childbirth. 2015;15:336.

10. Zhu L, Zhu R, Zhang S, et al. Chinese neonatal birth weight curve for different gestational age. Chin J Pediatr. 2015;53:97–103.

11. Liu J, Zhang S, Wang Q, et al. Seroepidemiology of hepatitis B virus infection in 2 million men aged 21–49 years in rural China: a population-based, cross-sectional study. Lancet Infect Dis. 2016;16:80–6.

12. Mardones F, Marshall G, Viviani P, et al. Estimation of individual neonatal survival using birthweight and gestational age: a way to improve neonatal care. J Health Popul Nutr. 2008;26:54–63.

13. Wennerstrom EC, Simonsen J, Melbye M. Long-term survival of individuals born small and large for gestational age. PLoS One. 2015;10:e0138594.

14. Fang J, Song Y, Liu H, Piao S. Vegetation-climate relationship and its application in the division of vegetation zone in China. Acta Bot Sin. 2002; 44:1105–22.

15. Blencowe H, Cousens S, Oestergaard MZ, et al. National, regional, and worldwide estimates of preterm birth rates in the year 2010 with time trends since 1990 for selected countries: a systematic analysis and implications. Lancet. 2012;379:2162–72.

16. Feng J, Yuan X, Zhu J, et al. Under-5-mortality rate and causes of death in China, 2000 to 2010. Chin J Epidemiol. 2012;33:558–61.

17. Ma L, Cao Y, Xu J, He J. The relationship between the stature and the geo-environmental factors of 102 populations in China. Acta Anthropologica Sinica. 2008;27:223–31.

18. Li Y, Zheng L, Xi H, et al. Body weight difference in Han Chinese populations. Acta Anatomica Sinica. 2015;46:270–4.

19. Zeitlin J, Saurel-Cubizolles MJ, De Mouzon J, Rivera L, et al. Fetal sex and preterm birth: are males at greater risk? Hum Reprod. 2002;17:2762–8.

20. De-Regil LM, Fernandez-Gaxiola AC, Dowswell T, Pena-Rosas JP. Effects and safety of periconceptional folate supplementation for preventing birth defects. Cochrane Database Syst Rev. 2010;6:CD007950.

21. Bukowski R, Malone FD, Porter FT, et al. Preconceptional folate supplementation and the risk of spontaneous preterm birth: a cohort study. PLoS Med. 2009;6:e1000061.

22. Kim MW, Ahn KH, Ryu KJ, et al. Preventive effects of folic acid supplementation on adverse maternal and fetal outcomes. PLoS One. 2014;9:e97273.

23. Central Technical Co-ordinating Unit ITC-oUI. Multicentric study of efficacy of periconceptional folic acid containing vitamin supplementation in prevention of open neural tube defects from India. Indian J Med Res. 2000; 112:206–11.

24. Jensen ET, Daniels JL, Sturmer T, et al. Hormonal contraceptive use before and after conception in relation to preterm birth and small for gestational age: an observational cohort study. BJOG. 2015;122:1349–61.

25. Chen XK, Wen SW, Sun LM, Yang Q, Walker MC, Krewski D. Recent oral contraceptive use and adverse birth outcomes. Eur J Obstet Gynecol Reprod Biol. 2009;144:40–3.

26. Mucci LA, Lagiou P, Hsieh CC, et al. A prospective study of pregravid oral contraceptive use in relation to fetal growth. BJOG. 2004;111:989–95.

27. Pelkonen S, Koivunen R, Gissler M, Nuojua-Huttunen S, et al. Perinatal outcome of children born after frozen and fresh embryo transfer: the Finnish cohort study 1995-2006. Hum Reprod. 2010;25:914–23.

28. Marino JL, Moore VM, Willson KJ, et al. Perinatal outcomes by mode of assisted conception and sub-fertility in an Australian data linkage cohort. PLoS One. 2014;9:e80398.

29. Jacobsen EA, Helmers RA, Lee JJ, Lee NA. The expanding role(s) of eosinophils in health and disease. Blood. 2012;120:3882–90.

30. Temmerman M, Gichangi P, Fonck K, et al. Effect of a syphilis control programme on pregnancy outcome in Nairobi, Kenya. Sex Trans Infect. 2000;76:117–21.

31. Costa MC, Bornhausen Demarch E, Azulay DR, Perisse AR, Dias MF, Nery JA. Sexually transmitted diseases during pregnancy: a synthesis of particularities. An Bras Dermatol. 2010;85:767–82. quiz 83-5

32. Qin JB, Feng TJ, Yang TB, Hong FC, Lan LN, Zhang CL. Maternal and paternal factors associated with congenital syphilis in Shenzhen, China: a prospective cohort study. Eur J Clin Microbiol Infect Dis. 2014;33:221–32.

33. Gomez GB, Kamb ML, Newman LM, Mark J, Broutet N, Hawkes SJ. Untreated maternal syphilis and adverse outcomes of pregnancy: a systematic review and meta-analysis. Bull World Health Organ. 2013;91:217–26.

34. Sinclair KD, Watkins AJ. Parental diet, pregnancy outcomes and offspring health: metabolic determinants in developing oocytes and embryos. Reprod Fertil Dev. 2013;26:99–114.

35. Otero-Ferrer F, Izquierdo M, Fazeli A, Holt WV. Sex-specific effects of parental diet during pregnancy on embryo development in the long snout seahorse. Reprod Fertil Dev. 2014;27:153.

36. Martin GB, Blache D, Miller DW, Vercoe PE. Interactions between nutrition and reproduction in the management of the mature male ruminant. Animal. 2010;4:1214–26.

Histologic chorioamnionitis does not modulate the oxidative stress and antioxidant status in pregnancies complicated by spontaneous preterm delivery

Laura Fernandes Martin[1], Natália Prearo Moço[1], Moisés Diôgo de Lima[2], Jossimara Polettini[3], Hélio Amante Miot[1], Camila Renata Corrêa[1], Ramkumar Menon[4] and Márcia Guimarães da Silva[1*]

Abstract

Background: Infection induced-inflammation and other risk factors for spontaneous preterm birth (PTB) and preterm premature rupture of membranes (pPROM) may cause a redox imbalance, increasing the release of free radicals and consuming antioxidant defenses. Oxidative stress, in turn, can initiate intracellular signaling cascades that increase the production of pro-inflammatory mediators.

The objective of this study was to evaluate the oxidative damage to proteins and antioxidant capacity profiles in amniochorion membranes from preterm birth (PTB) and preterm premature rupture of membranes (pPROM) and to determine the role of histologic chorioamnionitis in this scenario.

Methods: We included 27 pregnant women with PTB, 27 pPROM and 30 at term. Protein oxidative damage was assayed by 3-nitrotyrosine (3-NT) and carbonyl levels, using enzyme-linked immunosorbent assay (ELISA) and modified dinitrophenylhydrazine assay (DNPH), respectively. Total antioxidant capacity (TAC) was measured by ELISA.

Results: Protein oxidative damage determined by carbonyl levels was lower in PTB group than pPROM and term groups ($p < 0.001$). PTB group presented higher TAC compared with pPROM and term groups ($p = 0.002$). Histologic chorioamnionitis did not change either protein oxidative damage or TAC regardless of gestational outcome.

Conclusion: These results corroborates previous reports that pPROM and term birth exhibit similarities in oxidative stress- induced senescence and histologic chorioamnionitis does not modulate oxidative stress or antioxidant status.

Keywords: Oxidative stress, Antioxidant capacity, Histologic chorioamnionitis, Preterm birth

Background

Reactive oxygen and nitrogen species (ROS and RNS), collectively named free radicals, are generated spontaneously in all aerobic organisms [1–4]. The mechanism termed redox balance ensures that the production of free radicals is not harmful to biological systems by preventing the excessive formation and action of ROS and RNS or by favoring the repair and reconstruction of biological structures that have been affected by them [5, 6]. Antioxidant defense mechanisms essential to redox balance are composed of enzymatic and non-enzymatic antioxidants. Enzymatic antioxidants include catalase, glutathione peroxidase (GPx), glutathione reductase (GSR) and superoxide dismutase (SOD). Non-enzymatic antioxidants include antioxidant compounds, such as glutathione and vitamins A, C and E [7]. Oxidative stress is an imbalance in redox status, towards excess ROS and RNS generation [6, 8, 9]. When the total antioxidant capacity (TAC) decreases or free radical levels increase

* Correspondence: mgsilva@fmb.unesp.br
[1]Department of Pathology, Botucatu Medical School, São Paulo State University (UNESP), Distrito de Rubião Júnior, Botucatu, São Paulo CEP 18618-686, Brazil
Full list of author information is available at the end of the article

[10], these exacerbated ROS and RNS formations can damage lipids, proteins and nucleic acids by modifying their expression, structure and function [11–13].

Oxidative stress damage to cells and tissues plays an important role in several pathological processes, including cardiovascular disease [14, 15], cancer [16–18], chronic inflammation [19], neurological disorders [20], metabolic syndrome [21, 22] and pregnancy complications [1, 6, 9, 23, 24]. Recent reports have linked spontaneous preterm birth (PTB) and preterm premature rupture of membranes (pPROM) pathophysiology to oxidative stress damage, where the latter is associated with oxidative stress-induced inflammation and considered as the disease of the fetal membranes [25, 26].

Despite the multifactorial etiology of PTB, intra-amniotic infection followed by maternal inflammatory response activation is reported as the major risk factor for PTB and is present in approximately 40% of preterm pregnancies [27–30]. pPROM in labor is associated with approximately 75% of infection [31]. The inflammatory response in the amniochorion membranes in response to bacterial infection can be diagnosed using clinical or histological criteria. Histologic chorioamnionitis (HC) is defined by the presence of polymorphonuclear cell (PMN) infiltrate in the amniochorion membranes [32].

Bacterial phagocytosis by PMNs during an inflammatory process results in an oxidative burst that is an antimicrobial mechanism characterized by the rapid generation and release of ROS and RNS, leading to oxidative stress [33]. Oxidative stress, in turn, can initiate intracellular signaling cascades that increase the production of pro-inflammatory mediators [34, 35]. Recent reports suggest that a substantial number of PTB and pPROM are associated with sterile inflammation in the absence of documented intra-amniotic infection or histologic chorioamnionitis. This is indicative of an alternate pathophysiology that can lead to an inflammatory process. Oxidative stress-induced senescence and senescence associated with inflammation, termed as sterile inflammation, has been linked to both PTB and pPROM. Both infectious and sterile inflammation exhibit a similar set of biomarkers. This study was conducted to assess oxidative stress-induced damage by determining protein peroxidation and total antioxidant capacity of fetal membranes from pregnancies complicated by PTB and pPROM compared with normal term pregnancies and evaluate the role of histologic chorioamnionitis in this scenario.

Methods

The research project was approved by the Research Ethics Committee Board of the Federal University of Paraíba (UFPB), under protocol no. 1255858. Written informed consent was obtained from all the participants, and sociodemographic and behavioral data were acquired from patient medical records.

Study population

This cross-sectional study was conducted in the Obstetrics Unit of the UFPB Lauro Wanderley Hospital, Paraíba State, Brazil, and in the Laboratory of Immunopathology of the Maternal-Fetal Relationship of the Department of Pathology of Botucatu Medical School, São Paulo State University (UNESP), São Paulo State, Brazil, from January to December 2014. Eighty-four pregnant women were enrolled. The preterm group was composed of 27 pregnant women who presented PTB with intact membranes and 27 pregnant women who presented pPROM. All these pregnant women delivered before 37 weeks of gestation. The term group was composed of 30 normal pregnant women in labor. Normal pregnancy was defined as singleton full-term and uneventful pregnancy, with no chronic or gestational medical conditions. The PTB, pPROM and term groups were subdivided according to the presence or absence of histologic chorioamnionitis.

The exclusion criteria were as follows: BMI > 30 kg/m^2, preeclampsia, HELLP syndrome, gestational diabetes, hypertension, multiple pregnancies, cervical isthmus incompetence, placenta previa, placental abruption, RH-incompatibility, oligohydramnios or polyhydramnios, intrauterine growth restriction, malformation or fetal death, systemic infection, thyroid disease, HIV infection and drug and/or tobacco use.

Gestational age was calculated from the first day of the last menstrual period and/or by first-trimester ultrasound examination. Clinical diagnoses of PTB were made based on the following criteria: uterine contractions ≥4 per 20 min, cervical dilatation of at least 1 cm and cervical ripening [36]. pPROM was defined as the leakage of amniotic fluid prior to the onset of labor. This condition was confirmed with vaginal discharge pH ≥7 and/or positive result in an AmniSure test [37].

Sample collection and histopathological analyses

Amniochorion membranes were collected and cleaned of blood clots and decidua in sterile conditions after placental delivery, flash frozen in liquid nitrogen and stored at –80 °C until processing. Samples of the membranes were fixed in 10% formalin, embedded in paraffin, sectioned and stained with hematoxylin and eosin for histopathological analyses. Histologic chorioamnionitis was diagnosed by the presence of neutrophilic infiltration in amniochorion membranes, as described by Redline et al. [32].

Measurement of 3-nitrotyrosine levels

Protein peroxidation was determined using the 3-nitrotyrosine (3-NT) ELISA Kit, according to the manufacturer's instructions (Abcam, Cambridge, UK). 3-NT is a product of protein tyrosine nitration resulting from oxidative damage to proteins by peroxynitrite, which can result in changes in protein structure, function and catalytic activity.

Amniochorion membrane sections of 25 mg were prepared for the assay by grinding with liquid nitrogen and homogenization with 1 mL of PBS. Next, aliquots were prepared containing 60 µL of tissue homogenate to which 240 µL of extraction buffer containing protease inhibitor were added. The samples were incubated on ice for 20 min. Tissue homogenates were centrifuged at 16000 x g for 10 min at 4 °C and the supernatants were collected immediately and stored at −20 °C.

The total protein concentration of all samples was measured by the Bradford protein assay, according to the manufacturer's instructions (Bio-Rad, CA, USA), and then adjusted to 1 mg/mL.

A standard curve was obtained in parallel to each assay and the absorbance results were converted to pg/mL. At the end of the reaction, the absorbance was read spectrophotometrically at 450 nm in an automatic ELISA reader (Biotek Instruments Inc., Winooski, USA) and the concentration of 3-NT in each sample was determined by comparison with a standard curve. All the samples were tested in duplicate. The minimum detectable 3-NT level for assays was 0.053 ng/mL.

Measurement of carbonyl levels

Protein carbonylation represents the most frequent and usually irreversible oxidative modification affecting proteins. In this study, a modified dinitrophenylhydrazine (DNPH) assay was performed. The principal method used to evaluate protein carbonylation is protein carbonyl derivatization with 2,4 DNPH, followed by spectrophotometric measurement, in which NaOH is added to the protein solution after the addition of DNPH, triggering an increase of the maximum absorbance wavelength of derivatized proteins from 370 to 450 nm. This increase minimizes the background of free DNPH that are read at 366–370 nm [38].

Amniochorion membrane sections of 25 mg were prepared for the assay by grinding with liquid nitrogen and homogenization with 1 mL of PBS containing the anti-protease cocktail. Tissue homogenates were centrifuged at 1600 x g for 10 min at 4 °C and the supernatants were immediately collected and stored at −20 °C. The total protein concentration of all samples was measured by the Pierce BCA assay, according to the manufacturer's instructions (Thermo Fisher Scientific, MA, USA).

Aliquots of 100 µL were placed in a 96-well plate, and then 100 µL of DNPH solution (19.8 mg DNPH in 10 mL HCl2M) were added. The plate was incubated for 10 min at room temperature and then 50 µL of NaOH 6M were added to all wells. After exactly 10 min

incubation at room temperature, the absorbance was read spectrophotometrically at 450 nm in an automatic reader (Biotek Instruments Inc., Winooski, USA). All the samples were tested in duplicate. The concentration of protein carbonyls was quantified using the molar absorption coefficient of $22,000$ M^{-1} cm^{-1} [39].

Measurement of total antioxidant capacity

Total antioxidant capacity was assessed using the antioxidant assay kit, according to the manufacturer's instructions (Cayman Chemical, Ann Arbor, MI). This protocol assesses the combined activities of enzymatic and non-enzymatic compounds of the antioxidant system.

Amniochorion membrane fragments of 25 mg were prepared for the assay by grinding with liquid nitrogen and homogenization with 1 mL of PBS containing the anti-protease cocktail. The assay is based on the ability of the antioxidants presented in the homogenate to inhibit the oxidation of 2,2´-azino-di-[3-ethylbenzthiazoline sulfonate] (ABTS) to $ABTS^+$ by metmyoglobin. The amount of $ABTS^+$ produced was assessed spectrophotometrically at 405 nm. The antioxidant capacity in the sample to prevent ABTS oxidation was compared with Trolox, a water-soluble tocopherol analogue, and results were expressed as millimolar Trolox equivalent (mM Trolox). All the samples were tested in duplicate. The minimum detectable TAC level for assays was 0.004 mM.

Statistical analysis

The Kolmogorov-Smirnov test was used to check the normality of the data. Regarding sociodemographic and obstetric variables, ethnicity, parity and Apgar 1 were compared between the groups using the Fisher exact test, while the variables maternal age, gestational age and newborn weight were compared using the nonparametric Kruskall-Wallis test.

The levels of 3-NT, carbonyl and TAC were compared among PTB, pPROM and term groups using the nonparametric Kruskall-Wallis test and between presence and absence of HC in each group using the nonparametric Mann-Whitney test. A p value <0.05 was considered statistically significant. The software used was SigmaStat Software version 3.1.

Results

Sociodemographic characteristics

Sociodemographic, obstetric and neonatal characteristics of the patients included in the study are presented in Table 1. No statistically significant differences were verified in maternal age, ethnicity, parity and Apgar 1 among the groups studied. As expected, given the study design, gestational age at delivery ($p < 0.001$) and newborn weight

Table 1 Sociodemographic, obstetric and neonatal characteristics of the study population

Characteristics		PTB (n = 27)	pPROM (n = 27)	TERM (n = 30)	p-value
Maternal age (years)*		21 (19.25–24.0)	24 (17.5–32.0)	23 (20.0–27.25)	NS
Ethnicity	**White**	33.3% (9/27)	22.2% (6/27)	13.3% (4/30)	NS
	Non-white	66.7% (18/27)	77.8% (21/27)	86.7% (26/30)	NS
Gestational age (days)*		245 (165–256)[a]	238 (182–252)[a]	273 (259–294)[b]	<0.001
Newborn weight (g)*		2340 (630–3085)[a]	2255 (760–3550)[a]	3300 (2600–4690)[b]	<0.001
Parity	**Primiparous**	37% (10/27)	48.1% (13/27)	33.3% (10/30)	NS
Apgar 1° min	**<7**	18.5% (5/27)	14.8% (4/27)	3.33% (3/30)	NS

Values followed by the same letter do not differ
NS not significant
*Values expressed as median(min-max)

($p < 0.001$) were statistically higher in the term group compared with the PTB and pPROM groups.

Histopathological findings

Histologic chorioamnionitis was present in 22.2% (6/27) of the PTB group, 51.8% (14/27) of the pPROM group and 13.3% (4/30) of the term group. Following stratification according to histologic chorioamnionitis grading, moderate/severe cases were observed in 66% (4/6) in the PTB group, 21% (3/14) in the pPROM group and 25% (1/4) in the term group.

Oxidative stress and antioxidant capacity

Quantitation of protein damage markers and total antioxidant capacity in amniochorion membranes

3-NT concentrations, an indicator of protein peroxidation and oxidative stress, was not significantly different between the groups. However, protein oxidative damage determined by carbonyl levels was lower in the PTB group in comparison with the pPROM and term groups ($p < 0.001$). Furthermore, the PTB group had higher TAC compared with the pPROM and term groups ($p = 0.002$) (Fig. 1).

Quantitation of protein damage markers and total antioxidant capacity in amniochorion membranes based on histologic chorioamnionitis

Analyses of protein oxidative damage and total antioxidant capacity among the groups considering HC status are presented in Fig. 2. Protein oxidative damage assessed by 3-NT (Fig. 2a) and carbonyl (Fig. 2b) levels did not differ between the presence and absence of HC groups, regardless of gestational outcome. Similar data were obtained in relation to antioxidant capacity determined by TAC (Fig. 2c).

Discussion

Inflammation is the physiological effecter of term parturition and the pathological initiator of labor in both PTB and pPROM. Inflammatory changes in gestational tissues

result in the modification of membrane structural integrity, activation of myometrial contraction and cervical ripening that are simultaneous mechanisms responsible for the onset of labor [40]. Moreover, infection-induced inflammation and other risk factors for pPROM and PTB, including behavioral risks (e.g. cigarette smoking, alcohol and drug use), poor nutrition and obesity, can cause a redox imbalance, increasing the release of free radicals and consuming antioxidant defenses [6, 41, 42].

In this study, we demonstrated that amniochorion membranes from pregnancies complicated by pPROM showed higher protein oxidative damage and lower antioxidant capacity than those complicated by PTB. This is consistent with previous reports by Dutta et al. [25], who reported oxidative stress-induced damaged and damaged associated senescence as salient features of pPROM, but not in PTB when membranes were intact. Although there are etiological similarities between PTB and pPROM, our results also support mechanistic differences in pPROM and PTB pathways.

Menon et al. [6] reported that fetal membranes from pPROM have pronounced damage due to oxidative stress and proteolysis, whereas in PTB this oxidative damage is minimal. Compelling evidence suggests that pPROM may result from chronic oxidative stress in response to sustained exposure to risk factors, whereas PTB may be a consequence of acute oxidative stress [6, 43]. It has been suggested that an important mechanism associated with pPROM is the imbalance of redox status, where lower antioxidant status and higher oxidative stress-induced tissue damage triggers the weakening and rupture of fetal membranes. Alternately, better antioxidant capacity present in membranes from PTB can balance the acute oxidative stress allowing the cell to resist oxidative damage and membrane rupture. However, the risk factors may still cause host immune and inflammatory response sufficient to cause preterm labor. Thus, PTB pathophysiology shows a predominance of inflammatory process, while pPROM presents an intense oxidative damage of tissue, activation of senescence and senescence associated inflammation.

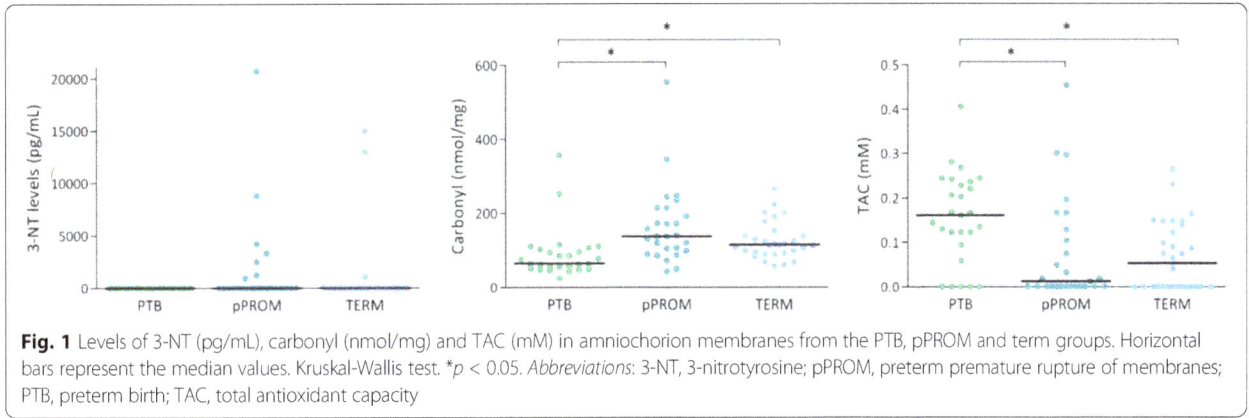

Fig. 1 Levels of 3-NT (pg/mL), carbonyl (nmol/mg) and TAC (mM) in amniochorion membranes from the PTB, pPROM and term groups. Horizontal bars represent the median values. Kruskal-Wallis test. *$p < 0.05$. *Abbreviations*: 3-NT, 3-nitrotyrosine; pPROM, preterm premature rupture of membranes; PTB, preterm birth; TAC, total antioxidant capacity

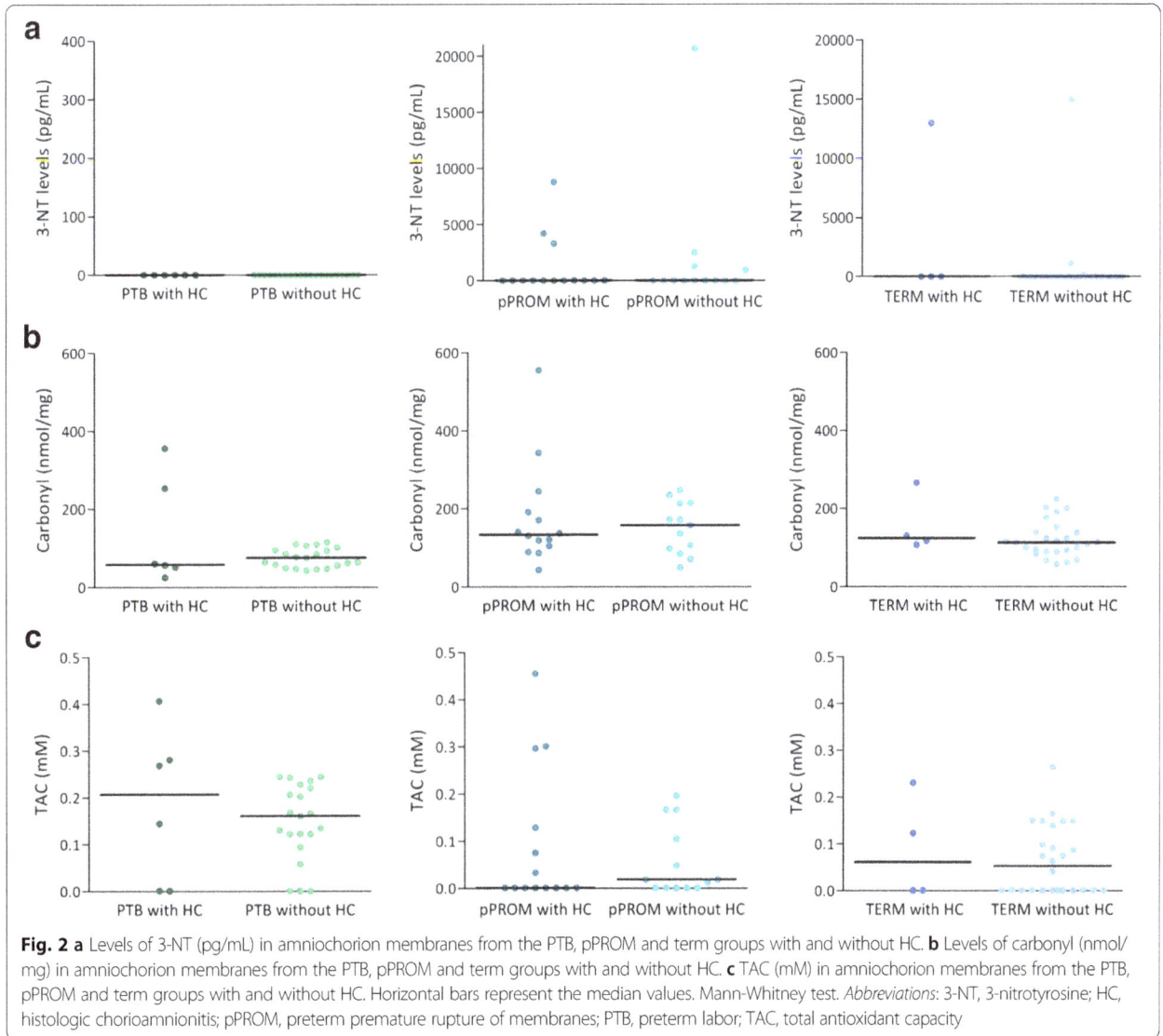

Fig. 2 a Levels of 3-NT (pg/mL) in amniochorion membranes from the PTB, pPROM and term groups with and without HC. **b** Levels of carbonyl (nmol/mg) in amniochorion membranes from the PTB, pPROM and term groups with and without HC. **c** TAC (mM) in amniochorion membranes from the PTB, pPROM and term groups with and without HC. Horizontal bars represent the median values. Mann-Whitney test. *Abbreviations*: 3-NT, 3-nitrotyrosine; HC, histologic chorioamnionitis; pPROM, preterm premature rupture of membranes; PTB, preterm labor; TAC, total antioxidant capacity

Infection in some cases of pPROM is likely secondary, resulting from membrane damage leading to its dysfunctional status, and reduced antimicrobial resistance allowing the ascendance of microbes. Reinforcing this idea, our results showed a predominance of moderate/severe cases of HC in 66% of the PTB group, whereas mild HC was predominant in 79% of the pPROM group.

At term, oxidative stress and fetal membrane senescence are a well-described condition, probably resulting from physiological aging of the placenta and membranes that lead to labor and delivery [44, 45]. Herein, we demonstrated that the protein oxidative damage observed in pPROM amniochorion membranes was similar to that observed in term membranes. This similarity corroborates the hypothesis that elevated oxidative stress in pregnancies complicated by pPROM accelerates the premature senescence and aging, senescence-associated inflammation and proteolysis in amniochorion membranes, predisposing these to membrane rupture and the onset of labor [25, 45].

Following the evaluation of protein oxidative damage and antioxidant status in amniochorion membranes, we further determined the role of HC in the oxidative stress profile in each gestational outcome. HC was diagnosed in approximately 13% of term pregnancies and over 37% of preterm pregnancies. These data are in agreement with other studies, which demonstrated that HC is diagnosed in approximately 20% of term pregnancies and over 50% of the PTB. The majority of these cases are not associated with clinical signs and symptoms of infection [46–48].

In our study, protein oxidative damage and antioxidant capacity in amniochorion membranes did not differ based on HC status, regardless of gestational outcome. These data corroborate the findings of Kacerovsky et al. [49] and Musilova et al. [50], who observed that oxidative stress markers in pregnancies complicated by pPROM were not influenced by intra-amniotic infection, nor by HC, when measured in amniotic fluid and umbilical cord blood, respectively. These results disagree with those reported by Temma et al. [51], who showed increased oxidative stress in human placenta with HC. Similarly, a recent study by Cháfer-Pericás et al. [52] demonstrated elevated oxidative stress in amniotic fluid in the presence of intra-amniotic infection. Additionally, Perrone et al. [53] observed that HC was associated with higher oxidative stress levels in umbilical cord blood. The apparent disagreement between studies may reflect differences in the definition of the phenotype studied, the biological samples analyzed and analytes measured, as well as methodologies used in each study. It is likely that HC is a secondary phenomenon that is risk exposure and mechanism dependent, where type of host inflammatory response and biochemical (cytokines/chemokines) may determine HC outcome and thus HC is a consequence of several pathological processes.

There are limitations in our study. The first of them is the small sample size of each group when subdivided by the histopathological status of amniochorion membranes. In addition, the discrepancy between the results of the methodologies used to determine protein oxidative damage may be explained by intrinsic differences present in each technique. Determining protein carbonyl content is the most general indicator of oxidative protein damage. In addition, due to its long lasting stability of the samples under the storage conditions described, measurement of protein carbonyl content is considered a reliable marker of protein oxidation [54–56]. 3-NT quantification, in turn, is used to evaluate the protein oxidative damage more specifically, since it is a product of protein tyrosine nitration [57]. Moreover, 3-NT quantification requires sensitive analytical methods because it is typically a low-yield process [57]. Endogenous levels of 3-NT are severely low and usually close to or below the limits of detection of the currently available analytical assays [57]. Future studies by our group will examine lipid, nucleic acid and other cellular elemental damage and independent determination of multiple antioxidants.

Conclusion

Taken together, our results suggest that increased oxidative stress and reduced antioxidant capacity are similar in amniochorion membranes from women who present pPROM and term pregnancies, reinforcing that accelerated premature senescence, senescence-associated inflammation and proteolysis predispose to pPROM. In this scenario, histologic chorioamnionitis does not modulate oxidative stress or antioxidant status profile.

Abbreviations

3-NT: 3-nitrotyrosine; ABTS: 2,2'-azino-di-[3-ethylbenzthiazoline sulfonate]; DNPH: modified dinitrophenylhydrazine assay; ELISA: enzyme-linked immunosorbent assay; GPx: glutathione peroxidase; GSR: glutathione reductase; HC: histologic chorioamnionitis; PBS: phosphate buffered saline; PMN: polymorphonuclear cell; pPRPM: preterm premature rupture of membranes; PTB: spontaneous preterm birth; RNS: reactive nitrogen species; ROS: reactive oxygen species; SOD: superoxide dismutase; TAC: total antioxidant capacity

Acknowledgments

This study was supported by São Paulo Research Foundation the São Paulo Research Foundation (FAPESP) (Grant 2012/17234-1) and National Council for Technological and Scientific Development (CNPq - 142419/2013-3). The funders had no role in study design, data collection and analysis, decision to publish, or preparation of the manuscript. We would also like to thank all the patients and participants of this study.

Funding

This study was supported by developmental funds granted to Dr. MGS of the Department of Pathology, Botucatu Medical School, São Paulo State University (UNESP), Brazil, by the São Paulo Research Foundation (FAPESP) (Grant 2012/17234-1) and granted to LFM, PhD student of Graduate Program in Pathology, Botucatu Medical School, UNESP, Brazil, by the National Council for Technological and Scientific Development (CNPq - 142,419/2013-3).

Authors' contributions

LFM, NPM and JP contributed to study design. LFM and NPM contributed to sample collection, execution of the study, data analysis, critical discussion and manuscript drafting. MDL and CRCC contributed to execution of the study. HAM and RM contributed to analysis of results. MGS contributed to the study design, supervision of study execution, critical discussion and manuscript analysis. All authors read and approved the final manuscript.

Competing interests

The authors declare that the research was conducted in the absence of any commercial or financial relationships that could be construed as a potential conflict of interest.

Author details

[1]Department of Pathology, Botucatu Medical School, São Paulo State University (UNESP), Distrito de Rubião Júnior, Botucatu, São Paulo CEP 18618-686, Brazil. [2]Department of Gynecology and Obstetrics, Federal University of Paraíba, UFPB, João Pessoa, Brazil. [3]The University of Western São Paulo, UNOESTE, Presidente Prudente, Brazil. [4]Department of Obstetrics & Gynecology, The University of Texas Medical Branch at Galveston, Galveston, TX, USA.

References

1. Longini M, Perrone S, Vezzosi P, Marzocchi B, Kenanidis A, Centini G, et al. Association between oxidative stress in pregnancy and preterm premature rupture of membranes. Clin Biochem. 2007;40:793–7.
2. Sies H. Oxidative stress: from basic research to clinical application. Am J Med. 1991;91
3. Finkel T. Signal transduction by reactive oxygen species. J Cell Biol. 2011. p. 7–15.
4. Cadenas E, Sies H. Oxidative stress: excited oxygen species and enzyme activity. Adv Enzym Regul. 1985;23:217–37.
5. Ďuračková Z. Some current insights into oxidative stress. Physiol Res. 2010; 59(4):459–69.
6. Menon R. Oxidative stress damage as a detrimental factor in preterm birth pathology. Front Immunol. 2014;5:567.
7. Chai M, Barker G, Menon R, Lappas M. Increased oxidative stress in human fetal membranes overlying the cervix from term non-labouring and post labour deliveries. Placenta. 2012;33:604–10.
8. Al-Gubory KH, Fowler PA, Garrel C. The roles of cellular reactive oxygen species, oxidative stress and antioxidants in pregnancy outcomes. Int J Biochem Cell Biol. 2010;42:1634–50.
9. Agarwal A, Gupta S, Sharma RK. Role of oxidative stress in female reproduction. Reprod Biol Endocrinol. 2005;3:28.
10. Halliwell B. Free radicals and antioxidants: updating a personal view. Nutr Rev. 2012;70:257–65.
11. Agarwal A, Aponte-Mellado A, Premkumar BJ, Shaman A, Gupta S. The effects of oxidative stress on female reproduction: a review. Reprod Biol Endocrinol. 2012;10:1–31.
12. Halliwell B, Whiteman M. Measuring reactive species and oxidative damage in vivo and in cell culture: how should you do it and what do the results mean? Br J Pharmacol. 2004;142:231–55.
13. Sies H. Strategies of antioxidant defense. Eur J Biochem. 1993;215:213–9.
14. de Vos LC, Lefrandt JD, Dullaart RPF, Zeebregts CJ, Smit AJ. Advanced glycation end products: an emerging biomarker for adverse outcome in patients with peripheral artery disease. Atherosclerosis. 2016;254:291–9.
15. Yeh J-K, Wang C-Y. Telomeres and telomerase in cardiovascular diseases. Genes (Basel). 2016;7:58. Available from: http://www.mdpi.com/2073-4425/7/9/58.
16. Katakwar P, Metgud R, Naik S, Mittal R. Oxidative stress marker in oral cancer: a review. J Cancer Res Ther. 2016;12:438–46.
17. Zhou L, Wen J, Huang Z, Nice EC, Huang C, Zhang H, et al. Redox proteomics screening cellular factors associated with oxidative stress in hepatocarcinogenesis. Prot Clin Appl. 2017;(11):1–49.
18. Udensi UK TP. Oxidative stress in prostate hypertrophy and carcinogenesis. Postepy Hig Med Dosw (Online). 2009;63:340–50.
19. Hussain T, Tan B, Yin Y, Blachier F, Tossou MCB, Rahu N. Oxidative Stress and Inflammation: What Polyphenols Can Do for Us? Oxid Med Cell Longev. 2016;2016. doi: 10.1155/2016/7432797.
20. Radi E, Formichi P, Battisti C, Federico A. Apoptosis and oxidative stress in neurodegenerative diseases; in : Journal of Alzheimer's Disease. 2014, pp S125–S152.
21. Moreto F, Kano HT, Torezan GA, de Oliveira EP, Manda RM, Teixeira O, et al. Changes in malondialdehyde and C-reactive protein concentrations after lifestyle modification are related to different metabolic syndrome-associated pathophysiological processes. Diabetes Metab Syndr 2015;9:218–222.
22. Bjørklund G, Chirumbolo S. Role of oxidative stress and antioxidants in daily nutrition and human health. Nutrition. 2017;33:311–21.
23. Poston L, Igosheva N, Mistry HD, Seed PT, Shennan AH, Rana S, et al. Role of oxidative stress and antioxidant supplementation in pregnancy. Am J Clin Nutr. 2011;94:1980–5.
24. Poston L, Raijmakers MTM. Trophoblast oxidative stress, antioxidants and pregnancy outcome - a review. Placenta. 2004;25:72–8.
25. Dutta EH, Behnia F, Boldogh I, Saade GR, Taylor BD, Kacerovský M, et al. Oxidative stress damage-associated molecular signaling pathways differentiate spontaneous preterm birth and preterm premature rupture of the membranes. Mol Hum Reprod. 2015;22(2):143–57.
26. Murtha AP, Menon R. Regulation of fetal membrane inflammation: a critical step in reducing adverse pregnancy outcome. Am J Obstet Gynecol. 2015; 213:447–8.
27. DiGiulio DB, Romero R, Amogan HP, Kusanovic JP, Bik EM, Gotsch F, et al. Microbial prevalence, diversity and abundance in amniotic fluid during preterm labor: a molecular and culture-based investigation. PLoS One. 2008;3:e3056.
28. Nguyen DP, Gerber S, Hohlfeld P, Sandrine G, Witkin SS. Mycoplasma hominis in mid-trimester amniotic fluid: relation to pregnancy outcome. J Perinat Med. 2004;32:323–6.
29. Perni SC, Vardhana S, Korneeva I, Tuttle SL, Paraskevas LR, Chasen ST, et al. Mycoplasma hominis and Ureaplasma urealyticum in midtrimester amniotic fluid: association with amniotic fluid cytokine levels and pregnancy outcome. Am J Obstet Gynecol. 2004;191:1382–6.
30. Yoon B, Romero R, Lim J-H, Shim S-S, Hong J-S, Shim J-Y, et al. The clinical significance of detecting Ureaplasma urealyticum by the polymerase chain reaction in the amniotic fluid of patients with preterm labor. Am J Obstet Gynecol. 2003;189:919–24.
31. Romero R, Quintero R, Oyarzun E, et al. Intraamniotic infection and the onset of labor in preterm premature rupture of the membranes. Am J Obstet Gynecol 1988;159:661–6.
32. Redline RW, Faye-Petersen O, Heller D, Qureshi F, Savell V, Vogler C. Amniotic infection syndrome: Nosology and reproducibility of placental reaction patterns. Pediatr Dev Pathol. 2003;6:435–48.
33. Biswas SK. Does the interdependence between oxidative stress and inflammation explain the antioxidant paradox? Oxidative Med Cell Longev. 2016;
34. Anderson MT, Staal FJ, Gitler C, Herzenberg LA. Separation of oxidant-initiated and redox-regulated steps in the NF-kappa B signal transduction pathway. Proc Natl Acad Sci U S A. 1994;91:11527–31.
35. Flohé L, Brigelius-Flohé R, Saliou C, Traber MG, Packer L. Redox regulation of NF-kappa B activation. Free Radic Biol Med. 1997;22:1115–26.
36. Bittar RE, Zugaib M. Indicadores de risco para o parto prematuro. Rev Bras Ginecol Obs. 2009;31:203–9.
37. Caughey AB, Robinson JN, Norwitz ER. Contemporary diagnosis and management of preterm premature rupture of membranes. Rev Obstet Gynecol. 2008;1:11–22.
38. Colombo G, Clerici M, Garavaglia ME, Giustarini D, Rossi R, Milzani A, et al. A step-by-step protocol for assaying protein carbonylation in biological samples. J Chromatogr B Anal Technol Biomed Life Sci. 2016;1019:178–90.

39. Mesquita CS, Oliveira R, Bento F, Geraldo D, Rodrigues JV, Marcos JC. Simplified 2,4-dinitrophenylhydrazine spectrophotometric assay for quantification of carbonyls in oxidized proteins. Anal Biochem. 2014;458:69–71.

40. Romero R, Espinoza J, Gonçalves LF, Kusanovic JP, Friel LA, Nien JK. Inflammation in preterm and term labour and delivery. Semin Fetal Neonatal Med. 2006;11:317–26.

41. Coughlan MT, Permezel M, Georgiou HM, Rice GE. Repression of oxidant-induced nuclear factor-??B activity mediates placental cytokine responses in gestational diabetes. J Clin Endocrinol Metab. 2004;89:3585–94.

42. Dietrich M, Block G, Norkus EP, Hudes M, Traber MG, Cross CE, et al. Smoking and exposure to environmental tobacco smoke decrease some plasma antioxidants and increase gamma-tocopherol in vivo after adjustment for dietary antioxidant intakes. Am J Clin Nutr. 2003;77(1):160–166.

43. Menon R, Polettini J, Syed TA, Saade GR, Boldogh I. Expression of 8-oxoguanine Glycosylase in human fetal membranes. Am J Reprod Immunol. 2014;72:75–84.

44. Behnia F, Taylor BD, Woodson M, Kacerovsky M, Hawkins H, Fortunato SJ, et al. Chorioamniotic membrane senescence: a signal for parturition? Am J Obstet Gynecol. 2015;213:359e1–359e16.

45. Menon R, Boldogh I, Hawkins HK, Woodson M, Polettini J, Syed TA, Fortunato SJ, et al. Histological evidence of oxidative stress and premature senescence in preterm premature rupture of the human fetal membranes recapitulated in vitro. Am J Pathol. 2014;184:1740–51.

46. Edwards RK. Chorioamnionitis and labor. Obstet Gynecol Clin North Am. 2005;32:287–96.

47. Conti N, Torricelli M, Voltolini C, Vannuccini S, Clifton VL, Bloise E, et al. Term histologic chorioamnionitis: a heterogeneous condition. Eur J Obstet Gynecol Reprod Biol. 2015;188:34–8.

48. Newton ER. Preterm labor, preterm premature rupture of membranes, and chorioamnionitis. Clin Perinatol. 2005;32:571–600.

49. Kacerovsky M, Tothova L, Menon R, Vlkova B, Musilova I, Hornychova H, et al. Amniotic fluid markers of oxidative stress in pregnancies complicated by preterm prelabor rupture of membranes. J Matern Fetal Neonatal Med. 2014;27:1–10.

50. Musilova I, Tothova L, Menon R, Vlkova B, Celec P, Hornychova H, et al. Umbilical cord blood markers of oxidative stress in pregnancies complicated by preterm prelabor rupture of membranes. J Matern Neonatal Med. 2016;29(12):1900–10.

51. Temma K, Shimoya K, Zhang Q, Kimura T, Wasada K, Kanzaki T, et al. Effects of 4-hydroxy-2-nonenal, a marker of oxidative stress, on the cyclooxygenase-2 of human placenta in chorioamnionitis. Mol Hum Reprod. 2004;10:167–71.

52. Cháfer-Pericás C, Stefanovic V, Sánchez-Illana Á, Escobar J, Cernada M, Cubells E, et al. Novel biomarkers in amniotic fluid for early assessment of intraamniotic infection. Free Radic Biol Med. 2015;89:734–40.

53. Perrone S, Tataranno ML, Negro S, Longini M, Toti MS, Alagna MG, et al. Placental histological examination and the relationship with oxidative stress in preterm infants. Placenta. 2016;46:72–8.

54. Butterfield DA, Castegna A. Proteomics for the identification of specifically oxidized proteins in brain: technology and application to the study of neurodegenerative disorders. Amino Acids. 2003;25:419–25.

55. Dalle-Donne I, Rossi R, Giustarini D, Milzani A, Colombo R. Protein carbonyl groups as biomarkers of oxidative stress. Clin Chim Acta. 2003;329(1–2):23–38.

56. Stadtman ER, Levine RL. Free radical-mediated oxidation of free amino acids and amino acid residues in proteins. Amino Acids. 2003;25(3–4):207–18.

57. Teixeira D, Fernandes R, Prudêncio C, Vieira M. 3-Nitrotyrosine quantification methods: current concepts and future challenges. Biochimie. 2016;125:1–11.

What is the safest mode of delivery for extremely preterm cephalic/non-cephalic twin pairs?

Catherine Dagenais[1], Anne-Mary Lewis-Mikhael[2], Marinela Grabovac[2], Amit Mukerji[3] and Sarah D. McDonald[1,2]*

Abstract

Background: Given the controversy around mode of delivery, our objective was to assess the evidence regarding the safest mode of delivery for actively resuscitated extremely preterm cephalic/non-cephalic twin pairs before 28 weeks of gestation.

Methods: We searched Cochrane CENTRAL, MEDLINE, EMBASE and http://clinicaltrials.gov from January 1994 to January 2017. Two reviewers independently screened titles, abstracts and full text articles, extracted data and assessed risk of bias. We included randomized controlled trials and observational studies. Our primary outcome was a composite of neonatal death (<28 days of life) and severe brain injury in survivors (intraventricular hemorrhage grade ≥ 3 or periventricular leukomalacia). We performed random-effects meta-analyses, generating odds ratios with 95% confidence intervals for the first and second twin separately, and for both twins together. We assessed the risk of bias using a modified Newcastle Ottawa Scale (NOS) for observational studies and used Grading of Recommendations Assessment, Development and Evaluation approach (GRADE).

Results: Our search generated 2695 articles, and after duplicate removal, we screened 2051 titles and abstracts, selecting 113 articles for full-text review. We contacted 36 authors, and ultimately, three observational studies met our inclusion criteria. In cephalic/non-cephalic twin pairs delivered by caesarean section compared to vaginal birth at 24^{+0}–27^{+6} weeks the odds ratio for our composite outcome of neonatal death and severe brain injury for the cephalic first twin was 0.35 (95% CI 0.00–92.61, two studies, $I^2 = 76\%$), 1.69 for the non-cephalic second twin (95% CI 0.04–72.81, two studies, $I^2 = 55\%$) and 0.83 for both twins (95% CI 0.05–13.43, two studies, $I^2 = 56\%$). According to the modified Newcastle Ottawa Scale we assessed individual study quality as being at high risk of bias and according to GRADE the overall evidence for our primary outcomes was very low.

Conclusion: Our systematic review on the safest mode of delivery for extremely preterm cephalic/non-cephalic twin pairs found very limited existing evidence, without significant differences in neonatal death and severe brain injury by mode of delivery.

Keywords: Twin, Extremely preterm, Extremely low birth weight, Vaginal delivery, Caesarean section, Breech presentation

* Correspondence: mcdonals@mcmaster.ca
[1]Department of Obstetrics & Gynecology, McMaster University, 1280 Main St W, HSC 3N52B, Hamilton, ON L8S 4K1, Canada
[2]Department of Health Research Methods, Evidence, and Impact, McMaster University, 1280 Main St W, Hamilton, ON L8S 4K1, Canada
Full list of author information is available at the end of the article

Background

Extreme prematurity, the birth of an infant before 28 weeks' gestation, contributes significantly to infant mortality [1] and childhood morbidity [2]. Extremely preterm births represent approximately 0.2% of singleton births [3, 4], but 4.1% of twins births [5]. In extremely preterm twins from 24 to 27 weeks, the most frequent combination of presentations is cephalic/non-cephalic (42.5%) followed by cephalic/cephalic (25.3%) and non-cephalic/non-cephalic (22.6%) which differs significantly from term proportions [6].

Controversy remains as to the influence of mode of delivery on neonatal outcomes in extremely preterm singletons and twins in general. Some [7, 8], but not all studies [9] have raised concerns about the safety of vaginal birth for extremely preterm breech singleton infants. In a recent meta-analysis, Grabovac et al. 2017 found that caesarean delivery was associated with a 40% decrease in the odds of mortality and 40% decrease in odds of severe intraventricular hemorrhage (IVH; grades ≥3) in extremely preterm breech singletons who were actively resuscitated [10].

In twins, determining the safest mode of delivery is more complex than in singletons, since beyond gestational age, birth order and various presentation combinations need to be considered. For cephalic/non-cephalic twins above 32 weeks, the 2013 randomized controlled trial by Barrett et al. found that trial of labor is safe [11], but due to their inclusion criteria, could not provide guidance on twin birth before 32 weeks.

While a caesarean section is typically performed when the first twin presents as non-cephalic, vaginal birth is generally attempted when both twins are cephalic [12–15]. When the first twin is cephalic and the second is non-cephalic, there is less clinical consensus, leading to variations in clinical practice depending on the clinicians' level of experience, training, and the prevailing obstetrical culture in their location of practice [12–15].

When the second twin is breech, the delivery involves a sequence of events which differs from a singleton breech delivery, including delivery through an already dilated cervix, potential for manoeuvres such as breech extraction and external cephalic version, precluding direct extrapolation of singleton data to the mode of delivery of twins. In face of all these considerations, we decided to perform a systematic review of the literature to assess the evidence regarding the safest mode of delivery of extremely preterm cephalic/non-cephalic twin pairs who were actively resuscitated.

Methods

We planned to follow the Cochrane Handbook for Systematic Reviews of Interventions (Version 5.1.0) for randomized studies and the PRISMA guidelines for observational studies [16, 17]. We registered this protocol on PROSPERO (CRD42017056295).

Information sources

We developed separate search strategies with the assistance of an experienced librarian for each database, consisting of medical subject headings (MeSH) and multipurpose terms (.mp), which we used to search Cochrane CENTRAL, MEDLINE and EMBASE from January 1,1994 - the year the guidelines for the use of antenatal corticosteroid were published -, until January 12, 2017, without language restriction (Additional file 1). We also searched for unpublished randomized controlled trials (RCT) on http://clinicaltrials.gov using the keywords "twin", "twins", "multiple pregnancy" and "multiple pregnancies". We imported all references into a bibliographic software (Endnote X8). We manually searched the references of included studies and relevant systematic reviews for additional articles. We consulted a Maternal Fetal Medicine expert for knowledge on other studies published in this area.

Eligibility

We planned to include all published randomized controlled trials and observational studies (cohort and case-control) comparing mode of delivery in extremely preterm (22^{+0} and 27^{+6} weeks) dichorionic or monochorionic-diamniotic twins presenting as a cephalic/non-cephalic pair who were actively resuscitated. If a study focused on mode of delivery in twins, but did not stratify the data according to gestational age or presentation, we contacted the authors to obtain these data. If the study population was defined by birth weight only, without data on gestational age, we included twins weighing ≤1000 g, which is approximately the 90th percentile for twins born at 27 weeks [18].

We excluded other types of publications (e.g. reviews, editorials, commentaries, case studies, conference proceedings, studies published only as abstracts, etc.). We excluded studies with insufficient data, such as <10 twin pairs total or less than five twin pairs per comparison group (i.e. caesarean and vaginal delivery). We excluded studies with data collected prior to 1994, regardless of publication date. If the data spanned 1994, we contacted the authors to confirm antenatal corticosteroid (ANCS) use was the standard of practice at the time of data collection, and included the study if either the authors confirmed that this was the case or were able to provide separate data for after 1994.

We focused on high-income countries, as they routinely provide active resuscitation for all infants ≥25 weeks, and variably offer resuscitation at 22, 23 or 24 weeks [19], while middle- and low-income countries typically do not. If data on active resuscitation were not provided in the study, we contacted the author to confirm that active resuscitation was planned for all included infants or to request separate data for the actively resuscitated infants only. If the author did not respond, but the study originated from a high-income country, we assumed that resuscitation was planned for all neonates ≥25 weeks. For middle and low incomes countries, if the author did not respond, we excluded the study.

We planned to exclude monochorionic-monoamniotic twins, conjoined twins, twins resulting from fetal reduction of a higher-order pregnancy, twin pairs with one or two fetal deaths before labour, twins with congenital anomalies and asynchronous delivery of the second twin where the aim was to prolong the pregnancy. We intended to exclude twins delivered by caesarean section as a result of an absolute contra-indication to vaginal delivery (e.g. fetal compromise before labour, fetal congenital anomaly, placenta or vasa praevia, uterine rupture, etc.).

Our primary outcome was a composite consisting of: 1) neonatal death defined as death in the first 28 days of life [20] and/or 2) severe brain injury (SBI) [21] among survivors, defined as severe intraventricular hemorrhage (IVH grades ≥3 based on Papile's grading) or periventricular leukomalacia (PVL).

Our main secondary outcomes were the components of our primary composite outcome examined individually: neonatal death, and in survivors, severe brain injury. Another main secondary outcome was overall perinatal mortality (intrapartum death and neonatal death). We examined these outcomes separately in each twin individually according to birth order, and in both twins as pairs together. Our other infant and maternal secondary outcomes are presented in Additional file 2.

Data collection

Two reviewers (CD and AMLM) independently reviewed the titles, abstracts, and full texts. As there are known issues with the kappa statistic (low kappa despite high agreement), we calculated percent agreement to assess inter-reviewer agreement on study inclusion. We used a piloted data collection form to extract data on baseline characteristics, exposures of interest, outcomes, and risk of bias assessment. Discrepancies between reviewers were resolved through discussion, with a third reviewer (SDM) available if necessary.

Risk of bias assessment

We planned to use the Cochrane Collaboration's Risk of Bias (RoB) tool for randomized control trials and the modified Newcastle-Ottawa Scale (NOS) for observational studies to assess risk of bias of our included studies [16, 22].

The Newcastle Ottawa Scale uses three categories, Selection, Comparability and Outcomes, to assess bias in observational studies. We modified the Selection and Outcomes categories by removing 1) ascertainment of exposure, since our exposures of interest (e.g. caesarean section or vaginal delivery) was only obtained through a secure medical record, 2) demonstration that the outcome of interest was not present at the beginning of the studies as the infant and maternal outcomes would not have been present at the time of the caesarean section or vaginal delivery, and 3) whether follow-up was long enough for the outcomes to occur because our outcomes of interest are assumed to have occurred after birth and before discharge from the hospital. We modified the Comparability category so that four points would be awarded for addressing key potential confounders. Those were identified in consultation with Maternal Fetal Medicine and Neonatology experts and were 1) caesarean section for fetal distress, 2) outborn status, 3) antenatal corticosteroid administration (ANCS) and 4) clinical chorioamnionitis. The study was awarded one point for each confounder it addressed for a maximum of four points. Hence, our modified scale awarded up to eight points in total. Since there are no validation studies on a modified scale, we determined that a study scoring eight points would be considered a high-quality study at low risk of bias. A study scoring seven points would be considered of moderate quality and at moderate risk of bias and a study scoring six points or less of low quality and at high risk of bias.

Data analysis

Since we expected between-study heterogeneity, we performed random-effects meta-analyses, generating odds ratios (OR) and 95% confidence intervals (95% CI). We assessed heterogeneity using I^2 statistic; we considered I^2 values 0–40% to be low, 30–60% moderate, 50–90% substantial and 75–100% considerable heterogeneity [16, 17]. We intended to analyze our primary composite and main secondary outcomes according to pre-planned gestational week categories $22^{+0}–23^{+6}$, $24^{+0}–25^{+6}$ and $26^{+0}–27^{+6}$ weeks and pooled together. We planned to separately pool RCT and observational data, to separately pool adjusted and unadjusted data, to separately analyze data from middle- and low-income countries, and to calculate the number needed to treat (NNT) for significant outcomes. All analyses were performed using Review Manager (RevMan) Version 5.3 [23].

Risk of bias across studies

We used the Grading of Recommendations, Assessment, Development, and Evaluation (GRADE) system to assess the overall quality of evidence for our primary outcome, i.e. the confidence that an outcome's effect size is close to the intervention's true effect [22].

We used the GRADE system to rate the quality of evidence for each outcome as high, moderate, low or very low. GRADE recommends that RCTs start as high-quality evidence and observational studies as low-quality evidence, which is then either downgraded (RCTs and observational) or upgraded (observational). The evidence is downgraded by the presence of risk of bias, inconsistency, indirectness, imprecision or publication bias. We assessed those in the following manner: 1) for RCTs, we planned to assess risk of bias using the Cochrane's RoB and for observational studies using the modified NOS; 2) Inconsistency was assessed by substantial heterogeneity as indicated by I^2 values above 50%; 3) Indirectness was assessed by differences in the population, intervention, or outcome, or indirect comparison; 4) Imprecision was assessed by checking whether 95% CIs overlap no effect and/or fail to exclude important benefit/harm; 5) Assessment of publication bias was planned with funnel plots for outcomes with 10 studies or more [24]. The evidence is upgraded in the presence of a large effect, dose-response effect and if all potential confounding would minimize the demonstrated effect.

Subgroup analyses

In addition to stratification by gestational age categories, we intended to separately analyze our main secondary outcomes by birth weight categories (<500 g, 500–999 g and <1000 g). We intended to include the infants who died intrapartum in the adjusted analysis if active resuscitation was planned for them, as excluding them could result in overestimation of the benefits of either mode of delivery.

Data permitting, we intended to address the a priori selected key confounders previously mentioned through subgroup analysis: caesarean section for fetal distress, outborn status, ANCS administration and clinical chorioamnionitis. We also intended to collect information on other potential confounders: cause of prematurity, gestational age at preterm premature rupture of the membranes (PPROM), presence of abruption, presence of growth restriction, weight discrepancy between twins, length of labour, length of birth interval between twins, magnesium sulfate administration before birth, surfactant administration after birth, exact presentation of second twin (breech vs transverse), and maneuvers required for vaginal delivery of the second twin (e.g. external cephalic version versus breech extraction).

We intended to perform a sensitivity analysis by removing low and moderate quality studies to obtain effect estimates using high quality studies only. We also planned to perform a sensitivity analyses by removing studies that excluded intrapartum fetal demise from their study population.

Results

Search strategy

Our search retrieved a total of 2695 abstracts (Cochrane CENTRAL = 193, MEDLINE = 611, EMBASE = 1881, Fig. 1). We identified an additional prospective cohort study from http://clinicaltrials.gov, with a planned subgroup analysis for twins less than 28 weeks, however the initial publication included solely data for twins more than 32 weeks [25], and the authors were unable to provide additional data after contact.

After removing duplicates, we screened 2051 titles and abstracts, selecting 113 full-text articles for review. The initial agreement between reviewers was 92% for full text review. We preliminarily included 36 studies, whose authors we contacted to obtain additional information (Fig. 1, Additional file 3). The response rate was 54%. Out of the 19 authors who responded, 14 could not provide the requested data [26–39], two authors contributed data we could not use [40, 41], and three authors provided data we included in our meta-analyses [42–44]. The main reasons for not being able to include studies without author response were absence of stratification of data by gestational age < 28 weeks or birth weight < 1000 g, by birth order or by presentation in the original paper (Additional file 3). For the 16 out of 19 authors (84%) who responded favorably to our request for additional information, the reason for not being able to provide data or include the provided data in the study were the same (Additional file 3).

Description of studies

We included three observational studies from high-income countries: France, Israel and Slovenia. The analyzed data were collected between 2003 and 2012 (Table 1). The comparison in all three studies was mode of delivery - caesarean section or vaginal delivery - for both twins.

Outcomes were not stratified for our population of interest in the original studies, namely cephalic/non-cephalic twin pairs <28 weeks, and hence the data were provided to us by all three authors upon request. Gestational age ranged from 22^{+0}–27^{+6} weeks across the three studies, and the outcomes were provided separately for each twin. One set of twins underwent a combined delivery, whereby the first twin was delivered vaginally and the second twin by caesarean section in Boukerrou 2011 [43]. The outcomes for this twin pair were included in the respective mode of delivery of each of the twin. We initially planned to include studies with at least 10 twin pairs, however, due to the paucity of studies meeting our inclusion criteria, and in order to maximize the number of twins, we included studies with eight or more twin pairs.

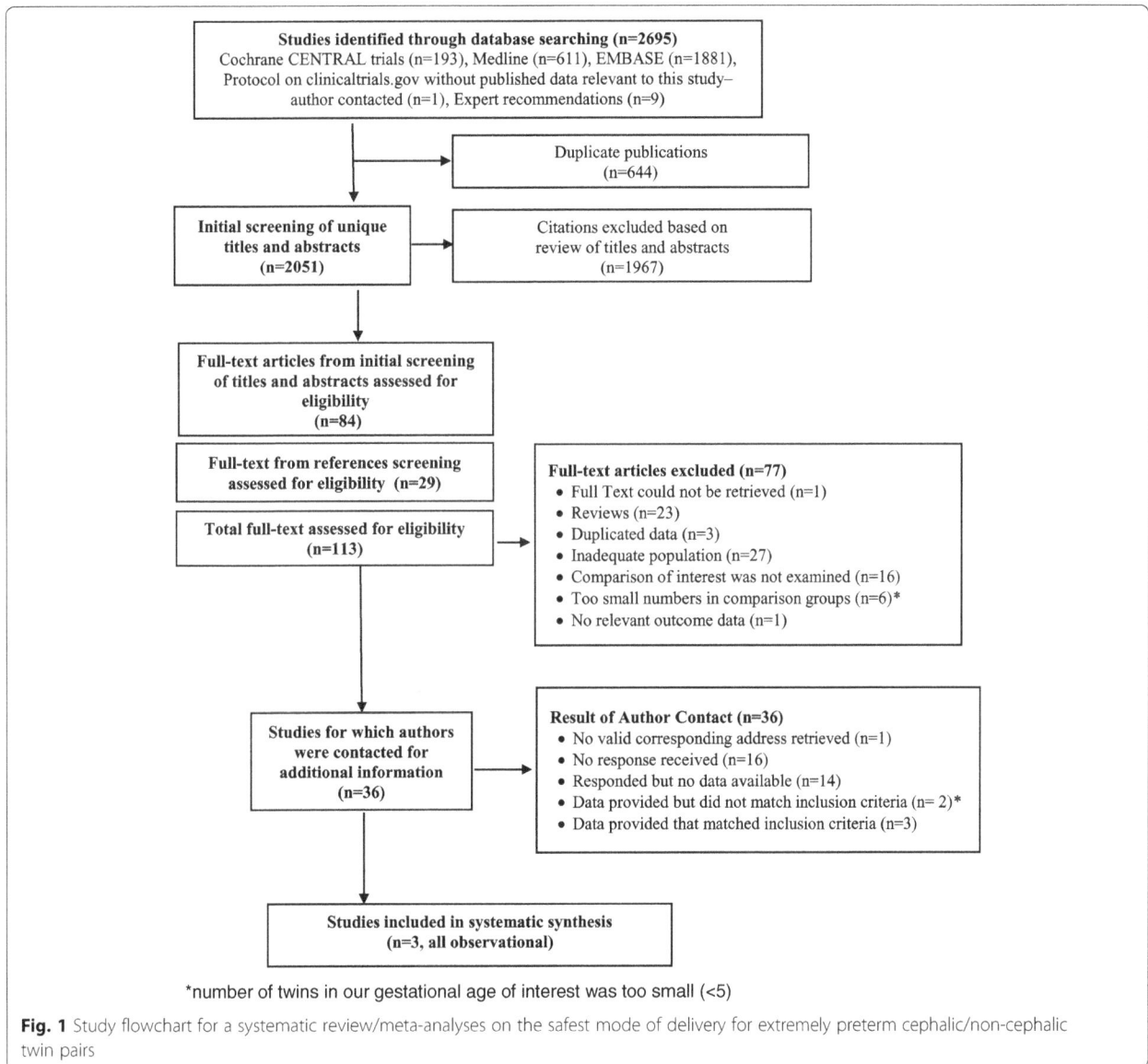

Fig. 1 Study flowchart for a systematic review/meta-analyses on the safest mode of delivery for extremely preterm cephalic/non-cephalic twin pairs

Risk of bias assessment

According to our modified NOS, all three studies were at high risk of bias, scoring three points out of the maximum of eight (Table 2). All studies lost one point in the Outcome category, as they did not account for loss to follow-up. None of the studies addressed any of the key confounders for our outcome of interest (i.e. caesarean section for fetal distress, outborn status, ANCS use and clinical chorioamnionitis), and hence no points were allotted for the Comparability criteria.

All twins from Boukerrou [43] and Barzilay [44] were planned for active resuscitation. Bricelj 2016 [42] could not confirm active resuscitation for all twins, and therefore we included their data only for twins born at $25^{+0}–27^{+6}$ weeks in our analysis.

Effects of mode of delivery

In cephalic/non-cephalic twin pairs delivered by caesarean section compared to vaginal birth at $24^{+0}–27^{+6}$ weeks the odds ratio for our composite outcome of neonatal death and severe brain injury for the cephalic first twin was 0.35 (95% CI 0.00–92.61, two studies, $I^2 = 76\%$, Fig. 2, Table 3), 1.69 for the non-cephalic second twin (95% CI 0.04–72.81, two studies, $I^2 = 55\%$) and 0.83 for both twins (95% CI 0.05–13.43, two studies, $I^2 = 56\%$).

The odds ratios of neonatal death were for twins delivered between $24^{+0}–27^{+6}$ weeks by caesarean section compared to vaginally were 0.36 for the cephalic first twins (95% CI 0.03–4.40, two studies, $I^2 = 0\%$, Fig. 3), 1.31 for the non-cephalic second twins (95% CI 0.02–79.60, two studies, $I^2 = 66\%$), and 0.73 for both twins together (95% CI 0.10–5.46, two studies, $I^2 = 26\%$).

Table 1 Study characteristics in a systematic review/meta-analyses on the safest mode of delivery for extremely preterm cephalic/non-cephalic twin pairs

Author, Publication Year, Country; Study Period; Study Design	Inclusion and exclusion criteria	Usual practice regarding twin delivery	Outcomes in original study*
Boukerrou, 2011 France; 2006–2011; Prospective cohort	**Inclusion:** All twin births during the study period **Exclusion:** HOM, stillbirths, births less 24 weeks	For non-cephalic second twin, breech extraction with or without internal podalic version is preferred.	**Neonatal death (0–28 days), graded IVH and PVL** (in provided data only)
Barzilay, 2015 Israel; 2004–2011; Retrospective cohort	**Inclusion:** All twin births with second twin birthweight less 1500 g **Exclusion:** Birth less 24 weeks, fetal death of one or both twins, major malformation in one or both twins	Allow vaginal delivery of cephalic-non-cephalic twin pairs regardless of EFW or GA if EFW of twin B is not 20% higher than that of twin A. Breech extraction is preferred for delivering non-cephalic twin B.	Apgar 5 min, Cord blood PH, **Neonatal death (not otherwise specified)**, Birth trauma, **RDS**, Sepsis, NEC, **IVH, Composite adverse neonatal outcome** (neonatal death, RDS, sepsis, NEC, or IVH grade ≥ 3)
Bricelj, 2016 Slovenia; 2003–2012; Retrospective cohort	**Inclusion:** All deliveries from 22 weeks or birth weight 500 g up to less than 37 weeks **Exclusion:** Delayed births, combined deliveries, stillbirths (in provided data only)	Not stated	TTN, **RDS, Ventilation need**

HOM high order multiple pregnancies, *EFW* estimated fetal weight, *GA* gestational age, *IVH* intraventricular hemorrhage, *PVL* periventricular leukomalacia, *RDS* respiratory distress syndrome, *NEC* necrotizing enterocolitis, *TTN* transient tachypnea of the newborn * Outcomes provided by the authors for twins less 28 weeks are **bolded**

The odds ratios of severe brain injury in survivors, for twins delivered between 24^{+0}–27^{+6} weeks by caesarean section compared to vaginally were 0.59 for the cephalic first twins (95% CI 0.00–154.35, two studies, I^2 = 74%, Fig. 4), 1.00 for the non-cephalic second twins (95% CI 0.02–40.28, two studies, I^2 = N/A), and 0.76 for both twins together (95% CI 0.03–17.34, two studies, I^2 = 48%). Data on severe brain injury were missing for five surviving twins out of fourteen (36%) in the data by Boukerrou 2011 [43] and for two surviving twins out of fourteen in the data from Barzilay 2015 [44].

For our secondary outcomes, the odds ratios of respiratory distress syndrome for twins delivered between 25^{+0}–27^{+6} weeks by caesarean section compared to vaginally were 0.23 for the cephalic first twins (95% CI 0.01–6.25, two studies, I^2 = N/A, Fig. 5), 1.60 for the non-cephalic second twins (95% CI 0.12–20.99, two studies, I^2 = N/A), and 0.77 for both twins together (95% CI 0.10–5.87, two studies, I^2 = 0%). Data for other secondary infant and maternal outcomes were not available.

We were unable to stratify any of our outcomes by gestational age categories, as the sample sizes were too small. We could not perform any of the planned subgroup analyses due to lack of data in primary studies. Since all studies were at high risk of bias, we could not perform the planned sensitivity analyses. We were unable to pool adjusted data, since that data was lacking for our population of interest in the primary studies.

Quality of the evidence (GRADE)
We downgraded the quality of evidence due to serious risk of bias and imprecision, but not due to inconsistency and

Table 2 Bias assessment in a systematic review/meta-analyses on the safest mode of delivery for extremely preterm cephalic/non-cephalic twin pairs

Study ID Author, Year, Country	Total	Selection		Outcome		Comparability			
		Representativeness of the exposed cohort	Selection of the non- exposed cohort	Assessment of outcome	Adequacy of follow up of cohorts	Emergent caesarean for fetal distress	Clinical Chorioamnionitis	Outborn Status	ANCS
Boukerrou, 2011 France	3/8	★	★	★	–	–	–	–	–
Barzilay, 2015 Israel	3/8	★	★	★	–	–	–	–	–
Bricelj, 2016 Slovenia	3/8	★	★	★	–	–	–	–	–

ANCS antenatal corticosteroids, ★ = 1 point awarded, "- "= no points awarded. Assessed risk of bias of observational studies using a modified Newcastle Ottawa Scale

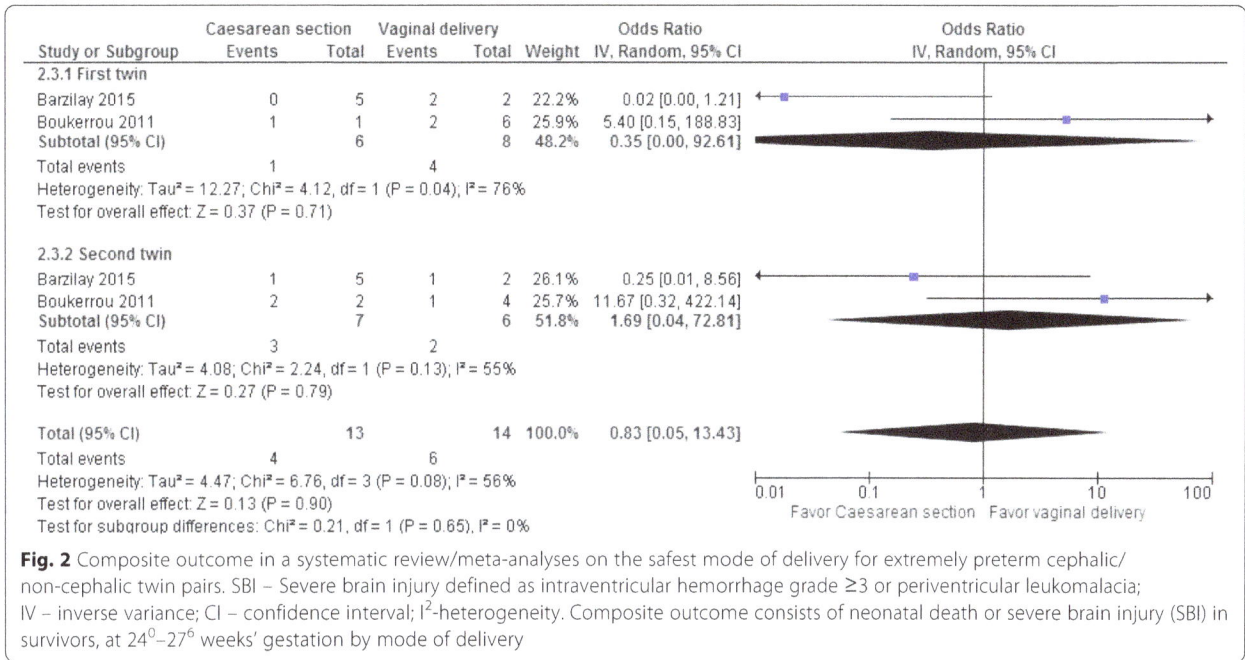

Fig. 2 Composite outcome in a systematic review/meta-analyses on the safest mode of delivery for extremely preterm cephalic/non-cephalic twin pairs. SBI – Severe brain injury defined as intraventricular hemorrhage grade ≥3 or periventricular leukomalacia; IV – inverse variance; CI – confidence interval; I²-heterogeneity. Composite outcome consists of neonatal death or severe brain injury (SBI) in survivors, at 24^0–27^6 weeks' gestation by mode of delivery

indirectness. Publication bias could not be assessed, as the number of studies was <10 per outcome. We could not upgrade the evidence, as a large effect was not present, and confounding was not accounted for; the dose-response was not applicable for our meta-analyses. The overall quality of evidence was very low for our primary composite outcome (neonatal death or SBI), for neonatal death and for respiratory distress syndrome (Table 3, Additional file 4).

Discussion
Main findings
In this systematic review on the safest mode of delivery for extremely preterm cephalic/non-cephalic twin pairs, we found scarce data. Analysis did not favour either caesarean section or vaginal birth. The confidence intervals were wide and encompassed one for our primary composite outcome of neonatal death and severe brain injury, as well as for neonatal death alone or severe brain

Table 3 Outcomes in a systematic review/meta-analyses on the safest mode of delivery for extremely preterm cephalic/non-cephalic twin pairs

Outcome	GA category (weeks)	Number of studies		CS (n/N)	VD (n/N)	OR (95% CI) for CS	I² (%)	GRADE Quality of the evidence*
Neonatal death or Severe Brain Injury in survivors	24^{+0}–27^{+6}	2	First twin (cephalic)	1/6	4/8	OR 0.35 (0.00–92.61)	76	Very Low
			Second twin (non-cephalic)	3/7	2/6	OR 1.69 (0.04–72.81)	55	
			Both twins	4/13	6/14	OR 0.83 (0.05–13.43)	56	
Neonatal death	24^{+0}–27^{+6}	2	First twin (cephalic)	0/7	2/10	OR 0.36 (0.03–4.40)	0	Very low
			Second twin (non-cephalic)	2/8	2/9	OR 1.31 (0.02–79.60)	66	
			Both twins	2/15	4/19	OR 0.73 (0.10–5.46)	26	
Severe Brain Injury in survivors	24^{+0}–27^{+6}	2	First twin (cephalic)	1/6	2/6	OR 0.59 (0.00–154.35)	74	Very low
			Second twin (non-cephalic)	1/5	0/4	OR 1.00 (0.02–40.28)	N/A	
			Both twins	2/11	2/10	OR 0.76 (0.03–17.34)	48	
Respiratory distress syndrome (RDS)	25^{+0}–27^{+6}	2	First twin (cephalic)	13/14	15/15	OR 0.23 (0.01–6.25)	N/A	Very low
			Second twin (non-cephalic)	13/14	13/15	OR 1.60 (0.12–20.99)	N/A	
			Both twins	26/28	28/30	OR 0.77 (0.10–5.87)	0	

GA gestational age, *CS* caesarean section, *VD* vaginal delivery, *n* number of cases within exposure group, *N* total number in exposure group, *OR* odds ratio, *CI* confidence interval, Severe Brain Injury defined as intraventricular hemorrhage grade ≥ 3 or periventricular leukomalacia, *N/A* not applicable. *Based on the Grading of Recommendations Assessment, Development and Evaluation quality of evidence assessment (GRADE) approach

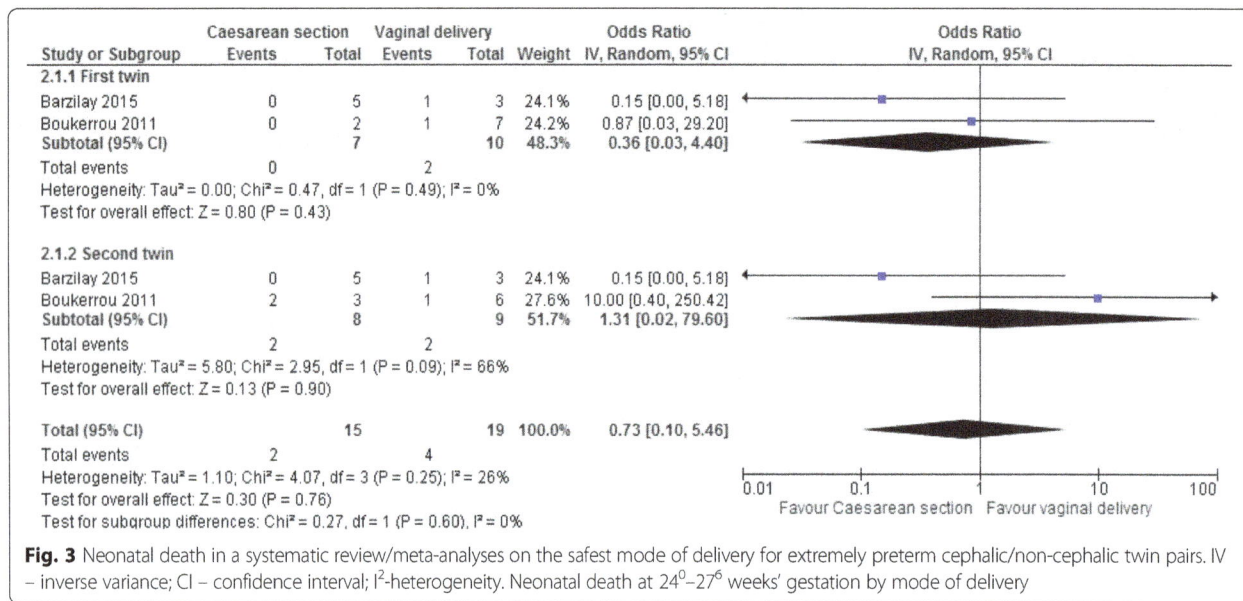

Fig. 3 Neonatal death in a systematic review/meta-analyses on the safest mode of delivery for extremely preterm cephalic/non-cephalic twin pairs. IV – inverse variance; CI – confidence interval; I^2-heterogeneity. Neonatal death at 24^0–27^6 weeks' gestation by mode of delivery

injury alone for the cephalic first twins, non-cephalic second twins and when both twins were considered together.

Strengths and limitations

This systematic review has some strengths, including its focus on a specific clinical dilemma for which consensus is lacking thus far. We strove to provide a clinically relevant assessment of the evidence regarding the safest mode of delivery for extremely preterm twins, and therefore we accounted for gestational age, birth order and presentation of each twin in our study design, as each of those could impact neonatal outcomes. We aimed at controlling the four major confounders of outcome in extremely preterm births (caesarean section for fetal distress, outborn status, ANCS use and clinical chorioamnionitis). Furthermore, the safest mode of delivery for twins cannot be inferred from singleton data as twinning itself may affect outcomes [45] and outcomes in both twins have to be looked at since the impact on both should be considered when choosing a mode of delivery.

Our systematic review also has limitations, the main one being the lack of primary randomized data on the safest mode of delivery of extremely preterm infants. Although the most ideal study design would be a randomized controlled trial, previous RCTs in singletons have failed [46–48], and hence it is unlikely that another large-enough RCT will be mounted in the near future.

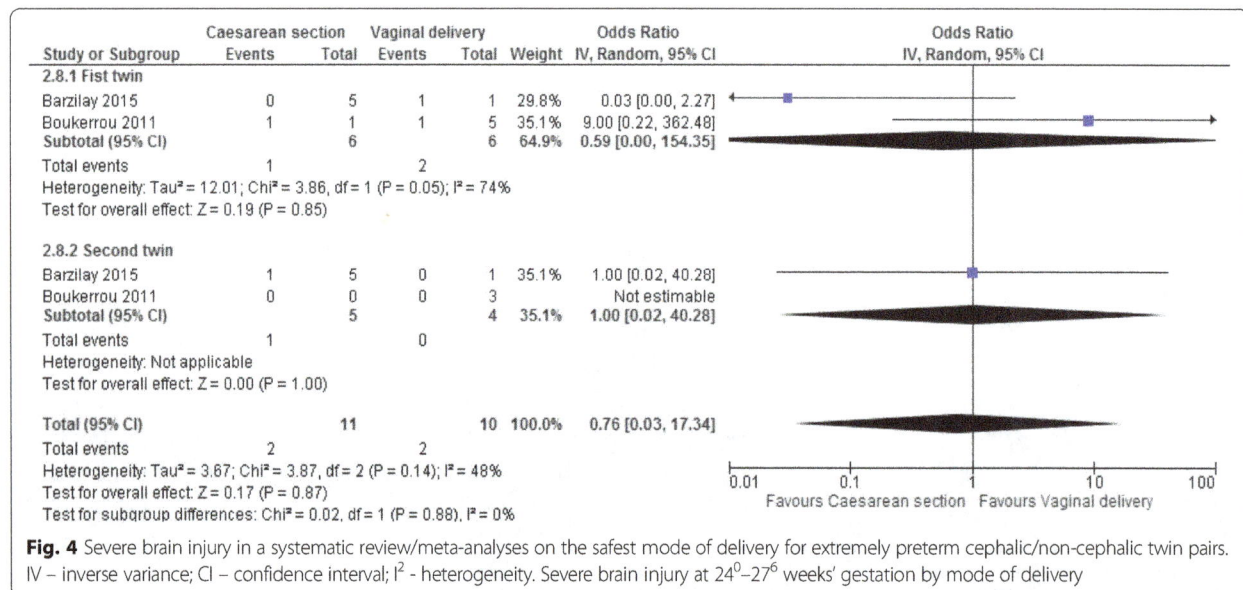

Fig. 4 Severe brain injury in a systematic review/meta-analyses on the safest mode of delivery for extremely preterm cephalic/non-cephalic twin pairs. IV – inverse variance; CI – confidence interval; I^2 – heterogeneity. Severe brain injury at 24^0–27^6 weeks' gestation by mode of delivery

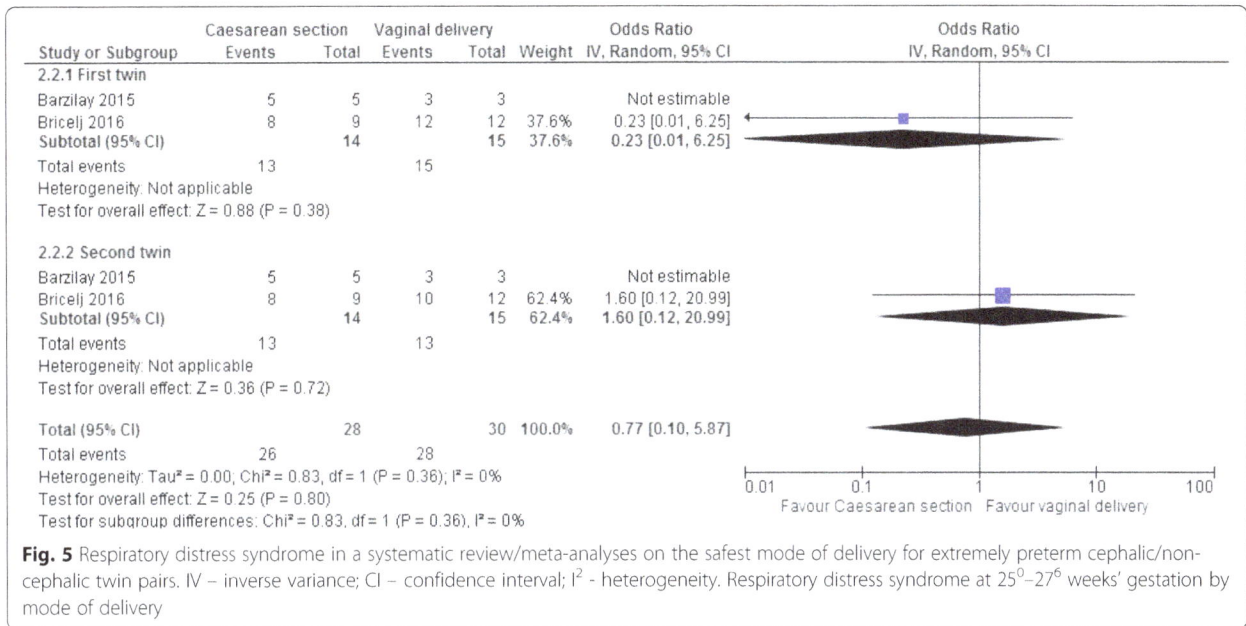

Fig. 5 Respiratory distress syndrome in a systematic review/meta-analyses on the safest mode of delivery for extremely preterm cephalic/non-cephalic twin pairs. IV – inverse variance; CI – confidence interval; I² - heterogeneity. Respiratory distress syndrome at 25^0–27^6 weeks' gestation by mode of delivery

We therefore must rely on alternative research methodology. The observational data were scarce in terms of the number of extremely preterm twins available for analyses, which may be the reason for lack of significant differences, even in our pooled data, between outcomes after caesarean and vaginal delivery. Moreover, although we addressed the most important confounder, active resuscitation, by requiring it for inclusion in the analysis, other key confounders were not available for our subpopulation in the primary studies, which may also contribute to the lack of significant differences. Additionally, over the 1994–2017 period, the quality and accuracy of ultrasound estimation of gestational age varied. It would have been preferable to have data according to planned mode of delivery, rather than actual, but this was not available.

Lastly, maybe the most striking limitation was the overall sparsity of available data from primary studies that met our inclusion criteria.

Comparing our findings to existing literature

In comparing our results to previous reviews on the impact of mode of delivery in twins, we found that some previous systematic reviews did not focus on the extreme preterm period, but rather on twins above 32 weeks of gestation or above 1500 g [49, 50], while others were unable to control for gestational age in their analysis [51]. To our knowledge, only narrative reviews have addressed the mode of delivery of extremely preterm twins. The first one included data from the 1980's and early 1990's, which are not as relevant to current clinical decision making given the subsequent advances in neonatal management and survival [52]. Nevertheless,

these authors concluded that: "*Management of low birth weight nonvertex second twins remains controversial... The retrospective nature and possibility for type II error of the majority of studies examining safety of vaginal delivery of the LBW nonvertex second twin makes definitive conclusions regarding vaginal delivery of these infants difficult.*" A more recent review encompassed three additional studies from the 2000's, but none of those stratified outcomes for twins below 1500 g or 34 weeks [53]. The authors concluded again that: "*The optimal mode of delivery in the preterm twin gestation (particularly those less than 2000 g) continues to be debated, data... remains limited.*"

Some individual cohort studies addressing the safest mode of delivery for first or second twins, with a birth weight below 1500 g or a gestational age less than 34 weeks have found a decrease in risk of death and/or morbidity with caesarean section [54–59] while others have not [28–30, 44, 60–65]. However, these studies neither stratified by gestational age less than 28 weeks nor by extremely low birth weight (< 1000 g), nor by presentation of the second twin.

In extremely preterm twins, prior to 1994 and hence advent of antenatal corticosteroid therapy and other advances in neonatal management, some studies had found a decrease in the risk of mortality with caesarean section in second twins weighing 601–999 g [66] and those weighing less than 1000 g [67]. More recently, Thomas 2016 [68] found an increase in survival with caesarean section for multiples from 24 to 26 weeks' gestation presenting as non-footling breech, but that difference was no longer significant after adjustment for gestational age, chorioamnionitis and maternal age.

This study did not stratify data by birth order, and included higher order multiples.

Garite 2004 [69] also found no significant difference in mortality according to mode of delivery in 24–26 week twins stratified by birth order but not by presentation. They hypothesized: *"It may also be that adverse outcomes, which tend to dominate most studies, in second twins that are seen in vaginal deliveries may be related primarily to term or near-term babies."* This would go along with our analyses, even though not significant, in which the point estimate favoured caesarean section for the cephalic first twins as well as when all twins were considered together but not for the second twin.

Yang 2005 [54] focused on non-cephalic second twins, and stratified for those weighing less than 500–1499 g, concluding that vaginal delivery increased the risk of mortality compared to caesarean section, even when comparing to caesarean section performed for the second twin in the context of a combined delivery. Wen 2004 [56], studying second twins in any presentation, found the same protective effect of caesarean section below 36 weeks, but not after 36 weeks, when the only increase in mortality for the second twin was in fact in the case of combined delivery. These observations suggest that in very preterm twins and likely extremely preterm twins, in contrast to higher gestational ages, the mode of delivery may interact in a different manner with birth order and presentation to influence mortality and morbidity. The exact gestational age at which such an interaction tips is unknown and warrants more research.

Conclusion

In this systematic review of the safest mode of delivery for extremely preterm cephalic/non-cephalic twin pairs, we did not find a significant reduction in the odds of our composite outcome, neonatal death and severe brain injury, with either mode of delivery. The extremely limited primary and clinically relevant data available highlights the need for further appropriately designed research regarding safest mode of delivery for extremely preterm twins. An appropriate method would have to include details relevant to clinical decision making in that field.

Future research should seek to understand the long term neurodevelopmental outcomes and maternal outcomes in relation to mode of delivery of extremely preterm twins.

Additional files

Additional file 1: Search strategy for a systematic review and meta-analysis on the safest mode of delivery for extremely preterm cephalic/non-cephalic twin pairs.

Additional file 2: Secondary infant and maternal outcomes included in a systematic review and meta-analyses on the safest mode of delivery for extremely preterm cephalic/non-cephalic twin pairs.

Additional file 3: Summary table of excluded studies in a systematic review and meta-analyses on the safest mode of delivery for extremely preterm cephalic/non-cephalic twin pairs - author contacted but could not provide the necessary data or did not respond.

Additional file 4: GRADE assessment for the primary composite outcome (neonatal death and severe brain injury), neonatal death and respiratory distress syndrome in a systematic review and meta-analyses for the safest mode of delivery for extremely preterm cephalic/non-cephalic twin pairs.

Acknowledgements
We are grateful to the authors of the primary studies who have provided additional data for the meta-analyses: Malik Boukerrou and Pierre-Yves Robillard (CHR de la Réunion, groupe hospitalier Sud-Réunion, Centre d'Études Périnatales de l'Océan Indien (CEPOI); Eran Barzilay (Sackler School of Medicine, Tel Aviv University); Katja Bricelj (University Medical Centre, Ljubljana,Slovenia) and Isaac Blickstein (Kaplan Medical Center and Hadassah- Hebrew University school of Medicine, Jerusalem, Israel); Norman Ginsberg (Northwestern University Medical School, Chicago) and Priyanka Gupta (University College of Medical Sciences, Delhi). We value the contribution of Ms. Neera Bhatnager, BSc, MLIS, Head of Systems, Coordinator of Research and Graduate Education Support, Health Sciences Library, McMaster University, for her assistance in developing the search strategies. We thank Simran Sharma and Kristen Viaje for supporting administrative aspects of the study.

Funding
The authors declare no source of financial support of the study, including provision of supplies or services from a commercial organization. SDM is supported by a CIHR Canada Research Chair (950–229,920). CIHR had no role in the design and conduct of the study; collection, management, analysis, and interpretation of the data; preparation, review, or approval of the manuscript; and decision to submit the manuscript for publication.

Authors' contributions
CD contributed to the study conception, performed the searches, reviewed titles and abstracts, reviewed full text articles, extracted data, performed data analyses and drafted the manuscript. AMLM contributed to the study conception, performed the duplicate review of titles and abstracts, review of full text articles, and data extraction, as well as reviewed the manuscript. MG contributed to the study conception and reviewed the manuscript for important intellectual content. AM contributed to the study conception, providing clinical expertise to neonatal aspects of the study and reviewed the manuscript for important intellectual content. SDM conceived the study idea, supervised the project and reviewed the manuscript for important intellectual content. All authors read and approved the final manuscript.

Competing interests
The authors declare that they have no competing interests.

Author details
[1]Department of Obstetrics & Gynecology, McMaster University, 1280 Main St W, HSC 3N52B, Hamilton, ON L8S 4K1, Canada. [2]Department of Health Research Methods, Evidence, and Impact, McMaster University, 1280 Main St W, Hamilton, ON L8S 4K1, Canada. [3]Department of Pediatrics, McMaster University, 1280 Main St W, Hamilton, ON L8S 4K1, Canada.

References

1. March of Dimes, PMNCH, Save the Children, World Health Organization. Born too soon: the global action report on preterm birth. World Health Organization. 2012.

2. Institute of Medicine. Preterm birth: causes, consequences, and prevention. In: Behrman RE, Butler AS, editors. Neurodevelopmental, health, and family outcomes for infants born preterm. Washington, D.C: National Academy Press; 2007.

3. Räisänen S, Gissler M, Saari J, Kramer M, Heinonen S. Contribution of risk factors to extremely, very and moderately preterm births–register-based analysis of 1,390,742 singleton births. PLoS One. 2013;8:e60660.

4. Shaw GM, Wise PH, Mayo J, Carmichael SL, Ley C, Lyell DJ, et al. Maternal prepregnancy body mass index and risk of spontaneous preterm birth. Paediatr Perinat Epidemiol. 2014;28:302–11.

5. Ananth CV, Chauhan SP. Epidemiology of Periviable births: the impact and neonatal outcomes of twin pregnancy. Clin Perinatol. 2017;44(2):333–45.

6. Chasen ST, Spiro SJ, Kalish RB, Chervenak FA. Changes in fetal presentation in twin pregnancies. J Matern Fetal Neonatal Med. 2005;17:45–8.

7. Bergenhenegouwen L, Meertens L, Schaaf J, Nijhuis J, Mol B, Kok M, et al. Vaginal delivery versus caesarean section in preterm breech delivery: a systematic review. J Obstet & Gynecol Reprod Biol. 2014;172:1–6.

8. Tucker-Edmonds B, McKenzie F, Macheras M, Srinivas SK, Lorch SA. Morbidity and mortality associated with mode of delivery for breech periviable deliveries. Am J Obstet Gynecol. 2015;213:70.e1–12.

9. Kayem G, Combaud V, Lorthe E, Haddad B, Descamps P, Marpeau L, et al. Mortality and morbidity in early preterm breech singletons: impact of a policy of planned vaginal delivery. J Obstet Gynecol Reprod Biol. 2015;192:61–5.

10. Grabovac M, Karim JN, Isayama T, Korale Liyanage S, McDonald SD. What is the safest mode of birth for extremely preterm breech singleton infants who are actively resuscitated? A systematic review and metaanalyses. BJOG. 2017. doi:10.1111/1471-0528.14938. [Epub ahead of print].

11. Barrett JFR, Hannah ME, Hutton EK, Willan AR, Allen AC, Armson BA, et al. A randomized trial of planned cesarean or vaginal delivery for twin pregnancy. N Engl J Med. 2013;369:1295–305.

12. Kilby MD, Bricker L on behalf of the Royal College of Obstetricians and Gynaecologists. Management of monochorionic twin pregnancy. BJOG. 2016;124:e1–e45.

13. Barrett J, Bocking A. The SOGC consensus statement: management of twin pregnancies. J SOGC. 2000;91:5–15.

14. Vayssiere C, Benoist G, Blondel B, Deruelle P, Favre R, Gallot D, et al. Twin pregnancies: guidelines for clinical practice from the French College of Gynaecologists and Obstetricians (CNGOF). J Obstet Gynecol Reprod Biol. 2011;156:12–7.

15. Hayes EJ. Practice bulletin no. 169: multifetal gestations: twin, triplet, and higher-order multifetal pregnancies. Obstet Gynecol. 2016;128:e131–46.

16. Higgins JPT, Altman DG, Gotzsche PC, Juni P, Moher D, Oxman AD, et al. The Cochrane Collaboration's tool for assessing risk of bias in randomised trials. BMJ. 2011;343:d5928.

17. Moher D, Liberati A, Tetzlaff J, Altman DG, Group P. Preferred reporting items for systematic reviews and meta-analyses: the PRISMA statement. Int J Surg. 2010;8:336–41.

18. Villar J, Cheikh Ismail L, Victora CG, Ohuma EO, Bertino E, Altman DG, et al. International standards for newborn weight, length, and head circumference by gestational age and sex: the newborn cross-sectional study of the INTERGROWTH-21st project. Lancet. 2014;384:857–68.

19. Lorenz JM. The outcome of extreme prematurity. Semin Perinatol. 2001;25:348–59.

20. Cunningham F, Leveno KJ, Bloom SL, Spong CY, Dashe JS, Hoffman BL, et al. Overview of obstetrics. In: Williams obstetrics, twenty-fourth edition. New York, NY: McGraw-Hill; 2013.

21. de Waal CG, Weisglas-Kuperus N, van Goudoever JB, Walther FJ, NeoNed Study G, Group LNFS. Mortality, neonatal morbidity and two year follow-up of extremely preterm infants born in The Netherlands in 2007. PLoS One. 2012;7:e41302.

22. Guyatt G, Oxman AD, Akl EA, Kunz R, Vist G, Brozek J, et al. GRADE guidelines: 1. Introduction-GRADE evidence profiles and summary of findings tables. J Clin Epidemiol. 2011;64:383–94.

23. Cochrane Community. RevMan 5 Download. [http://community.cochrane.org/tools/review-production-tools/revman-5/revman-5-download]. Accessed Jun 8.

24. Sterne JA, Sutton AJ, Ioannidis JP, Terrin N, Jones DR, Lau J, et al. Recommendations for examining and interpreting funnel plot asymmetry in meta-analyses of randomised controlled trials. BMJ. 2011;343:d4002.

25. Schmitz T, Prunet C, Azria E, Bohec C, Bongain A, Chabanier P, et al. Association between planned cesarean delivery and neonatal mortality and morbidity in twin pregnancies. Obstet Gynecol. 2017;129:986–95.

26. Smith GC, Pell JP, Dobbie R. Birth order, gestational age, and risk of delivery related perinatal death in twins: retrospective cohort study. BMJ. 2002;325:1004.

27. Marttila R, Kaprio J, Hallman M. Respiratory distress syndrome in twin infants compared with singletons. Am J Obstet Gynecol. 2004;191:271–6.

28. Shinwell ES, Blickstein I, Lusky A, Reichman B. Effect of birth order on neonatal morbidity and mortality among very low birthweight twins: a population based study. Arch Dis Child Fetal Neonatal Ed. 2004;89: F145–8.

29. Vidovics M, Jacobs VR, Fischer T, Maier B. Comparison of fetal outcome in premature vaginal or cesarean breech delivery at 24-37 gestational weeks. Arch Gynecol Obstet. 2014;290:271–81.

30. Sheay W, Ananth CV, Kinzler WL. Perinatal mortality in first- and second-born twins in the United States. Obstet Gynecol. 2004;103:63–70.

31. Smith GCS, Fleming KM, White IR. Birth order of twins and risk of perinatal death related to delivery in England, Northern Ireland, and Wales, 1994-2003: retrospective cohort study. BMJ. 2007;334:576.

32. Malloy MH. Impact of cesarean section on neonatal mortality rates among very preterm infants in the United States, 2000-2003. Pediatrics. 2008;122:285–92.

33. Jain NJ, Kruse LK, Demissie K, Khandelwal M. Impact of mode of delivery on neonatal complications: trends between 1997 and 2005. J Matern Fetal Neonatal Med. 2009;22:491–500.

34. Markestad T, Kaaresen PI, Ronnestad A, Reigstad H, Lossius K, Medbo S, et al. Early death, morbidity, and need of treatment among extremely premature infants. Pediatrics. 2005;115:1289–98.

35. Hogberg U, Hakansson S, Serenius F, Holmgren PA. Extremely preterm cesarean delivery: a clinical study. Acta Obstet Gynecol Scand. 2006;85: 1442–7.

36. Usta IM, Nassar AH, Awwad JT, Nakad TI, Khalil AM, Karam KS. Comparison of the perinatal morbidity and mortality of the presenting twin and its co-twin. J Perinatol. 2002;22:391–6.

37. Usta IM, Rechdan JB, Khalil AM, Nassar AH. Mode of delivery for vertex-nonvertex twin gestations. Int J Gynecol Obstet. 2005;88:9–14.

38. Tadic E, Stefanic-Mitrovic D, Milic N, Kulisic D, Baraka K. Should we increase the number of cases of cesarean sections?. [Croatian]. Gynaecologia et Perinatologia. 2003;12:33–6.

39. Sbeiti N, Ziedeh F, Ramadan M, Lababidi H, Rajab M. Outcomes of premature and very-low-birth-weight infants from 1991 to 2002. J Med Liban. 2005;53:162–7.

40. Gupta P, Faridi MM, Goel N, Zaidi ZH. Reappraisal of twinning: epidemiology and outcome in the early neonatal period. Singap Med J. 2014;55:310–7.

41. Ginsberg NA, Levine EM. Delivery of the second twin. Int J Gynecol Obstet. 2005;91:217–20.

42. Bricelj K, Tul N, Lasic M, Bregar AT, Verdenik I, Lucovnik M, et al. Respiratory morbidity in twins by birth order, gestational age and mode of delivery. J Perinat Med. 2016;44:899–902.

43. Boukerrou M, Robillard PY, Gerardin P, Heisert M, Kauffmann E, Laffitte A, et al. Modes of deliveries of twins as a function of their presentation. A study of 371 pregnancies. Gynecol Obstet Fertil. 2011;39:76–80.

44. Barzilay E, Mazaki-Tovi S, Amikam U, de Castro H, Haas J, Mazkereth R, et al. Mode of delivery of twin gestation with very low birthweight: is vaginal delivery safe? Am J Obstet Gynecol. 2015;213(219):e211–8.

45. Shinwell ES. Neonatal morbidity of very low birth weight infants from multiple pregnancies. Obstet Gynecol Clin N Am. 2005;32:29–38. viii

46. Viegas OA, Ingemarsson I, Sim LP, Singh K, Cheng M, Ratnam SS, et al. Collaborative study on preterm breeches: vaginal delivery versus caesarean section. Asia Oceania J Obstet Gynaecol. 1985;11:349–55.

47. Zlatnik FJ. The Iowa premature breech trial. Am J Perinatol. 1993;10:60–3.

48. Penn ZJ, Steer PJ, Grant A. A multicentre randomised controlled trial comparing elective and selective caesarean section for the delivery of the preterm breech infant. Br J Obstet Gynaecol. 1996;103:684–9.

49. Hogle KL, Hutton EK, McBrien KA, Barrett JF, Hannah ME. Cesarean delivery for twins: a systematic review and meta-analysis. Am J Obstet Gynecol. 2003;188:220–7.

50. Steins Bisschop CN, Vogelvang TE, May AM, Schuitemaker NWE. Mode of delivery in non-cephalic presenting twins: a systematic review. Arch Gynecol Obstet. 2012;286:237–47.

51. Rossi AC, Mullin PM, Chmait RH. Neonatal outcomes of twins according to

birth order, presentation and mode of delivery: a systematic review and meta-analysis. BJOG. 2011;118:523–32.

52. Boggess KA, Chisholm CA. Delivery of the nonvertex second twin: a review of the literature. Obstet Gynecol Surv. 1997;52:728–35.

53. Hui D, Barrett JFR. Mode of delivery in term and preterm twins: a review. Fetal Matern Med Rev. 2014;25:1–11.

54. Yang Q, Wen SW, Chen Y, Krewski D, Fung Kee Fung K, Walker M. Neonatal death and morbidity in vertex-nonvertex second twins according to mode of delivery and birth weight. Am J Obstet Gynecol. 2005;192:840–7.

55. Wen SW, Fung Kee Fung K, Oppenheimer L, Demissie K, Yang Q, Walker M. Neonatal morbidity in second twin according to gestational age at birth and mode of delivery. Am J Obstet Gynecol. 2004;191:773–7.

56. Wen SW, Fung Kee Fung K, Oppenheimer L, Demissie K, Yang Q, Walker M. Neonatal mortality in second twin according to cause of death, gestational age, and mode of delivery. Am J Obstet Gynecol. 2004;191:778–83.

57. Ziadeh SM, Badria LF. Effect of mode of delivery on neonatal outcome of twins with birthweight under 1500 g. Arch Gynecol Obstet. 2000;264:128–30.

58. Herbst A, Kallen K. Influence of mode of delivery on neonatal mortality in the second twin, at and before term. BJOG. 2008;115:1512–7.

59. Chervenak FA, Johnson RE, Youcha S, Hobbins JC, Berkowitz RL. Intrapartum management of twin gestation. Obstet Gynecol. 1985;65:119–24.

60. Doyle LW, Hughes CD, Guaran RL, Quinn MA, Kitchen WH. Mode of delivery of preterm twins. Aust N Z J Obstet Gynaecol 1988;28:25-28.

61. Rydhstrom H. Prognosis for twins with birth weight less than 1500 gm: the impact of cesarean section in relation to fetal presentation. Am J Obstet Gynecol. 1990;163:528–33.

62. Davison L, Easterling TR, Jackson JC, Benedetti TJ. Breech extraction of low-birth-weight second twins: can cesarean section be justified? Am J Obstet Gynecol. 1992;166:497–502.

63. Winn HN, Cimino J, Powers J, Roberts M, Holcomb W, Artal R, et al. Intrapartum management of nonvertex second-born twins: a critical analysis. Am J Obstet Gynecol. 2001;185:1204–8.

64. Caukwell S, Murphy DJ. The effect of mode of delivery and gestational age on neonatal outcome of the non-cephalic- presenting second twin. Am J Obstet Gynecol. 2002;187:1356–61.

65. Sentilhes L, Oppenheimer A, Bouhours AC, Normand E, Haddad B, Descamps P, et al. Neonatal outcome of very preterm twins: policy of planned vaginal or cesarean delivery. Am J Obstet Gynecol. 2015; 213(73):e71–73.e77.

66. Barrett JM, Staggs SM, Van Hooydonk JE, Growdon JH, Killam AP, Boehm FH. The effect of type of delivery upon neonatal outcome in premature twins. Am J Obstet Gynecol. 1982;143:360–7.

67. Zhang J, Bowes WA Jr, Grey TW, McMahon MJ. Twin delivery and neonatal and infant mortality: a population-based study. Obstet Gynecol. 1996;88:593–8.

68. Thomas PE, Petersen SG, Gibbons K. The influence of mode of birth on neonatal survival and maternal outcomes at extreme prematurity: a retrospective cohort study. Aust N Z J Obstet Gynaecol. 2016;56:60–8.

69. Garite TJ, Clark RH, Elliott JP, Thorp JA. Twins and triplets: the effect of plurality and growth on neonatal outcome compared with singleton infants. Am J Obstet Gynecol. 2004;191:700–7.

Influence of weight gain, according to Institute of Medicine 2009 recommendation, on spontaneous preterm delivery in twin pregnancies

Paola Algeri[1*], Francesca Pelizzoni[1], Davide Paolo Bernasconi[2], Francesca Russo[1], Maddalena Incerti[1], Sabrina Cozzolino[1], Salvatore Andrea Mastrolia[1] and Patrizia Vergani[1]

Abstract

Backgrounds: Maternal total weight gain during pregnancy influences adverse obstetric outcomes in singleton pregnancies. However, its impact in twin gestation is less understood. Our objective was to estimate the influence of total maternal weight gain on preterm delivery in twin pregnancies.

Methods: We conducted a retrospective cohort study including diamniotic twin pregnancies with spontaneous labor delivered at 28 + 0 weeks or later. We analyzed the influence of total weight gain according to Institute of Medicine (IOM) cut-offs on the development of preterm delivery (both less than 34 and 37 weeks). Outcome were compared between under and normal weight gain and between over and normal weight gain separately using Fisher's exact test with Holm-Bonferroni correction.

Results: One hundred seventy five women were included in the study and divided into three groups: under (52.0%), normal (41.7%) and overweight gain (6.3%). Normal weight gain was associated with a reduction in the rate of preterm delivery compared to under and over weight gain [less than 34 weeks: under vs. normal OR 4.97 (1.76–14.02), over vs. normal OR 4.53 (0.89–23.08); less than 37 weeks: OR 3.16 (1.66–6.04) and 6.51 (1.30–32.49), respectively].

Conclusions: Normal weight gain reduces spontaneous preterm delivery compared to over and underweight gain.

Keywords: Twin pregnancy, Preterm delivery, Preterm labor, Weight gain, Institute of medicine recommendation

Background

Pre-gestational body mass index (pBMI), gestational body mass index (gBMI) and total weight gain influence the incidence of preterm delivery and other adverse obstetric outcomes in singletons [1, 2] but their effect on twins is poorly understood, although multiple pregnancies appear to have similar associations between these outcomes, pBMI or weight gain compared to singletons [1, 2]. Indeed, studies evaluating the role of both total and weekly weight gain in twin pregnancies identified a strong correlation between low total weight gain during pregnancy and preterm delivery (PD) [3, 4]. In 1990, the Institute of Medicine (IOM) proposed ranges of recommended total weight gain correlated to pBMI for singleton pregnancy and an optimal total weight gain between 15.9 and 20.5 kg not related to pBMI for twin pregnancy [5, 6].

In 2009, the IOM revised these guidelines and defined pBMI specific weight gain cut-off, also for twin pregnancies. Optimal ranges proposed for weight gain at term (≥ 37 weeks) are: 17–25 kg for normal weighted women (pBMI 18.5–24.9), 14–23 kg for over weighted women (pBMI 25–29.9) and 11–19 kg for obese women (pBMI 30 or more). No recommendations were given for underweighted women (pBMI less than 18.5) [7].

This is of higher importance due to the rise in the incidence of twin pregnancies in the last three decades because of the older age at childbearing and of the diffusion

* Correspondence: p.algeri@campus.unimib.it
[1]Department of Obstetrics and Gynecology, University of Milano-Bicocca, S. Gerardo Hospital, MBBM Foundation, Via Pergolesi 33, Monza, 20900 Monza, Monza e Brianza, Italy
Full list of author information is available at the end of the article

of assisted reproductive technology [8]. Today, approximately 1 of 80 pregnancies is a multiple gestation, corresponding to 2.6% of all newborns (1–3% in Italy) and they are more frequently diamniotic. Multiple pregnancies present a higher incidence of maternal and fetal adverse outcomes compared to singleton ones [3, 9–13]. Twin pregnancies account for 12.2% of preterm births and 15.4% of neonatal deaths [14–16].

In literature, both pBMI and total weight gain were reported as important influencing factors in pregnancies outcomes. However, the studies took into consideration only one of these parameters at a time. New cut-offs proposed by IOM allowed an easier evaluation of maternal weight influence on obstetrics outcomes, not only in singleton pregnancies but also in twins.

Few studies evaluated the role of the new IOM guidelines in influencing preterm delivery in twins, also considering that IOM gave cut-offs only for gestational age at delivery ≥ 37 weeks [17–19].

In 2010, Fox et al. conducted a study on a cohort of twins divided into subgroups considering pBMI. They show that patients whose weight gain during pregnancy met or exceeded the revised 2009 IOM guidelines had significantly improved pregnancy outcomes such as longer gestation, less overall PD, less spontaneous PD and larger neonates compared to lower weight gain [18]. In 2012, also Quintero et al. found that a weight gain below recommended guidelines was associated with higher rates of spontaneous PD at less than 35 weeks in twin pregnancies [19].

A recent review tried to define the role of absolute total weight gain in the development of adverse pregnancy outcomes. The authors suggested that a higher incidence of PD was correlated with underweight gain and underlined a positive correlation between total weight gain and gestation length [20].

Gestational gain weight and pBMI have been proven to influence not only the risk of PD but also other obstetric outcomes, such as birth weight, hypertensive disorders, gestational diabetes and neonatal adverse outcomes [17].

Contrasting results were instead reported about hypertensive disorders: while some authors described higher incidence of gestational hypertension and preeclampsia in women with excessive weight gain, others showed no differences among different weight gain groups in a series of twin pregnancies delivering at term [5, 17, 20].

In light of the above and due to the scarcity of data available in the literature about this topic, we designed a study with the aim to estimate the influence of total weight gain according to the 2009 IOM recommendations on preterm delivery before 37 and 34 weeks in twin pregnancies with spontaneous onset of labor. Secondary outcomes were the possible correlation with small for gestational age (SGA) and large for gestational age (LGA), pregnancy hypertensive disorders, gestational diabetes, and neonatal adverse outcomes.

Methods

We performed a retrospective cohort study on diamniotic twin pregnancies delivered at more or equal 28 + 0 weeks after spontaneous onset of labor at our Institution (Fondazione MBBM, San Gerardo Hospital, University of Milano Bicocca, Monza, Italy), between January 2010 and December 2013.

Exclusion criteria of our study were induction of labor (15% of all twin pregnancies at our Institution), elective cesarean section (4% of all twin pregnancies at our Institution), monoamniotic twins, intrauterine demise, fetal malformations, twin-to-twin transfusion syndrome, and gestational age at delivery < 28 weeks. We decided to set a gestational age < 28 weeks at delivery as an exclusion criteria in order to have a better definition of the weight gain trend for each patient. A shorter pregnancy duration could be a confounding factor in defining the maternal weight gain.

Patients with pBMI < 18.5 were also excluded since there are no IOM recommendations for underweight patients in case of multiple pregnancies.

All twin gestations were followed according to national guidelines for management of twin pregnancy [21]. The protocol included maternal clinical assessment and ultrasound monitoring every 2 weeks, from 16 weeks, for monochorionic diamniotic pregnancies and every 4 weeks, starting from 20 weeks, for dichorionic diamniotic gestations.

At our Maternal-Fetal Unit, women undergo their first access at obstetric booking that is usually performed during the first trimester after a positive pregnancy test (<8 weeks of gestation). At the first visit we collect patient's medical and obstetric history, define gestational age (calculated based on the last menstrual period and confirmed by ultrasound assessment), as well as chorionicity. Baseline characteristics and pregnancy outcomes were entered into our database by an assigned physician at every patient's access and periodically reviewed by a senior consultant. pBMI was recorded at the first visit, and maternal weight was measured at each obstetric control until delivery.

Since self-report of pBMI can be affected by recall bias, we attempted to reduce the risk of bias with an early assessment of pregnant women as described above.

Total weight gain was calculated as the difference between maternal weight at delivery and pre-gestational weight. This parameter was used to classify women who delivered at 37 weeks or more according to IOM guidelines [7]. In case of preterm delivery (between 28 and 36 + 6 weeks), we calculated a weekly weight gain cut-off as total weight gain during pregnancy in kg/gestational weeks at delivery. We compared this weekly weight gain to a hypothesized weekly IOM cut-off, calculated as IOM cut-off at term/37 weeks, as previously reported, represented for normal-weight women, this was 1.0 lb. per week (37 lbs. over 37 weeks); for overweight women, this was 0.84 lb. per week (31 lbs. over 37 weeks); for obese women, this was 0.68 lb. per week (25 lbs. over 37 weeks) [18].

The data used for the analysis were already available for every patient as part of the clinical report of the Obstetric Department.

SGA and LGA were defined, respectively, as neonatal weight at birth < 10° centile and > 90° centile compared to Italian Neonatal Study (INeS) charts [22]. We considered as separate outcomes the occurrence of at least one twin SGA/LGA and both twins SGA/LGA.

We defined "gestational hypertensive disorders" as the presence of at least one among gestational hypertension, preeclampsia or eclampsia, diagnosed according to American Congress of Obstetricians and Gynecologists (ACOG) criteria [23].

Gestational diabetes was defined as any degree of glucose intolerance with onset or first recognition during pregnancy [24].

We defined composite adverse neonatal outcome as the presence of at least one among: need for neonatal resuscitation, respiratory distress syndrome, disseminated intravascular coagulation, intra-ventricular hemorrhage, leucomalacia, sepsis, necrotizing enteritis, retinopathy of prematurity and neonatal death.

The present work was exempt from IRB approval as per Institutional policy on retrospective studies. At our medical center, women provide a written consent to the use of their clinical anonymized and de-identified data upon admission.

Statistical analysis

Population characteristics were compared among IOM weight gain groups using Chi Square test (categorical variables) or One Way ANOVA (continuous variables). Primary and secondary outcomes rates were compared between under and normal gain and between over and normal gain separately using Fisher's exact test with Holm-Bonferroni correction. Logistic regression analysis was carried out in order to evaluate the independent effect of weight gain adjusted for pBMI on the outcomes. A separate model was built for each primary and secondary outcome. All the analyses were performed using the R software, version 3.0.2. A p value of less than 0.05 was considered significant.

Results

The incidence of twin pregnancies at our Institution was 2.5–3% during the study period.

A cohort of 175 diamniotic twin pregnancies was included in our study, considering exclusion criteria: 91 (52.0%) presented underweight gain, 73 (41.7%) normal weight gain and 11 (6.3%) over weight gain, according to IOM recommendations.

Table 1 shows general population characteristics in the three study groups, considering the IOM classification for total weight gain. The normal weight gain group had a higher mean gestational age at delivery compared with the under and over gain weight ones (respectively 36.5 ± 2.0, 35.3 ± 3.0, 35.3 ± 2.0 weeks). Normal and overweight gain patients presented higher neonatal weight at birth for both twins compared to the under gain ones (respectively 2494.11, 2974.55, 2196.54 g). The over weight gain group presented a higher incidence of pre–gestational over weighted patients (45.5%). The study groups did not differ for other characteristics.

The incidence of primary and secondary adverse outcomes was compared among the three groups, and the results are presented in Tables 2 and 3.

We found that the normal weight gain group presented a significant lower incidence of spontaneous PD compared to both under and over weight gain groups [respectively 39.7% vs 67.0% (p: 0.002); 39.7% vs 81.8% (p: 0.04)]. Underweight gain women presented significantly higher rates of early preterm spontaneous delivery compared to normal weight gain ones; a trend was also reported when overweight gain was compared to normal weight gain group [respectively 25.3% vs. 6.8% (p: 0.005); 27.3% vs. 6.8% (p: 0.13)].

No differences in the occurrence of SGA in one or both twins were observed among the three study groups. In addition, no cases of LGA were recorded. Gestational hypertensive disorders occurred in our population included 1 case of gestational hypertension and seven cases of preeclampsia in the underweight group, five and eight respectively in the normal weight, and one and six in the overweight one. No cases of eclampsia were reported. In the normal weight gain group, women presented a trend toward a higher incidence of hypertensive gestational diseases compared to underweight gain patients, even if not significant (17.8% vs. 7.7%, $p = 0.06$). This complication was significantly less frequent in the normal weight gain group compared with the over weight gain one (17.8% vs. 63.6%, $p = 0.006$). No difference in the incidence of gestational diabetes mellitus and neonatal adverse composite outcomes were reported in the three study groups, and we had no neonatal deaths.

The results of the bivariate analysis on both primary and secondary outcomes were confirmed in the multivariate logistic regression analysis, adjusting for the effect of pBMI (Tables 4 and 5, respectively). Both under and over weight gain increased the risk of PD compared to normal weight gain: ORs were 4.97 (1.76–14.02) and 4.53 (0.89–23.08) for early preterm and 3.16 (1.66–6.04) and 6.51 (1.30–32.49) for PD at less than 37 weeks

Table 1 Population general characteristics, according to weight gain groups

	Under (91)	Normal (73)	Over (11)	P value
Maternal age	34 ± 5.55	34 ± 5.86	34 ± 5.03	0.99
Nulliparity	52 (57.1%)	44 (60.3%)	8 (72.7%)	0.32
Smoker	3 (3.9%)	5 (6.8%)	1 (9.1%)	0.38
Chronic Hypertension	1 (1.1%)	1 (1.4%)	0	0.93
pBMI[a]	22.75 ± 4.44	23.00 ± 3.29	23.97 ± 2.50	0.70
18.5 ≤ pBMI[a] ≤ 24.9	74 (81.3%)	54 (74.0%)	6 (54.5%)	0.11
25 ≤ pBMI[a] ≤ 29.9	10 (11.0%)	15 (20.5%)	5 (45.5%)	*0.01*
pBMI[a] ≥ 30	7 (7.7%)	4 (5.5%)	0	0.57
Medically assisted procreation	16 (17.6%)	18 (24.7%)	4 (36.4%)	0.26
Mono- Chorionicity	13 (14.3%)	11 (15.1%)	2 (18.2%)	0.94
Clinical chorionamnionitis	1 (1.1%)	0	0	0.63
Preterm rupture of membranes[b]	30 (33.0%)	13 (17.8%)	3 (27.3%)	0.09
Gestational age at delivery (weeks)	35.3 ± 3.0	36.5 ± 2.0	35.3 ± 2.0	*0.002*
Vaginal delivery	34 (37.4%)	23 (31.5%)	4 (36.4%)	0.73
1st twin birth weight (gr)	2196.54 ± 592.16	2494.11 ± 426.87	2374.55 ± 471.63	*0.002*
2nd twin birth weight (gr)	2154.89 ± 499.41	2392.95 ± 413.94	2443.50 ± 334.47	*0.002*

Results are reported as means and standard deviations (continuous factors) or numbers and percentages (categorical factors). The p-value of an overall test comparing the three groups is also provided (One-way ANOVA for continuous factors and Chi-square test for categorical factors)
Italic data are statistically significant
[a]pBMI = pre-gestational Body Mass Index; [b]Preterm rupture of membrane = rupture before 37 weeks

(Table 4). Women in the underweight gain group had a lower risk of developing hypertensive gestational disorders compared to the women of the normal weight gain group, even if it was not significant, but only a trend (OR = 0.39, 0.15–1.05). The over weight gain group, instead, presented a significantly higher risk of hypertensive gestational disorders compared to the normal weight gain group (OR = 7.69, 1.94–30.47).

Discussion
Principal findings of the study
In this study, we evaluated the influence of total maternal weight gain, according to the revised IOM recommendations, on the development of spontaneous PD in diamniotic twin gestations [7]. Our results show that 1) normal weight gain is associated with a significant reduction in preterm parturition; and 2) when taking into consideration gestational age at delivery, both under and overweight gain groups presented an increased risk of early

preterm parturition compared to normal weight gain women; and 3) a significantly increased risk for preterm parturition before 37 weeks (three and six times respectively) was present in underweight and overweight women respectively, compared with normal weight gain women.

IOM recommendations for weight gain in twin pregnancies
The important novelty of 2009 IOM recommendations was to give pBMI correlated cut-offs in twin pregnancies. On the other side, a limitation on the clinical use of these guidelines was to refer only to term twin pregnancies, excluding a twin group that delivered before 37 weeks [7, 17]. Therefore, just because IOM guidelines may be used limitedly to term twin pregnancies, we wanted to value how to apply them also in preterm gestations. Thus, we used a weekly gain weight cut-off (IOM cut-off at term/37 weeks), as already done by Fox et al. in a previous study [18].

Table 2 Incidence of the primary outcomes in the weight gain groups

	Under (n. 91)	Normal (n. 73)	p-value§	Over (n. 11)	Normal (n. 73)	p-value§
Preterm delivery < 37 weeks	61 (67.0%)	29 (39.7%)	P = .002	9 (81.8%)	29 (39.7%)	P = .04
Early preterm delivery < 34 weeks	23 (25.3%)	5 (6.8%)	P = .005	3 (27.3%)	5 (6.8%)	P = .13

Results are reported as numbers and percentages. The p-value of an overall test (Chi-square test) correlating the three groups for the two by two comparison
Italic data are statistically significant
§Fisher' exact test with Holm-Bonferroni correction

Table 3 Incidence of the secondary outcomes in the weight gain groups

	Under (n. 91)	Normal (n. 73)	Over (n. 11)	P value[c]
At least one twin SGA[a]	16 (17.6%)	13 (17.8%)	0 (0%)	0.31
Both twins SGA[a]	4 (4.4%)	1 (1.4%)	0 (0%)	0.43
Hypertensive disorders	7 (7.7%)	13 (17.8%)	7 (63.6%)	*< 0.001*
Gestational diabetes	15 (16.5%)	7 (9.6%)	0	0.18
1st twin adverse outcomes[b]	20 (22.0%)	6 (8.2%)	2 (18.2%)	0.06
2nd twin adverse outcomes[b]	20 (22.0%)	8 (11.0%)	2 (18.2%)	0.18

Results are reported as numbers and percentages
Italic data are statistically significant
[a]SGA = small for gestational age; [b]Adverse outcomes = neonatal resuscitation, respiratory distress syndrome, disseminated intravascular coagulation,
intra-ventricular hemorrhage, leucomalacia, sepsis, necrotic enteritis, retinopathy of prematurity; [c]Fisher's exact test with Holm-Bonferroni correction, for all comparison; ns, not significant

Available literature assessing the influence of weight gain on pregnancy outcomes, in twin gestations

Several studies [17–19] analyzed the influence of IOM recommendations on pregnancy outcomes in twin pregnancies. The available literature on the topic is presented herein: 1) Fox et al. [18] collected 297 twin women divided into four groups based on their pBMI (underweight, normal weight, overweight, and obese). They compared pregnancy outcomes for women whose weight gain per week equaled or exceeded the IOM recommendations to women whose weight gain per week was lower than IOM cut-off, in three pBMI-based subgroups (underweight patients were excluded). They found that weight gain was associated with the gestational age at delivery and birth weight of the larger and smaller twin. Specifically, their study showed that, in women with a normal pBMI, patients whose weight gain met or exceeded the IOM recommendations had significantly improved outcomes, such as increment in birthweight of the larger twin and a lower rate of PD before 32 weeks (3.4% vs. 11.5%). In women with an overweight pBMI, if the weight gain met or exceeded the IOM recommendations, they reported higher gestational age at delivery, larger birth weight, and less preterm birth. In pre-gestational obese women, no statistically significant differences were noted; 2) The same authors [17] retrospectively studied a cohort of 170 women restricted to

Table 4 Effect of weight gain on the primary outcomes estimated by logistic regression

	Early preterm delivery OR (95%CI)	Preterm delivery < 37 weeks OR (95%CI)
Under vs normal	4.97 (1.76; 14.02)	3.16 (1.66; 6.04)
Over vs normal	4.53 (0.89; 23.08)	6.51 (1.30; 32.49)

The models were adjusted for pre-pregnancy BMI

twin pregnancies at 37 weeks or more. Their analysis valued pregnancy outcomes in three groups based on IOM recommendations defined as poor, normal, and excessive weight gain. The rate of newborns weighing more than 2500 g was 40%, 60.5% and 79.5% in the three groups, respectively. No differences in gestational hypertension, pre-eclampsia, gestational diabetes or neonatal intensive care unit admission across groups were observed; 3) Gonzalez-Quintero et al. [19], aimed to determine the validity of IOM recommendations for weight gain in twin pregnancies in terms of impact on perinatal outcomes comparing women with mean weight gain per week meeting or exceeding recommendations versus patients who did not meet the suggested weight gain. There was a significantly higher number of both infants weighing > 2500 g or > 1500 g for women gaining weight at or above guidelines. Of interest, women whose gain was below recommended guidelines were 50% more likely to deliver spontaneously at < 35 weeks.

What do our study adds compared to the available literature

Our study follows, in line with the available literature, the idea of assessing whether changes in weight gain during pregnancy in twin gestations, may have an impact on maternal and perinatal outcomes. Moreover, our study design shows several peculiarities, which differentiate it from the previous reports.

Specifically, 1) considering that IOM recommendations were already pBMI correlated, we simplified our analysis and divided our population considering if patients met, exceeded, or presented lower gain weight according to pBMI IOM cut-offs, without performing further stratification of the study groups. The rationale for it was to make the influence of weight gain on PD clearer and useful in clinical practice. Indeed, our analysis showed that a normal weight gain, was correlated with better perinatal and maternal outcomes; 2) Compared with the analysis by Fox et al. [17], our study population also included twins delivered preterm at 28 weeks or more. This was done in order not to lose the effect of prematurity on the analyzed outcomes, since prematurity is common in twin gestations and different outcomes such as preeclampsia and SGA are more frequent in women delivering preterm; 3) In line with Quintero et al., we found that a weight gain below the recommended guidelines was associated with higher rates of spontaneous PD. Moreover, we compared normal weight gain both with under and over gain weight and did not associate patients who met or exceeded IOM recommendations. Of interest, we hypothesized that, both lower and excessive weight gain were associated with worse outcomes; our results confirmed the idea that pregnant women whose weight gain was over recommendation, are at higher risk of hypertensive disorder and PD.

Table 5 Effect of weight gain on the secondary outcomes estimated by logistic regression

	At least one twin SGA[a] OR(95%CI)	Hypertensive gestational disorders OR(95%CI)	Gestational diabetes mellitus OR(95%CI)	Neonatal adverse outcomes[b] OR(95%CI)
Under vs. normal	1.01 (0.45; 2.28)	0.39 (0.15; 1.05)	1.98 (0.75; 5.22)	0.94 (0.29; 3.05)
Over vs. normal	–	7.69 (1.94; 30.47)	–	0.44 (0.05; 3.82)

The model for "neonatal adverse outcomes" was adjusted for pre-pregnancy BMI and gestational age. All the other models were adjusted only for pre-pregnancy BMI
[a]SGA = small for gestational age; [b]Adverse outcomes = neonatal resuscitation, respiratory distress syndrome, disseminated intravascular coagulation, intra-ventricular hemorrhage, leucomalacia, sepsis, necrotic enteritis, retinopathy of prematurity

Strengths and limitations of the study

The novelty of our work was to evaluate if there is an effect of IOM guidelines on the development of spontaneous PD in a cohort of twins at both term and preterm.

Moreover, our study has some limitations, mainly related to its retrospective design and to the small sample size as well as on the fact that it is built on a database registry.

Another possible weakness is the potential for missing data. To minimize this, at our hospital, data is reported by the obstetrician directly after delivery and skilled personnel routinely reviews the information before entering it into the database thereby minimizing recall bias. Coding was done after assessing the medical and prenatal care records together with the routine hospital documents. In addition, since there were no data regarding weekly weight gain cut-offs for twin pregnancies in IOM recommendations, we decided to apply linearity to weekly gain cut-offs as performed within IOM recommendations for single pregnancies [25].

Conclusions

Our findings suggest that normal weight gain, according to revised IOM recommendations, is associated with a reduction of spontaneous PD and, in a selected population, with better pregnancy course and better obstetrics outcomes. This information could be useful for early counseling in twin pregnancy.

Abbreviations

IOM: Institute of medicine; LGA: Large for gestational age; pBMI: Pre-gestational body mass index; PD: Preterm delivery; SGA: Small for gestational age

Acknowledgments
None.

Funding
None.

Authors' contributions

PA Protocol/project development; manuscript writing/editing; data collection or management; data analysis. FP Protocol/project development; manuscript writing/editing; data collection or management. DPB data analysis; manuscript writing/editing. FR manuscript writing/editing. MI Protocol/project development; manuscript writing/editing. SC manuscript writing/editing. SAM/manuscript editing. PV Protocol/project development; manuscript writing/editing. All authors have read and approved the final version of the manuscript.

Competing interests
The authors declare that they have no competing interests.

Author details
[1]Department of Obstetrics and Gynecology, University of Milano-Bicocca, S. Gerardo Hospital, MBBM Foundation, Via Pergolesi 33, Monza, 20900 Monza, Monza e Brianza, Italy. [2]Department of Health Sciences, Center of Biostatistic for Clinical Epidemiology, University of Milan-Bicocca, Via Pergolesi 33, Monza, 20900 Monza, Monza e Brianza, Italy.

References

1. Abenhaim HA, Kinch RA, Morin L, Benjamin A, Usher R. Effect of prepregnancy body mass index categories on obstetrical and neonatal outcomes. Arch. Gynecol. Obstet. 2007;**275**(1):39–43.
2. Menacker F, Hamilton BE. Recent trends in cesarean delivery in the United States. NCHS Data Brief. 2010;35:1–8.
3. Brown JE, Carlson M. Nutrition and multifetal pregnancy. J Am Diet Assoc. 2000;100(3):343–8.
4. Kanadys WM, Oleszczuk J. Maternal weight gain during twin pregnancy. Its relationship to the incidence of preterm delivery. Ginekol Pol. 2000;71(11): 1355–9.
5. Yeh J, Shelton JA. Association of pre-pregnancy maternal body mass and maternal weight gain to newborn outcomes in twin pregnancies. Acta Obstet Gynecol Scand. 2007;86(9):1051–7.
6. Institute of Medicine. Subcommittee on nutritional status and weight gain during pregnancy. Washington, DC: National Academy Press; 1990.
7. Institute of Medicine. Weight gain during pregnancy: reexamining the guidelines. Washington, DC: National Academies Press; 2009.
8. Vayssiere C, Benoist G, Blondel B, Deruelle P, Favre R, Gallot D, Jabert P, Lemery D, Picone O, Pons JC, et al. Twin pregnancies: guidelines for clinical practice from the French College of Gynaecologists and Obstetricians (CNGOF). Eur J Obstet Gynecol Reprod Biol. 2011;156(1):12–7.
9. Luke B, Gillespie B, Min SJ, Avni M, Witter FR, O'Sullivan MJ. Critical periods of maternal weight gain: effect on twin birth weight. Am J Obstet Gynecol. 1997;177(5):1055–62.
10. Lantz ME, Chez RA, Rodriguez A, Porter KB. Maternal weight gain patterns and birth weight outcome in twin gestation. Obstet Gynecol. 1996;87(4):551–6.
11. Luke B, Minogue J, Witter FR, Keith LG, Johnson TR. The ideal twin pregnancy: patterns of weight gain, discordancy, and length of gestation. Am J Obstet Gynecol. 1993;169(3):588–97.
12. Luke B. The evidence linking maternal nutrition and prematurity. J Perinat Med. 2005;33(6):500–5.
13. Russo FM, Pozzi E, Pelizzoni F, Todyrenchuk L, Bernasconi DP, Cozzolino S, Vergani P. Stillbirths in singletons, dichorionic and monochorionic twins: a comparison of risks and causes. Eur J Obstet Gynecol Reprod Biol. 2013; 170(1):131–6.
14. Ghai V, Vidyasagar D. Morbidity and mortality factors in twins. An epidemiologic approach. Clin Perinatol. 1988;15(1):123–40.
15. Gardner MO, Goldenberg RL, Cliver SP, Tucker JM, Nelson KG, Copper RL. The origin and outcome of preterm twin pregnancies. Obstet Gynecol. 1995;85(4):553–7.

16. Lee CM, Yang SH, Lee SP, Hwang BC, Kim SY. Clinical factors affecting the timing of delivery in twin pregnancies. Obstet Gynecol Sci. 2014;57(6):436–41.

17. Fox NS, Saltzman DH, Kurtz H, Rebarber A. Excessive weight gain in term twin pregnancies: examining the 2009 Institute of Medicine definitions. Obstet Gynecol. 2011;118(5):1000–4.

18. Fox NS, Rebarber A, Roman AS, Klauser CK, Peress D, Saltzman DH. Weight gain in twin pregnancies and adverse outcomes: examining the 2009 Institute of Medicine guidelines. Obstet Gynecol. 2010;116(1):100–6.

19. Gonzalez-Quintero VH, Kathiresan AS, Tudela FJ, Rhea D, Desch C, Istwan N. The association of gestational weight gain per institute of medicine guidelines and prepregnancy body mass index on outcomes of twin pregnancies. Am J Perinatol. 2012;29(6):435–40.

20. Bodnar LM, Pugh SJ, Abrams B, Himes KP, Hutcheon JA. Gestational weight gain in twin pregnancies and maternal and child health: a systematic review. J Perinatol. 2014;34(4):252–63.

21. Nicola C, Mariarosaria DT, Giovanni BLS, Anna MM, Antonio R, Nicola R, Tamara S, Alessandro S, Bianiamino T, Patrizia V. In collaborations with: Pietro A, Maria EB, Giuseppe C, Giancarlo C, Marzia M, Stefano P, Giuliana S. Revised by: Paolo S, Vito T, Nicola C, Fabio S. Gestione della gravidanza multipla - Linee guida italiane, Fondazione Confalonieri Ragonese su mandato SIGO, AOGOI, AGUI. 2016. Online at http://www.sigo.it/wp-content/uploads/2016/03/Gestione-della-Gravidanza-Multipla.pdf.

22. Bertino E, Spada E, Occhi L, Coscia A, Giuliani F, Gagliardi L, Gilli G, Bona G, Fabris C, De Curtis M, et al. Neonatal anthropometric charts: the Italian neonatal study compared with other European studies. J Pediatr Gastroenterol Nutr. 2010;51(3):353–61.

23. ACOG Committee on Obstetric Practice. ACOG practice bulletin. Diagnosis and management of preeclampsia and eclampsia. Number 33, January 2002. American College of Obstetricians and Gynecologists. Int J Gynaecol Obstet. 2002;77(1):67-75.

24. American Diabetes Association (2004). Gestational diabetes mellitus. Diabetes Care. Jan;27 Suppl 1:S88–90.

25. Weight Gain During Pregnancy: Reexamining the guidelines. Editors Institute of Medicine (US) and National Research Council (US) committee to reexamine IOM pregnancy weight guidelines; Rasmussen KM, Yaktine AL, editors. Source Washington (DC): National Academies Press (US); 2009. The National Academies Collection: Reports funded by National Institutes of Health.

14

Prevalence and factors associated with preterm birth at kenyatta national hospital

Peter Wagura[1*], Aggrey Wasunna[1], Ahmed Laving[1], Dalton Wamalwa[1] and Paul Ng'ang'a[2]

Abstract

Background: The World Health Organization estimates the prevalence of preterm birth to be 5–18% across 184 countries of the world. Statistics from countries with reliable data show that preterm birth is on the rise. About a third of neonatal deaths are directly attributed to prematurity and this has hindered the achievement of Millennium Development Goal-4 target. Locally, few studies have looked at the prevalence of preterm delivery and factors associated with it. This study determined the prevalence of preterm birth and the factors associated with preterm delivery at Kenyatta National Hospital in Nairobi, Kenya.

Methods: A cross-sectional descriptive study was conducted at the maternity unit of Kenyatta National Hospital in Nairobi, Kenya in December 2013. A total of 322 mothers who met the eligibility criteria and their babies were enrolled into the study. Mothers were interviewed using a standard pretested questionnaire and additional data extracted from medical records. The mothers' nutritional status was assessed using mid-upper arm circumference measured on the left. Gestational age was assessed clinically using the Finnstrom Score.

Results: The prevalence of preterm birth was found to be 18.3%. Maternal age, parity, previous preterm birth, multiple gestation, pregnancy induced hypertension, antepartum hemorrhage, prolonged prelabor rupture of membranes and urinary tract infections were significantly associated with preterm birth ($p = < 0.05$) although maternal age less < 20 years appeared to be protective. Only pregnancy induced hypertension, antepartum hemorrhage and prolonged prelabor rupture of membranes remained significant after controlling for confounders. Marital status, level of education, smoking, alcohol use, antenatal clinic attendance, Human Immunodeficiency Virus status, anemia, maternal middle upper arm circumference and interpregnancy interval were not associated with preterm birth.

Conclusions: The prevalence of preterm birth in Kenyatta National Hospital was 18.3%. Maternal age ≤ 20 years, parity > 4, twin gestation, maternal urinary tract infections, pregnancy induced hypertension, antepartum hemorrhage and prolonged prelabor rupture of membranes were significantly associated with preterm birth. The latter 3 were independent determinants of preterm birth. At-risk mothers should receive intensified antenatal care to mitigate preterm birth.

Keywords: Preterm birth, Prematurity, Preterm delivery

Background

Of the estimated 130 million babies born each year globally, approximately 15 million are born preterm. Prematurity is a major cause of neonatal mortality and morbidity as well as a significant contributor to long term adverse health outcomes. Prematurity is a major hindrance to the attainment of the Millennium Development Goals (MDG)-4 target given its high contribution to neonatal mortality. The survival chances of babies born preterm vary significantly depending on where they are born. The risk of neonatal death due to complications of preterm birth is at least 12 times higher for an African baby than for a European baby. Preterm birth (PTB) is a global problem with prevalence ranging between 5 and 18% across 184 countries. The highest rates of preterm birth are in Sub-Saharan Africa and Asia which account for half the world's births, more than 60% of the world's preterm babies and over 80% of the world's 1.1

* Correspondence: wagurapmwangi@gmail.com
[1]Department of Paediatrics and Child Health, College of Health Sciences, University of Nairobi, P.O. Box 19676-00202, Nairobi, Kenya
Full list of author information is available at the end of the article

million neonatal deaths annually due to complications related to preterm birth. Though most countries especially the low and middle income ones lack reliable data on preterm birth, nearly all of those with reliable trend data show an increase in preterm birth rates over the past 20 years. Indeed, all but 3 out of 65 countries in the world with reliable trend show an increase in preterm birth rates in the last 20 years. Significant progress has been made in the care of premature infants but not in reducing the prevalence of preterm birth which is generally on the rise. Causes of preterm birth are unknown in over 50% of spontaneous preterm labor while mechanisms of preterm labor remain poorly understood [1–7]. Identifying and understanding the risk factors for preterm birth has the potential to help address this problem.

Kenya like most developing countries lacks reliable data on the burden of preterm delivery. Kenyatta National Hospital (KNH) is the largest regional referral and handles many high risk pregnancies some of which result in preterm birth. Despite this, few published studies on the burden of preterm birth and the factors associated with it exist locally. This study aimed to determine the prevalence of preterm birth and the factors associated with PTB. The findings of the study are presented in this article.

Methods
Study design
A hospital based descriptive cross-sectional study was conducted using interviewer administered questionnaire. Additional information was obtained from medical records of the mothers and babies.

Study area
KNH is the largest referral hospital in Kenya and Eastern and Central Africa and also serves as a teaching hospital for the University of Nairobi and the Kenya Medical Training College. It is located in Nairobi which is the capital city of Kenya with a population of about 4 million. The hospital has a busy maternity unit registering over 10,000 deliveries annually. It also has a busy newborn unit (NBU) which offers specialised neonatal care. Being a teaching and referral hospital, KNH handles many high risk pregnancies whose outcomes often include preterm birth.

Participants
The study population comprised of all mothers who had live births at Kenyatta National Hospital and their newborns. A total of 322 mothers who met the eligibility criteria were enrolled into the study. These mothers delivered a total of 331 babies 18 of which were twins.

Data collection
All mothers who had live births at KNH in December 2013 were identified using the birth register within 24 h of delivery. Systematic sampling was used to recruit mother-baby pairs. Mothers were traced to the postnatal wards. Informed consent was obtained from the mothers and babies admitted to the newborn unit were also traced. A standard pretested questionnaire was administered to the mothers while additional data was obtained from the mothers' and babies' medical records as required. The records examined for additional data included the mothers' antenatal and admission records and the babies' medical records for those admitted in the NBU after delivery. Information collected from the mother included maternal age, marital status, level of education, occupation, smoking and alcohol use during pregnancy, parity, date of last normal menstrual period, date of current and preceding delivery (for calculation of interpregnancy interval) and history of previous preterm birth. Information obtained from medical records included antenatal clinic (ANC) attendance and number of visits, Human Immune Deficiency (HIV) status, hemoglobin level, mode of delivery, onset of labor (spontaneous or medically indicated), pregnancy outcome (singleton or multiple), birthweight (to nearest 10 g), baby's gender, prelabor rupture of membranes (PROM) for > 18 h, pregnancy induced hypertension (PIH), antepartum hemorrhage (APH), history of burning sensation during pregnancy or treatment for urinary tract infection (UTI). Anemia was defined as hemoglobin level of < 10 g/dl. PIH was defined clinically as a blood pressure of > 140/90 mmHg after 20 weeks of gestation with or without proteinuria and/or edema as diagnosed and documented by the attending clinician. APH was defined as any vaginal bleeding in the mother after 24 weeks of gestation as documented in the records by the attending clinician. UTI was defined as a documented clinical/laboratory diagnosis of UTI any time during the pregnancy and/or a positive history of treatment of burning sensation with micturition as reported by the mother. Maternal nutritional status was assessed by measuring the left mid-upper arm circumference (MUAC) using non-stretchable World Food Program MUAC tapes used for screening pregnant mothers. A low MUAC was defined as a measurement of less than 24 cm. Gestational age was calculated using a standard obstetric wheel based on menstrual dates and confirmed within 24 h of birth by clinical assessment using the Finnstrom Score. This method was developed by Finnstrom et al. in 1977. Seven (7) physical parameters which are scalp hair, skin opacity, length of fingernails, breast size, nipple formation, ear cartilage and plantar skin creases were used. This tool is not only easy to use but is also sensitive with an accuracy of +/− 2 weeks when administered within

24 h of birth [8, 9]. To limit observer bias, gestational assessment of all babies was done by only one research assistant trained by the principal investigator and aided by a printed pictorial scoring chart. For uniformity, gestational age used for analysis was based on Finnstrom score and not on menstrual dates. Preterm birth was defined as a gestation of less than 37 completed weeks. Prematurity was further categorized as extreme (less than 28 weeks), severe (28–31 weeks), moderate (32–33 weeks) and late preterm or near term (34–36 weeks).

Data analysis

Data was entered into Microsoft Access database, cleaned and stored in a password protected external storage device. Data was analyzed using Stata 11.0. Mean, median, frequencies and percentages were reported to describe the variables and inferential statistics were used to establish associations between prematurity and the various risk factors using a chi-square analysis. Multivariate logistic regression was used to determine the factors independently associated with preterm birth.

Results

Background characteristics of participants

The mean maternal age was 26 ± 5 years with majority (89%) being aged 20 years and above. Most of the mothers (83%) were married. About 85% of the mothers had attained post-primary level of education. About 97% of the enrolled mothers had singleton deliveries while 82% delivered at term. Fifty three percent of all the babies in the study were males. The mean birth weight of term babies was 3059 ± 538 g. The median weight of preterm babies was 2110 g (IQR 1650–2400). The mean gestation was 39 ± 3 weeks and 33 ± 3 weeks for term and preterm babies respectively. Of the preterm births, 62% were late preterms (34–36 weeks), 19% were moderate preterms (32-33 weeks), 16% were severe preterm (28–31 weeks) and 3% were extreme preterm (< 28 weeks).

Prevalence of preterm birth

The prevalence of preterm birth among live births was 18.3% (95% Confidence Interval (CI) of 14.1–22.5%).

Socio-demographic characteristics

About 80% of mothers in the term and 90% in the preterm group were aged 20–34 years. Thirteen percent of mothers aged less than 20 years delivered at term compared to 3.4% who had preterm delivery and this was significant ($p = 0.034$). The proportions of mothers aged 35 years and above were similar in the two groups. There was no difference between the preterm and term groups in terms of marital status ($p = 0.133$), maternal level of education ($p = 0.330$), occupation ($p = 0.823$),

smoking ($p = 0.728$), antenatal alcohol use ($p = 0.501$) and maternal MUAC ($p = 0.651$). None of the socio-demographic factors was significantly associated with preterm birth except maternal age less than 20 years which was negatively associated with preterm delivery (OR 0.236). Table 1 shows the relationship between the socio-demographic characteristics and preterm delivery.

Previous pregnancy characteristics

Most mothers had a parity of less than four. Women with a parity of 4 or more were nearly 5 times more likely to deliver preterm compared to those whose parity was < 4 ($p = 0.019$; OR 4.709). About 35% of mothers who delivered before term had a history of previous preterm delivery compared to 16% of those who delivered at term and this was significant ($p = 0.010$). Approximately 6% of mothers in the preterm group and 11% in the term group had an interpregnancy interval of < 24 months but this was not statistically significant ($p = 0.357$)). The relationship between previous pregnancy characteristics and preterm birth is summarized in Table 2.

Antenatal factors

The proportion of mothers who did not attend ANC in the term and preterm groups was 2.3 and 3.4% respectively and this was not significant ($p = 0.621$). Mothers who had not had any antenatal care were one and a half times more likely to deliver preterm (OR 1.503). About 29% of mothers in term and 37% in preterm group had less than 3 antenatal visits but this was statistically insignificant ($p = 0.256$). Approximately 13% of preterm mothers and 12% of term mothers were HIV positive. There was no association between HIV status and preterm delivery ($p = 0.834$). The proportion of women who had anemia during pregnancy was the same for the two groups ($p = 0886$). Table 3 shows the relationship between the antenatal characteristics and preterm delivery.

Delivery factors

Approximately 40% of preterm deliveries were via Caesarean section (C/S) compared to 26% among those who delivered vaginally. Women who delivered via Caesarean section were nearly two times (OR 1.832) more likely to deliver preterm than those who delivered vaginally. Delivery via Caesarean section had significant but marginal association with preterm birth ($p = 0.049$). About 28 and 36% of mothers in the term and preterm group respectively had induced labor or medically indicated C/S. However, there was no association between onset of labour and preterm birth ($p = 0.231$). The proportion of twin pregnancy among women who delivered at term and preterm was 2 and 7% respectively and this was significant ($p = 0.040$). Twin pregnancy conferred nearly a 4-fold increase in the risk of preterm birth (OR 3.753).

Table 1 Socio-demographic characteristics

Factors	Term (n = 263) (%)	Preterm (n = 59) (%)	OR (95% CI)	P-value
Maternal age (years)				
< 20	34 (13.0)	2 (3.4)	0.236 (0.054–1.001)	0.034
20–34	210 (79.8)	53 (89.8)	Ref	
≥ 35	19 (7.2)	4 (6.8)	0.834 (0.272–2.555)	0.751
Marital status				
Unmarried	48 (18.3)	6 (10.2)	0.507 (0.206–1.248)	0.133
Married	215 (81.7)	53 (89.8)		
Level of education				
No formal/Primary	36 (13.7)	11 (18.6)	1.445 (0.687–3.039)	0.330
Post-primary	227 (86.3)	48 (81.4)		
Maternal occupation				
Unemployed	169 (64.3)	37 (62.7)	0.935 (0.521–1.679)	0.823
Employed/business	94 (35.7)	22 (37.3)		
Smoking during pregnancy				
Yes	3 (1.1)	1 (1.7)	1.494 (0.153–14.623)	0.728
No	260 (98.9)	58 (98.3)		
Alcohol in pregnancy				
Yes	16 (6.1)	5 (8.5)	1.429 (0.502–4.070)	0.501
No	247 (93.9)	54 (91.5)		
MUAC (cm)				
< 24	10 (3.8)	3 (5.1)	1.391 (0.369–5.252)	0.651
≥ 24	253 (96.2)	56 (94.9)		

Table 4 shows the relationship between the delivery characteristics and preterm delivery.

Obstetric factors

About 32 and 8% of mothers in the preterm and term groups had PIH while 13 and 5% of mothers in the two groups had APH respectively. Mothers with PIH and those with APH had a 5-fold and 3-fold increase in risk of preterm birth (OR 5.203 and 2.790). Approximately 27% of mothers who had preterm delivery and 8% of those who delivered at term had a history of PROM for more

than 18 h while 47.5% of mothers in preterm group and 32% of those in the term group respectively reported having had UTI or burning sensation with micturition during pregnancy. As shown in Table 5, all these factors were significantly associated with preterm birth ($p < 0.05$).

Independent determinants of preterm birth

Maternal age, parity, previous preterm birth, twin gestation, UTI, PIH, prolonged PROM and APH were found to be significantly associated with preterm birth. However, on multivariate logistic regression only PIH, APH

Table 2 Previous pregnancy characteristics

Factors	Term (n = 263) (%)	Preterm (n = 59) (%)	OR (95% CI)	P-value
Parity				
≥ 4	4 (1.5)	4 (6.8)	4.709 (1.143–19.407)	0.019
< 4	259 (98.5)	55 (93.2)		
Previous preterm				
Yes	20 (15.6)	12 (35.3)	2.945 (1.259–6.891)	0.010
No	108 (84.4)	22 (64.7)		
Interpregnancy interval (months)				
< 24	14 (10.9)	2 (5.7)	0.506 (0.110–2.342)	0.357
≥ 24	114 (89.1)	33 (94.3)		

Table 3 Antenatal characteristics

Factors	Term n (%)	Preterm n (%)	OR (95% CI)	P-value
ANC attendance				
Yes	257 (97.7)	57 (96.6)	1.503 (0.296–7.639)	0.621
No	6 (2.3)	2 (3.4)		
No. of ANC visits				
< 3	75 (29.2)	21 (36.8)	1.416 (0.776–2.584)	0.256
≥ 3	182 (70.8)	36 (63.2)		
HIV status				
Seropositive	29 (11.5)	7 (12.5)	1.099 (0.455–2.652)	0.834
Seronegative	223 (88.5)	49 (87.5)		
Hemoglobin (g/dl)				
< 10	65 (29.0)	14 (28.0)	0.951 (0.481–1.880)	0.886
≥ 10	159 (71.0)	36 (72.0)		

and prolonged PROM remained significant. The risk of preterm birth increased 8-fold with PIH (OR 7.805), 5-fold if the mother had prolonged PROM (OR 5.319) and 4-fold with APH (OR 4.264) after controlling for confounders. The multivariate logistic regression is summarized in Table 6.

Discussion

Most developing countries lack reliable data on the prevalence of preterm birth [2, 4]. This study aimed to determine the prevalence of preterm birth and associated factors at the largest teaching and referral hospital in Nairobi, Kenya. Our findings demonstrate that preterm birth is a significant health problem in this population with a hospital based prevalence rate of 183 per 1000 live births and that PIH, APH and prolonged PROM are independently associated with PTB. The high rate of preterm birth in this study is in agreement with World Health Organization (WHO) estimates that show that the highest rates are in sub Saharan Africa and South Asia and similar to the finding of other studies in India, Zimbabwe and Malawi [2, 10–12]. However, this PTB rate is higher than would be expected for community based studies.

Compared to low and medium level health facilities in which most normal and uncomplicated deliveries are conducted, KNH being a major referral hospital handles more complicated deliveries, a significant proportion of which are preterm. Consequently, when estimating the PTB rate, the numerator is higher in relation to the denominator for the tertiary hospital resulting in a higher prevalence. The prevalence of preterm birth in the current study is much higher than that reported by Olugbenga and others in a study in a teaching hospital in Nigeria [13]. The difference in PTB rates between our study and the study done by Olugbenga et al. in almost similar setting in the sense of both being teaching hospitals could be explained by the distinct approaches in estimating the gestational age of the babies. While their study excluded mothers who were unsure of dates, those who had a discrepancy of more than 2 weeks between gestation by dates and Ballard's assessment as well as those who had multiple gestation, our study relied wholly on the clinical gestational age assessment based on Finnstrom score. It is likely that our approach overestimated the prevalence of PTB while that of Olugbenga et al. may have underestimated the same.

Table 4 Delivery characteristics

Factors	Term n (%)	Preterm n (%)	OR (95% CI)	P-value
Mode of delivery				
C/S	68 (25.9)	23 (39.0)	1.832 (1.014–3.310)	0.049
Vaginal	195 (74.1)	36 (61.0)		
Onset of labour				
Induced/Medical C/S	73 (27.8)	21 (35.6)	1.438 (0.791–2.614)	0.231
Spontaneous	190 (72.2)	38 (64.4)		
Pregnancy outcome				
Twins	5 (1.9)	4 (6.8)	3.753 (1.016–14.427)	0.040
Singleton	258 (98.1)	55 (93.2)		

Table 5 Obstetric characteristics

Factors	Term (n = 263) (%)	Preterm (n = 59) (%)	OR (95% CI)	P-value
Pre-eclampsia				
Yes	22 (8.4)	19 (32.2)	5.203 (2.586–10.4690)	< 0.001
No	241 (91.6)	40 (67.8)		
APH				
Yes	14 (5.3)	8 (13.6)	2.790 (1.112–6.997)	0.023
No	249 (94.7)	51 (86.4)		
PROM>18Hrs				
Yes	22 (8.4)	16 (27.1)	4.059 (1.974–8.349)	< 0.001
No	240 (91.6)	43 (72.9)		
History of UTI				
Yes	84 (31.9)	28 (47.5)	1.925 (1.085–3.414)	0.024
No	179 (68.1)	31 (52.5)		

The current study did not show any association between the maternal socio-demographic factors except maternal age < 20 years that appeared to be marginally protective. Though our findings showed a marginal negative association between maternal age < 20 years and PTB (p value =0.034, OR = 0.236), this is both unexpected and different from other studies [11–14]. Although about 11% of all mothers were aged < 20 years, less than 1% had preterm birth. The number of women who delivered prematurely in this regard was too small to authoritatively detect significant association with preterm birth and may have inadvertently resulted in the negative association in our study. Previous preterm delivery was associated with preterm birth and this was similar to the findings of other studies [13, 14]. Though the exact mechanism for this is not well established, it may be due to persistence of unidentified factors such as subclinical infections as well as underlying disorders such as hypertension, obesity or diabetes in some women precipitating preterm delivery [1, 15]. The current study demonstrated that mothers with a parity of ≥4 were 4 times more likely to deliver prematurely. This finding is similar to that of previous studies which had shown that multiparaous women were more likely to deliver preterm

Table 6 Multivariate logistic regression of significant factors

Variables	AOR (95% Confidence Interval)	P value
Maternal age < 20 years	0.183 (0.032–1.055	0.057
Parity	0.716 (0.118–4.336)	0.716
Twin gestation	1.908 (0.482–7.552)	0.358
UTI	1.775 (0.657–4.795)	0.258
Prolonged PROM	5.319 (2.320–12.195)	< 0.001
Pregnancy induced hypertension	7.805 (3.686–16.525)	< 0.001
APH	4.264 (1.517–11.986)	< 0.001
Previous preterm birth	1.407 (0.721–2.746)	0.317

[13, 14]. High parity is likely to increase the risk of preterm delivery due to uterine changes such as myometrial stretching from previous pregnancies. Some of the mothers with high parity may also have had a bad obstetric history which may be due to unidentified factors that may persist in subsequent pregnancies. Interpregnancy interval had no association with preterm birth. This was different from the findings of Gordon and colleagues and Agustin Conde and others but similar to that of J Etuk and others in Nigeria [14, 16, 17]. It is possible that women in our setting recover faster from the effect of previous pregnancy and this may be due to intensified nutritional care of mothers soon after delivery which is a common practice locally.

Delivery via Caesarean Section was significantly associated with preterm birth but onset of labor was not. This was similar to the finding of Olugbenga et al. [13]. Operative delivery has no causal relationship with preterm birth but rather is as a result of indicated delivery for maternal or fetal reasons occasioned by obstetric complications such as PIH and APH as observed in this study.

Twin gestation was significantly associated with preterm birth in this study. This is similar to the findings of J Etuk and others [14]. Mutiple gestation is associated with uterine overdistension and this may result in spontaneous preterm labour. In addition other complications such as pre-eclampsia and polyhydramnios are more likely to occur with multiple gestations and thus contribute to iatrogenic preterm birth [1].

ANC attendance as well as number of antenatal visits was not associated with preterm birth in our study. This is different from what Feresu A et al. had reported in Zimbabwe [11]. This may have been due to the Focused Antenatal Care (FANC) approach in Kenya which has emphasized the need to have four targeted antenatal visits which ensures women start ANC attendance much earlier [18]. Maternal HIV status was not associated with preterm delivery in the current study. This finding was similar to that of J Coley and colleagues in Tanzania and J Ndirangu and others in South Africa [19, 20]. It is possible that with increasing availability and use of antiretroviral drugs for prophylaxis and treatment of HIV in pregnancy, the impact of HIV on pregnancy outcomes including risk of preterm birth may have been reduced. Anemia in pregnancy had been associated with preterm birth in some studies but not in others [13, 14, 21]. Our study did not show any association between preterm birth and anemia. With the FANC approach, all pregnant mothers receive iron and folate supplements as early as possible and this reduces the risk of complications related to anemia including preterm birth. A low maternal MUAC was not associated with preterm birth. This finding was different from that of Sebayang et al. in Indonesia and Kalanda et al. in Malawi [21, 22]. One possible reason for this difference is that most women in the current study were from an urban setting compared with the rural setting of the other two studies. UTI in pregnancy was associated with premature birth. This was similar to the findings of studies in Iran and Nigeria [9, 15]. Due to morphological and functional changes that occur in pregnancy, stasis of urine favors UTI. Like other infections, UTI stimulate production of cytokines which may induce preterm labor through release of prostaglandins.

Results of the current study demonstrated that after controlling for confounders, prolonged PROM, PIH and APH remained significantly associated with preterm birth. These findings are similar to those reported in other studies. PROM has been associated with chorioamnionitis which may be subclinical and chlamydial vaginitis. Microorganisms that cause bacterial vaginosis can easily ascend in prolonged PROM and cause intrauterine infections. It is postulated that subclinical chorioamnionitis and other unidentified infections may trigger the release of inflammatory mediators such as interleukin 1 leading to release of prostaglandins from the uterine decidua that ultimately induce preterm labor. PIH which is one of the major obstetric complications was significantly associated with PTB in the current study. Though the pathophysiology of this condition remains poorly understood, uteroplacental ischemia is a plausible explanation for the poor pregnancy outcomes associated with PIH including preterm delivery and low birthweight. Furthermore, PIH is a common reason for indicated preterm deliveries and this may explain its association with PTB even though this may not be causal in nature. Like PIH, APH is also a major contributor to indicated preterm deliveries whether vaginally or operatively without necessarily having a temporal relationship with PTB [1, 9, 15]. This study identifies mothers with prolonged PROM, PIH and APH as a high risk group for PTB. These are largely modifiable factors and should form a good basis for prenatal interventions and better management geared towards reducing the burden of PTB.

Limitations of the study

Only mothers who had live births were interviewed and their babies assessed for gestational age. The study did not address factors associated with preterm stillbirth. UTI in pregnancy was partly based on mothers' self report of symptoms and not on laboratory confirmation and therefore over-reporting was likely. Clinical assessment of gestation using the Finnstrom method that solely relied on physical characteristics is also a limitation of this study. Use of secondary data for some variables is another limitation of our study.

Conclusions

Preterm birth among women delivering at KNH in Nairobi Kenya is a significant problem. Prolonged PROM, PIH and APH are independent determinants of preterm birth. Better management of these obstetric complications and research to elucidate the mechanisms by which they cause preterm birth, offers a practical approach of reducing the high preterm birth rates.

Abbreviations

ANC: Antenatal clinic; AOR: Adjusted odds ratio; APH: Antepartum hemorrhage; C/S: Caesarean section; CI: Confidence interval; DOMC: Division of Malaria Control; DRH: Division of Reproductive Health; FANC: Focused antenatal care; HIV: Human immunodeficiency virus; JHPIEGO: John Hopkins Program for International Education in Gynecology and Obstetrics; KNH: Kenyatta national hospital; MDG: Millennium development goal; MOH: Ministry of Health; MUAC: Mid upper arm circumference; NBU: Newborn unit; OR: Odds ratio; PIH: Pregnancy induced hypertension; PROM: Prelabor rupture of membranes; PTB: Preterm Birth; SVD: Spontaneous vertex delivery; UTI: Urinary tract infection; WHO: World Health Organization

Acknowledgements

The authors would like acknowledge all the mothers who participated in the study as well as their babies. We also thank Steve Mwendwa and Mercy Nafula who were the research assistants for the valuable role they played in data collection and the health personnel in the maternity and newborn units. The authors also acknowledge Kenyatta National Hospital for funding the study. The results and conclusions are those of the authors and are independent from the funding source.

Funding

This study was partially funded by Kenyatta National Hospital through its Research and Programs department as part of the hospital's initiative to support research. The funding body did not play any role in the design of the study, collection, analysis and interpretation of data or in writing of manuscript. The conclusions of this study are solely those of the authors.

Authors' contributions

All authors were involved in the development of the study design and the implementation plan. PW was the principal investigator for the study and wrote the manuscript. AW, AL and DW were co-investigators and contributed in the writing of the manuscript. PN did data analysis and contributed to the writing of the manuscript. All authors critically reviewed the manuscript and approved the final version.

approval was number P116/03/2013 issued on 19th July, 2013. Written informed consent was obtained for participation in the study. No inducements or rewards were given to participants to join the study. Confidentiality was maintained at all times. Data collected as part of the study were not linked to individual or personal identifiers.

Competing interests
The authors declare that they have no competing interests.

Author details
[1]Department of Paediatrics and Child Health, College of Health Sciences, University of Nairobi, P.O. Box 19676-00202, Nairobi, Kenya. [2]Division of Neglected Tropical Diseases, Ministry of Health, P.O. Box 20750-00202, Nairobi, Kenya.

References
1. Goldenberg RL, Culhane JF, Iams JD, Romero R. Epidemiology and causes of preterm birth. Lancet. 2008;371:75–84.
2. March of Dimes/WHO. Born too soon-the global action report on preterm birth 2012.
3. Lawn JE, Cousens S, Zupan J. 4 million neonatal deaths: when? Where? Why? Lancet. 2008;365(Suppl 9462):891–900.
4. Blencowe H, Cousens S, Oestergaard M, et al. National, regional and worldwide estimates of preterm birth rates in the year 2010 with time trends for selected countries since 1990: a systematic analysis. Lancet. 2012; 379(9832):2162–72.
5. United Nations General Assembly. United Nations millennium declaration. New York: United Nations; 2000.
6. Martines J, Paul VK, Bhutta ZA, Koblinsky M, Soucat A, Walker N, Bahl R, Fogstad H, Costello A. Neonatal survival: a call for action. Lancet. 2005; 365(Suppl 9465):1189–97.
7. Lawn JE, Kerber K, Enweronu-Laryea C, Bateman O. Newborn survival in low resource settings–are we delivering? BJOG. 2009;116(Suppl 1):49–59.
8. Finnström O. Studies on maturity in newborn infants. ActaPaediatrScand. 1977;66:601–4.
9. Goyal SC, Tak SK, Bhandari B. Determination of gestational age: comparative accuracy of different methods. Indian J Pediatr. 1989;56(1):115–9.
10. Shubhada A, Kambale SV, Phalke BD. Determinants of preterm labour in a rural medical college hospital in western Maharashtra. NJOG. 2013; 8(Suppl 1):31–3.
11. Feresu SA, Harlow SD, Welch K, Gillespie RW. Incidence of and socio-demographic risk factors for stillbirth, preterm birth and low birthweight among Zimbabwean women. Paediatr Perinat Epidemiol. 2004;18(Suppl 2):154–63.
12. van den Broek NR, Jean-Baptiste R, Neilson JP. Factors associated with preterm, early preterm and late preterm birth in Malawi. PLoS One. 2014; 9(Suppl 3):e90128.
13. Olugbenga A, Mokuolu BM, Suleiman OO, Adesiyun A, Adeniyi B. Prevalence and determinants of pre-term deliveries in the University of Ilorin Teaching Hospital, Ilorin, Nigeria. Pediatric Report. 2010;2(Suppl 3):11–3.
14. Etuk SJ, Etuk IS, Oyo-Ita AE. Factors influencing the incidence of preterm birth in Calabar, Nigeria. Niger J Physiol Sci. 2005;20(Suppl 1–2):63–8.
15. Muglia LJ, Katz M. The enigma of spontaneous preterm birth. N Engl J Med. 2010;362:529–35.
16. Smith GCS, Pell JP, Dobbie R. Interpregnancy interval and risk of preterm birth and neonatal death: retrospective cohort study. BMJ. 2003;327:313–7.
17. Conde-Agudelo A, Rosas-Bermãdez A, Kafury-Goeta A. Birth spacing and risk of adverse perinatal outcomes. JAMA. 2006;295(Suppl 15):1809–23.
18. MOH-DRH, DOMC, JHPIEGO. Focused antenatal care and malaria in pregnancy: orientation package. Nairobi: Ministry of Health; 2002.
19. Coley JL, Kapiga S, Hunter D, et al. The association between maternal HIV-1 infection and pregnancy outcomes in Dar es Salaam, Tanzania. BJOG. 2001; 108:1125–33.
20. Ndirangu J, Newell M-L, Bland RM, Thorne C. Maternal HIV infection associated with small-for-gestational age infants but not preterm births: evidence from rural South Africa. Hum Reprod. 2012;27(Suppl 6):1846–56.
21. Sebayang S, Dibley M, Kelly P, Shanka A, Anuraj H. Determinants of low birth weight, and small-for-gestational-age and preterm birth in Lombok, Indonesia: analyses of the birth weight cohort of the SUMMIT trial. Trop Med Int Health. 2012;17(Suppl 8):938–50.
22. Kalanda BF. Maternal anthropometry and weight gain as risk factors for poor pregnancy outcomes in a rural area of southern Malawi. Malawi Med J. 2007;19(Suppl 4):149–53.

15

Cerclage is associated with the increased risk of preterm birth in women who had cervical conization

Geum Joon Cho[1†], Yung-Taek Ouh[1†], Log Young Kim[2], Tae-Seon Lee[2], Geun U. Park[3], Ki Hoon Ahn[1], Soon-Cheol Hong[1], Min-Jeong Oh[1] and Hai-Joong Kim[1*]

Abstract

Background: The aim of this study was to determine the effect of cerclage in women who underwent cervical conization.

Methods: Study data were collected from the Korea National Health Insurance Claims Database of the Health Insurance Review and Assessment Service for 2009–2013. Women who had a conization in 2009 and a subsequent first delivery between 2009 and 2013 in Korea were enrolled.

Results: Among the women who had conization in 2009, 1075 women had their first delivery between 2009 and 2013. A cerclage was placed in 161 of the women who were treated by conization. The rate of preterm birth was higher in the women who were treated with cerclage following a conization compared with those without cerclage (10.56 vs 4.27, $p < 0.01$, respectively). The multivariate regression analysis revealed that the women who were treated cerclage following a conization had an increased risk of preterm delivery compared with women without cerclage (odds ratio (OR), 2.6, 95% confidence interval (CI), 1.4–4.9).

Conclusion: Our study showed that cerclage associated with an increased risk of preterm birth and preterm premature rupture of membranes in women who underwent conization. Further studies are required to clarify the mechanism by which cerclage affects the risk of preterm birth.

Keywords: Cerclage, Preterm birth, Conization, Preterm premature rupture of membrane

Background

Preterm birth is defined as delivery before 37 weeks, and it has been implicated in approximately two thirds of infant deaths [1–3]. Although the infant mortality rate has declined over the past century, it has remained a major health problem. Screening for the risk of preterm labor is not beneficial in the general population. However, a short cervix is one of the poorest predictors of preterm birth [4, 5]. Cervical incompetence is a clinical diagnosis characterized by recurrent, painless cervical dilatation and shortening. Since the 1950s, a cervical cerclage has been a relatively common procedure performed for the treatment of cervical incompetence [6].

A large study from Norway evaluated 15,108 births that occurred in women who had previously undergone cervical conization, and 57,136 who gave birth before conization [7]. The researchers reported the proportion of preterm deliveries in each group, 17.2% versus 6.7%. Even if the cause of cervical incompetence is obscure, previous trauma to the cervix, such as dilatation and curettage or conization, has been implicated. Conization may lead to cervical insufficiency, and cerclage is a treatment option.

The efficacy of prophylactic cerclage for prevention of a preterm birth remains controversial. It has been reported that cervical cerclage cannot only prevent preterm birth but also may be an independent risk factor in women following conization [8]. In a retrospective study of 25 patients with a prior conization who underwent prophylactic cerclage, the treatment did not prevent preterm birth [9].

* Correspondence: haijkim@gmail.com
†Geum Joon Cho and Yung-Taek Ouh contributed equally to this work.
[1]Department of Obstetrics and Gynecology, Korea University College of Medicine, Seoul, Republic of Korea
Full list of author information is available at the end of the article

The aim of this study was to determine the effect of cerclage in women who had cervical conization.

Methods

We collected the data from the Korea National Health Insurance (KNHI) Claims Database of the Health Insurance Review and Assessment Service (HIRA) for 2009–2013. We have mentioned about KNHI Claims Database [10]. Briefly, 97% of the Korean population is required to enroll in the KNHI program. The remaining 3% of the population is treated under the Medical Aid Program. Thus, this centralized database contained nearly all contents about the occurrence of disease except the disease or treatment that are not covered by insurance. According to the Act on the Protection of Personal Information Maintained by Public Agencies, HIRA possess the claims data by concealing individual identities. The database included an unidentifiable code representing each individual, together with age, diagnosis, and a list of prescribed procedures. Therefore, studies using data from HIRA can be exempt from institutional board reviews. The datasets used and/or analysed during the current study are available from the corresponding author on reasonable request.

All women who underwent conization in 2009 and gave birth during 2009 to 2013 were identified by using the International Classification of Diseases, Tenth Revision (ICD-10) diagnosis and procedure codes. A first pregnancy was linked to conization during the study period. Women who had undergone conization in 2009 and then had their first delivery between 2009 and 2013 were only included in our study. Using procedure code for cerlcage, it was confirmed whether or not cerclage was performed during pregnancy.

To identify women with preterm delivery and preterm premature rupture of membrane (pPROM) from the HIRA database, ICD-10 codes O60.1 for preterm delivery and ICD-10 code O42.x with code for preterm delivery for pPROM were used.

Data about the women's characteristics, such as age, delivery mode (vaginal delivery or cesarean section), multiple pregnancies (defined as twin or higher-order gestation), and the number of years between conization and delivery, were obtained.

We used the Student's t-test to compare continuous variables between groups and chi-square test to compare categorical variables. To evaluate risk the risk of preterm delivery, a model of multivariate logistic regression analysis was performed with preterm delivery or pPROM in the second pregnancy.

A P value < 0.05 was considered statistically significant. Statistical analyses were performed using SPSS software, version 12.0 (SPSS Inc., Chicago, IL, USA).

Results

Among the 23,553 women who had conization in 2009, 1075 had their first delivery between 2009 and 2013. Cerclage was placed in 161 of the women who had been treated by conization.

Table 1 shows the basic characteristic of the study population treated by cerclage following conization. Compared to women without cerclage, women with cerclage following conization had higher rates of pre-eclampsia in the first pregnancy. However, there were no differences in age, rates of multiple pregnancy, or years from conization to delivery between the two groups. The rate of preterm birth was higher in women who underwent cerclage following a conization compared with women without cerclage (10.56 vs 4.27, $p < 0.01$, respectively). The rate of pPROM was also higher in women with cerclage following a conization than in women without cerclage (6.21 vs 2.41, $p < 0.01$, respectively).

The multivariate regression analysis (Table 2) revealed that women with cerclage following a conization had an increased risk of preterm delivery compared with women without cerclage (OR 2.64, 95% CI 1.43–4.87). Women with cerclage following a conization also had an increased risk of pPROM compared with women without cerclage (Table 3) (OR 2.60, 95% CI 1.19–5.64).

Discussion

In our study, cervical cerclage could not prevent preterm birth among women who had been treated by conization; cerclage was associated with an increased risk of preterm birth compared with that among patients who did not undergo a cerclage. On the basis of previous studies that reported cerclage significantly prevents preterm birth and perinatal mortality and morbidity in women with previous spontaneous preterm birth [11], we hypothesized that cervical cerclage would also prevent preterm birth among women who had been treated by conization. Thus, it is interesting to note that cervical cerclage was actually associated with an increased risk of preterm birth in this study. The reason for this unexpected association is unclear, but there are some plausible explanations. First, suture materials placed in the uterine cervix are a foreign body and can cause inflammation after cervical cerclage. In this study, the rate of pPROM in the preventive cervical cerclage group was higher compared with control group. pPROM is a complex autotoxic disease that involves activation and interaction of the cytokine, MMP, and apoptosis pathways, although it was originally thought to be due to a direct action of bacteria [12]. It has been reported that the 42% of patients with total intra-amniotic inflammation were associated with pPROM even in the absence of intra-amniotic infection, and it was applied to manage pPROM [13]. It can be assumed that cerclage induced

Table 1 Basic characteristics of the study participants

	Pregnant women		P-value
	Without cerclage (n = 914)	With cerclage (n = 161)	
Age (years)	30.69 ± 2.32	30.79 ± 2.41	0.481
Cesarean section (%)	185 (20.24)	63 (39.13)	< 0.001
Multiple pregnancy (%)	22 (2.41)	6 (3.73)	0.320
Years since delivery from conization (years)	2.14 ± 1.05	2.07 ± 1.03	0.733
Preterm delivery (weeks)	39 (4.27)	17 (10.56)	< 0.001
pPROM (%)	22 (2.41)	10 (6.21)	0.867

pPROM, preterm premature rupture of membranes

cervical inflammation and consequent intraamniotic inflammation, and elevated the preterm birth rate even in the absence of infection. Sakai [13] compared the risk of preterm birth according to cervical mucus interleukin-8 (IL-8) among patients who underwent cervical cerclage for shortening. Their study showed that cerclage may be harmful to patients with elevated cervical mucus IL-8, but that cerclage reduced the risk of preterm delivery in patients with normal cervical mucus IL-8 [13]. Whereas cerclage was effective in patients with a short cervix without cervical inflammation, it was deleterious in patients with inflammation; this finding suggested that cerclage causes preterm delivery by inducing inflammation and chorioamnionitis. Moreover, as pregnant women who had undergone conization were enrolled in this study, cerlcage, repeated trauma may attribute to reduction of tension threshold of cervical tissue, which causes preterm birth. Thus, cervical cerclage itself may influence the development of preterm birth. Another reason for this effect may be that treatment with cerclage was targeted at patients who already had other risk factors of preterm birth, since cervical incompetence can be caused by anatomical defect or uterine abnormities, as well as a short cervix. Moreover, pregnancy outcomes including preterm delivery and pPROM may be different in women who underwent between prophylactic and emergent cerclage. However, as the indication of cerclage and gestational age at cerclage were not available in this study, further studies are needed to evaluate the exact mechanisms by which cerclage may affect development of preterm birth in women who underwent cervical conization.

Our results have implications that might be clinically relevant. In our study, cerclage did not prevent preterm birth; moreover, cervical cerclage was associated with a higher rate of preterm birth. In addition, when compared with the incidence of preterm birth in South Korea, the risk of preterm birth is not higher among women with conization. This finding suggests that in pregnant women who have undergone conization, prophylactic cerclage is not essential for preventing preterm birth; this conclusion is consistent with the results of other recent studies [9, 14]. Rather, our results show that pregnancy after conization is not an absolute indication for prophylactic cerclage, and other risk factors should be considered confounding factors. Several studies have examined the association of cone depth with the risk of preterm birth. The risk of preterm birth increased 6–20% per millimeter of cervical excision [15, 16]. It has been also reported that a depth thicker than 12 mm and larger than 6 cm^3 carried a 3-fold risk for preterm birth [17]. Because gynecologists who perform conizations and obstetricians providing prenatal care may be different providers in most cases in Korea, clinicians should share the clinical data about conization to avoid unnecessary prophylactic cerclage that could be harmful.

Several limitations should be considered when interpreting the present findings. First, this study was based on insurance claim data in the KNHI Claims Database, which was designed for cost claim issues, not research. Thus, the cause of the preterm births was not available. It has been reported that preeclampsia, fetal distress, small-for-gestational age, and placental abruption were the most common indications for a medical intervention resulting in preterm birth [18]. Therefore, in our study,

Table 2 Adjusted odds ratios (OR) and 95% confidence interval (CI) for the risk of preterm birth

	OR	95% CI
Age (years)	1.0	0.9, 1.0
Cerclage (yes)	2.6	1.4, 4.9
Multiple pregnancy (yes)	10.5	4.4, 25.2
Years since delivery from conization (years)	0.9	0.7, 1.2

The model is adjusted for variables in the Table; 95% CI, 95% confidence interval

Table 3 Adjusted odds ratios (OR) and 95% confidence interval (CI) for the risk of pPROM

	OR	95% CI
Age (years)	1.0	0.9, 1.1
Cerclage (yes)	2.6	1.2, 5.64
Multiple pregnancy (yes)	5.8	1.9, 18.3
Years since delivery from conization (years)	0.8	0.6, 1.2

The model is adjusted for variables in the Table, 95% CI, 95% confidence interval

other potential causes of preterm birth cannot be excluded. However, in this study, the definition of preterm birth was limited to ICD-10 code, O60.1 (preterm spontaneous labor with preterm delivery) to exclude preterm birth by other causes.

Another limitation of our study is that we were not able to access information such as cervical status before conization, and depth of conization, all of which are known factors of preterm delivery [19–21], because these data were not available in the database.

Nevertheless, the strength of the present study lies in the large population-based cohort, with very few patients lost to follow-up. Although there have been several studies about the effectiveness of cerclage on preterm birth, they recruited fewer than 100 patients because of the infrequency of cervical cerclage following conization [9, 14]. By contrast, we evaluated 161 patients who had undergone a cerclage with previous conization and 914 without cerclage. This large study group strengthens the result of our study. Moreover, biochemical characteristics of the cervix have reported to be different according to patient's parity [22, 23]. Thus, another strength of our study is that we enrolled only women who delivered their first child during the same period to minimize the effect of parity.

Conclusions

In conclusion, our study revealed that the incidence of preterm birth was not significantly different between the group that underwent conization and the group that did not. Prophylactic cerclage during pregnancy is not necessary for women who have undergone conization. Further studies are needed to add information about the effect of the sonographic cervical length, the time interval between conization and delivery, gestational weeks at cerclage, and cone size, to inform the current guidelines for prophylactic cervical cerclage after conization.

Abbreviations

HIRA: Health insurance review and assessment service; IL-8: Interleukin-8; KNHI: Korea National Health Insurance; pPROM: Preterm premature rupture of membrane

Funding

This research was supported by a grant from the Korea Health Technology R&D Project through the Korea Health Industry Development Institute, funded by the Ministry of Health and Welfare, Republic of Korea (Grant No. HI14C0306 and H15C0810).

Authors' contributions

GJC, YTO and HJK conceptualized the study. LYK and GUP participated in study design. GJC, LYK and TSL collected the data. LYK, GUP and MJO participated in the analysis and interpretation of results. GJC wrote the first draft. KHA, SCH and HJK critically revised the manuscript. All authors read and approved the final version.

Competing interests

The authors declare that they have no competing interests.

Author details

[1]Department of Obstetrics and Gynecology, Korea University College of Medicine, Seoul, Republic of Korea. [2]The Health Insurance Review and Assessment Service of Korea, Seoul, South Korea. [3]Department of applied statistics, Chung-Ang University, Seoul, South Korea.

References

1. Dollfus C, Patetta M, Siegel E, Cross AW. Infant mortality: a practical approach to the analysis of the leading causes of death and risk factors. Pediatrics. 1990;86(2):176–83.
2. McCormick MC. The contribution of low birth weight to infant mortality and childhood morbidity. N Engl J Med. 1985;312(2):82–90.
3. Rush RW, Keirse MJ, Howat P, Bau JD, Anderson AB, et al. Contribution of preterm delivery to perinatal mortality. Br Med J. 1976;2(6042):965–8.
4. Papastefanou I, Pilalis A, Eleftheriades M, Souka AP. Prediction of Preterm Delivery by Late Cervical Length Measurement after 24 Weeks. Fetal DiagnTher. 2015;38(3):200–4.
5. Berghella V, Baxter JK, Hendrix NW. Cervical assessment by ultrasound for preventing preterm delivery. Cochrane Database Syst Rev. 2009;3:CD007235.
6. Suhag A, Berghella V. Cervical cerclage. ClinObstet Gynecol. 2014;57(3):557–67.
7. Albrechtsen S, Rasmussen S, Thoresen S, Irgens LN, Iversen OE. Pregnancy outcome in women before and after cervical conisation: population based cohort study. BMJ. 2008;337:a1343.
8. Rafaeli-Yehudai T, Kessous R, Aricha-Tamir B, Sheiner E, Erez O, et al. The effect of cervical cerclage on pregnancy outcomes in women following conization. J Matern Fetal Neonatal Med. 2014;27(15):1594–7.
9. Shin MY, Seo ES, Choi SJ, Oh SY, Kim BG, et al. The role of prophylactic cerclage in preventing preterm delivery after electrosurgical conization. J Gynecol Oncol. 2010;21(4):230–6.
10. Kang EJ, Seo JH, Kim LY, et al. Pregnancy-Associated Risk Factors of Postpartum Breast Cancer in Korea: A Nationwide Health Insurance Database Study. PLoS One. 2016;11:e0168469.
11. Berghella V, Odibo AO, Tolosa JE. Cerclage for Short Cervix on Ultrasonography in Women With Singleton Gestations and Previous Preterm Birth. Obstet Gynecol. 2011;117(3):663–71.
12. Menon R, Fortunato SJ. Infection and the role of inflammation in preterm premature rupture of the membranes. Best Pract Res Clin Obstet Gynaecol. 2007;21(3):467–78.
13. Sakai M, Shiozaki A, Tabata M, Sasaki Y, Yoneda S, et al. Evaluation of effectiveness of prophylactic cerclage of a short cervix according to interleukin-8 in cervical mucus. Am J Obstet Gynecol. 2006;194(1):14–9.
14. Nam KH, Kwon JY, Kim YH, Park YW. Pregnancy outcome after cervical conization: risk factors for preterm delivery and the efficacy of prophylactic cerclage. J Gynecol Oncol. 2010;21(4):225–9.
15. Jakobsson M, Gissler M, Sainio S, Paavonen J, Tapper AM. Preterm delivery after surgical treatment for cervical intraepithelial neoplasia. Obstet Gynecol. 2007;109(2 Pt 1):309–13.
16. Noehr B, Jensen A, Frederiksen K, Tabor A, Kjaer SK. Depth of cervical cone removed by loop electrosurgical excision procedure and subsequent risk of spontaneous preterm delivery. Obstet Gynecol. 2009;114(6):1232–8.
17. Khalid S, Dimitriou E, Conroy R, Paraskevaidis E, Kyrgiou M, et al. The thickness and volume of LLETZ specimens can predict the relative risk of pregnancy-related morbidity. BJOG. 2012;119(6):685–91.
18. Ananth CV, Vintzileos AM. Maternal-fetal conditions necessitating a medical intervention resulting in preterm birth. Am J Obstet Gynecol. 2006;195(6):1557–63.
19. Pils S, Eppel W, Seemann R, Natter C, Ott J. Sequential cervical length screening in pregnancies after loop excision of the transformation zone conisation: a retrospective analysis. BJOG. 2014;121(4):457–62.
20. Berretta R, Gizzo S, Dall'Asta A, Mazzone E, Monica M, et al. Risk of preterm

delivery associated with prior treatment of cervical precancerous lesion according to the depth of the cone. Dis Markers. 2013;35(6):721–6.

21. Jakobsson M, Gissler M, Paavonen J, Tapper AM. Loop electrosurgical excision procedure and the risk for preterm birth. Obstet Gynecol. 2009; 114(3):504–10.

22. Zorzoli A, Soliani A, Perra M, Caravelli E, Galimberti A, et al. Cervical changes throughout pregnancy as assessed by transvaginal sonography. Obstet Gynecol. 1994;84(6):960–4.

23. Oxlund BS, Ørtoft G, Brüel A, Danielsen CC, Bor P, et al. Collagen concentration and biomechanical properties of samples from the lower uterine cervix in relation to age and parity in non-pregnant women. Reprod Biol Endocrinol. 2010;8:82.

Nausea and vomiting during pregnancy associated with lower incidence of preterm births: the Japan Environment and Children's Study (JECS)

Naomi Mitsuda[1*], Masamitsu Eitoku[1], Keiko Yamasaki[2], Masahiko Sakaguchi[2,5], Kahoko Yasumitsu-Lovell[1], Nagamasa Maeda[3], Mikiya Fujieda[4], Narufumi Suganuma[1] and Japan Environment & Children's Study (JECS) Group

Abstract

Background: Nausea and vomiting during pregnancy (NVP) is considered to be associated with favorable fetal outcomes, such as a decreased risk for spontaneous abortion. However, the relationship between NVP and preterm births remains unknown. This study was conducted to evaluate the association between NVP and the risk of preterm births.

Methods: The dataset of a birth cohort study, the Japan Environment and Children's Study (JECS), was retrospectively reviewed. Participants' experience of NVP prior to 12 gestational weeks were evaluated by a questionnaire administered from 22 weeks of pregnancy to 1 month before delivery. NVP responses were elicited against four choices based on which the study population was divided into four subcohorts. Preterm birth was the main study outcome. Logistic regression analysis was used to quantify an association between NVP and risk of preterm birth.

Results: Of 96,056 women, 79,460 (82.7%) experienced some symptoms of NVP and 10,518 (10.9%) experienced severe NVP. Compared to those who did not experience NVP, women with severe NVP had lower odds for preterm birth [adjusted odds ratio (aOR) 0.84, 95% confidence interval (95% CI) 0.74–0.95]. An even lower OR was found among very preterm birth and extremely preterm birth (aOR 0.44, 95% CI 0.29–0.65).

Conclusion: An inverse association exists between NVP and preterm births, especially, very preterm births and extremely preterm births.

Keywords: Nausea and vomiting during pregnancy, Preterm birth, JECS

Background

Nausea and vomiting during pregnancy (NVP) is among the most common clinical complaints in the first trimester of pregnancy. NVP affects up to 70% of pregnant women, but there is considerable variation among reported frequencies (35–91%) [1]. NVP has been posited to have multifactorial causation, including genetic, endocrine, and gastrointestinal factors [2–4]. However, a clear etiopathogenesis of NVP has not been established. Some studies have shown that NVP represents a favorable hormonal milieu, accompanied by larger placentas and elevated levels of chorionic gonadotrophin and estrogens in pregnant women [5, 6]. Another hypothesis asserts that the role of NVP is to protect pregnant women and embryos from foodborne pathogens and dietary toxins [7, 8].

In the context of these hypotheses, NVP is associated with favorable fetal outcomes [9, 10]. A number of past studies linked NVP with a decreased risk for spontaneous abortion [11–14]. Some studies have shown that women who experience NVP have a lower risk of preterm birth than those without such symptoms [15, 16], although other studies have shown no association or

* Correspondence: jm-nmitsuda@kochi-u.ac.jp
[1]Department of Environmental Medicine, Kochi Medical School, Kochi University, Kohasu, Oko-cho, Nankoku, Kochi 783-8505, Japan
Full list of author information is available at the end of the article

reported the opposite [17–19]. This study was conducted to evaluate the association between maternal NVP and preterm birth from the data of the Japan Environment and Children's Study (JECS).

Methods
Study design
We retrospectively analyzed the dataset of the JECS, a long-term birth cohort study to elucidate the influence of chemical exposures during the fetal period and early childhood on children's health with follow-up until age 13. The protocol and baseline data of this study are available elsewhere [18].

For the JECS, pregnant women were recruited between January 31, 2011 and March 31, 2014. Eligibility criteria for study participants (expectant mothers) were as follows: 1) residing in the study areas at the time of recruitment and attending collaborating healthcare providers; 2) expected delivery date after August 1, 2011; and 3) capable of comprehending Japanese and completing self-administered questionnaires. Details of the JECS project have been described in a previous article [20].

With regards to exposure measurement, lifestyle and other background information was collected using a self-administered questionnaire distributed to participating pregnant women from the first trimester up to 21 weeks and 6 days of pregnancy (M-T1) and from 22 weeks of pregnancy to 1 month before delivery (M-T2). Medical histories of past and present pregnancies, and physical status of participants and their offspring, were collected from an obstetrician's medical chart at registration (Dr-T1) and at delivery (Dr-0 m). Study analyses were based on M-T2, Dr-T1, and Dr-0 m.

Sample selection
The present study was based on the "jecs-ag-20,160,424", which was released in June, 2016. The JECS dataset included 104,102 births. We excluded miscarriage ($n = 1250$) and multiple births ($n = 1929$). We also excluded women who had delivered before 26 weeks of gestation because they may have delivered before the M-T2 questionnaire was provided ($n = 271$). Moreover, we excluded cases with missing data on gestational age ($n = 2323$), and cases with missing data on NVP ($n = 2273$). In total, 96,056 births were included in the final study sample (Fig. 1).

Variables
Information on NVP, maternal education, and maternal smoking habits during pregnancy were obtained from M-T2. In M-T2, participants were asked whether they experienced NVP in the first 12 gestational weeks (1. did not experience NVP; 2. nausea only; 3. experienced NVP but could have meals; and 4. experienced NVP and could not have meals).

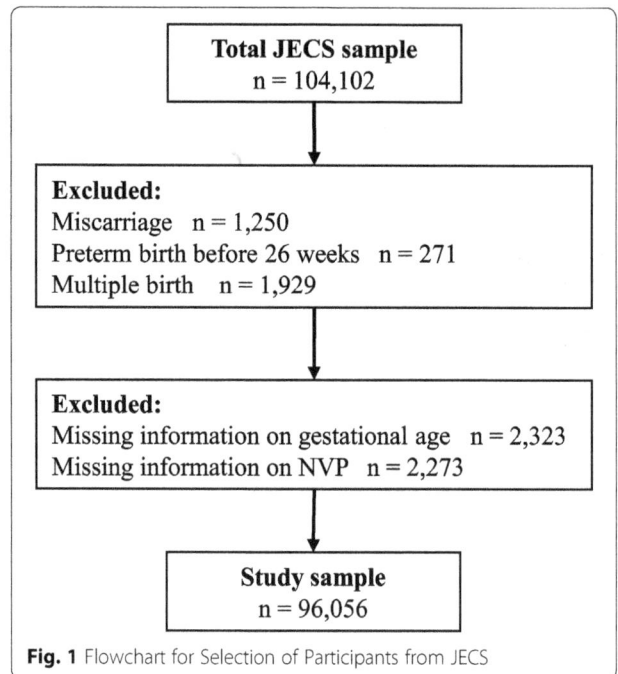

Fig. 1 Flowchart for Selection of Participants from JECS

Information on parity, maternal height, and pre-pregnancy weight was obtained from Dr-T1, and data on maternal age, gestational age, birth outcomes, and prenatal complications were obtained from Dr-0 m. Participants underwent ultrasound examinations during the first trimester, and these results were used to determine the expected date of delivery if there was more than a 7-day difference between this date and the date calculated from the last menstrual period.

Maternal age was categorized into six groups: younger than 20 years, 20–24 years, 25–29 years, 30–34 years, 35–39 years, and 40 years or older. By data on parity, the cohort was classified into nullipara and multipara. A proxy for socioeconomic status, maternal length of education, was categorized into ≤12 years and > 12 years. Body mass index (BMI) was calculated from the information on pre-pregnancy height and weight and categorized into three groups: underweight (< 18.5 kg/m^2), normal (18.5–24.9 kg/m^2) and overweight (≥ 25 kg/m^2). Maternal smoking habits were categorized into smoking during pregnancy and others.

Gestational age, defined as an outcome variable, was categorized as post term (≥42 weeks), term (37–41 weeks) and preterm (< 37 weeks). Further, preterm birth was subdivided into moderately preterm (32–36 weeks), very preterm (28–31 weeks), and extremely preterm (26–27 weeks) [21].

Statistical analyses
The study population was divided into four groups, based on the answers to the questionnaire for NVP symptoms as follows: those who did not experience NVP (no NVP); those who experienced nausea only

(mild NVP); those who experienced NVP but could have meals (moderate NVP); and those who experienced NVP and could not have meals (severe NVP). Maternal characteristics and pregnancy outcomes were compared among the four NVP groups. Gestational age was compared employing Kruskal–Wallis test for non-normally distributed data. Categorical variables were compared using a chi-squared test. P-values < 0.05 indicated statistical significance.

Logistic regression analysis was used to estimate the association between NVP and the risk of preterm birth. For analysis of the odds ratio (OR) of preterm birth, we used a dichotomized outcome variable: preterm birth (< 37 weeks) and others (≥ 37 weeks). For analysis of OR of very preterm birth and extremely preterm birth, we used another dichotomized outcome variable: very preterm birth and extremely preterm birth (born at < 32 weeks of gestation) and others (born at ≥ 32 weeks). ORs were adjusted for maternal age, parity, maternal education, maternal pre-pregnancy BMI, and smoking habits during pregnancy. Results are presented as crude odds ratios (cOR) and adjusted odds ratios (aOR), or as mean differences with 95% confidence intervals (95% CI). All analyses were conducted using Stata 13.1 (Stata Corp, Texas).

Table 1 Maternal characteristics according to NVP status

	Total	No NVP	Mild NVP	Moderate NVP	Severe NVP	P value
	$n = 96,056$	$n = 16,596$	$n = 41,198$	$n = 27,744$	$n = 10,518$	
	n	n (%)	n (%)	n (%)	n (%)	
Maternal Age (years)						
< 20	814	190 (1.2)	256 (0.6)	256 (0.9)	112 (1.1)	< 0.001
20–24	8630	1678 (10.1)	3026 (7.4)	2787 (10.1)	1139 (10.8)	
25–29	26,528	4487 (27.0)	10,775 (26.2)	8111 (29.2)	3155 (30.0)	
30–34	34,075	5432 (32.7)	14,997 (36.4)	9967 (35.9)	3679 (35.0)	
35–39	21,622	3861 (23.3)	10,038 (24.4)	5636 (20.3)	2087 (19.8)	
≥ 40	4383	945 (5.7)	2106 (5.1)	986 (3.6)	346 (3.3)	
Missing[a]	4					
Parity						
Nullipara	37,800	8244 (51.4)	15,404 (38.2)	10,040 (36.9)	4112 (40.1)	< 0.001
Multipara	56,005	7804 (48.6)	24,875 (61.8)	17,170 (63.1)	6156 (60.0)	
Missing[a]	2251					
Education (years)						
≤ 12	34,790	6398 (38.7)	14,118 (34.4)	10,320 (37.3)	3954 (37.8)	< 0.001
> 12	60,893	10,126 (61.3)	26,931 (65.6)	17,315 (62.7)	6521 (62.3)	
Missing[a]	373					
BMI (kg/m²)						
< 18.5	15,500	2859 (17.2)	6834 (16.6)	4167 (15.0)	1640 (15.6)	< 0.001
18.5–24.9	70,221	12,141 (73.2)	30,216 (73.4)	20,351 (73.4)	7513 (71.5)	
≥ 25	10,272	1584 (9.6)	4122 (10.0)	3209 (11.6)	1357 (12.9)	
Missing[a]	63					
Smoking during pregnancy						
No	90,887	15,325 (93.3)	39,155 (95.8)	26,294 (95.5)	10,113 (97.0)	< 0.001
Yes	4386	1106 (6.7)	1724 (4.2)	1239 (4.5)	317 (3.0)	
Missing[a]	783					
Pregnancy Complications						
Threatened abortion	11,428	1695 (10.2)	4885 (11.9)	3451 (12.4)	1397 (13.3)	< 0.001
Threatened premature labor	18,715	2896 (17.5)	7990 (19.4)	5566 (20.1)	2263 (21.5)	< 0.001
Premature rupture of membrane	7932	1549 (9.3)	3374 (8.2)	2218 (8.0)	791 (7.5)	< 0.001
Pregnancy-induced hypertension	2964	622 (3.8)	1189 (2.9)	841 (3.0)	312 (3.0)	< 0.001

Chi-squared test
[a] Not included in percentage distribution

Table 2 Distribution of gestational week according to NVP status

	Total	No NVP	Mild NVP	Moderate NVP	Severe NVP	P value
	n = 96,056	n = 16,596	n = 41,198	n = 27,744	n = 10,518	
Gestational week, Median (p5–p95), weeks						
	39.4 (37.0–41.1)	39.4 (36.9–41.3)	39.4 (37.0–41.1)	39.4 (37.0–41.1)	39.4 (37.0–41.3)	0.006[a]
Gestational week, n(%)						
26–27 week	88	16 (0.10)	46 (0.11)	20 (0.07)	6 (0.06)	< 0.001[b]
28–31 week	364	94 (0.6)	152 (0.4)	93 (0.3)	25 (0.2)	
32–36 week	3929	743 (4.5)	1674 (4.1)	1089 (3.9)	423 (4.0)	
37–41 week	91,454	15,694 (94.6)	39,224 (95.2)	26,495 (95.5)	10,041 (95.5)	

[a] Kruskal-Wallis test
[b] Chi-squared test

Results

As shown in Table 1, the 96,056 pregnant women were categorized into no NVP (n = 16,596; 17.3%), mild NVP (n = 41,198; 42.9%), moderate NVP (n = 27,744; 28.9%), and severe NVP (n = 10,518; 10.9%). Higher rates of no symptoms of NVP were seen among women with older age, nullipara, higher education, low pre-pregnancy BMI, and smoking during pregnancy.

The prevalence of pregnancy-related complications possibly causing preterm birth were also significantly different among the four groups. In women without NVP, the prevalence of threatened abortion and threatened premature labor were lowest, whereas rates of preterm rupture of membrane and pregnancy-induced hypertension were highest (Table 1).

The overall rate of preterm births (< 37 weeks) was 4.6% (4397/96,056). Rates of extremely (26–27 weeks), very (28–31 weeks), and moderately (32–36 weeks) preterm births were 0.09% (88/96,056), 0.38% (364/96,056), and 4.1% (3929/96,056), respectively. Median gestational age was not statistically influenced by NVP status. However, the prevalence of preterm birth was slightly higher in women without NVP (Table 2). When compared to women without NVP, women with mild or moderate NVP had lower odds for overall preterm births (aOR 0.87, 95% CI 0.80–0.95 and aOR 0.85, 95% CI 0.78–0.93, respectively), and women with severe NVP had the lowest odds (aOR 0.84, 95% CI 0.74–0.95; Table 3). Differences between women with and without NVP were more obvious when the risk of very preterm birth and extremely preterm birth was analyzed. When compared to women without NVP, women with mild or moderate NVP had lower

odds for very preterm birth and extremely preterm birth (aOR 0.74, 95% CI 0.58–0.94 and aOR 0.62, 95% CI 0.47–0.82, respectively), and women with severe NVP had the lowest odds (aOR 0.44, 95% CI 0.29–0.67; Table 4).

Discussion

In our nationwide cohort study of approximately 100,000 births, we found that NVP symptoms were associated with decreased risk of preterm birth. An even lower OR was found for very preterm birth and extremely preterm birth. Furthermore, pregnancy complications such as preterm rupture of membrane and pregnancy-induced hypertension were less frequent in women who experienced at least some symptoms of NVP than in women with no NVP.

These findings are similar to the results of a Norwegian large cohort study showing higher prevalence of preterm births in women who did not experience NVP than in women who did experience NVP [15]. Czeizel showed that women who had medically recorded NVP and were treated for it had longer gestational age and a lower proportion of preterm birth than women who had mild NVP without any treatment or hospitalization due to hyperemesis gravidarum [16]. Klebanoff reported lower rates of preterm births in women who reported vomiting during pregnancy [13]. These two results are also similar to our findings, whereas Naumann and Weigel reported no association between NVP and rate of preterm births [18, 19], and Temming reported higher rates of preterm births in women who reported NVP [17].

As Czeizel indicated, these previous inconsistent results may be attributed to the difference in the

Table 3 Odds ratio of preterm birth in relation to NVP status

	No NVP	Mild NVP			Moderate NVP			Severe NVP		
		OR	95% CI	P value	OR	95% CI	P value	OR	95% CI	P value
Crude Odds ratio	1(reference)	0.88	0.81–0.95	0.002	0.84	0.76–0.91	< 0.001	0.83	0.74–0.94	0.002
Adjusted Odds ratio[a]	1(reference)	0.87	0.80–0.95	0.002	0.85	0.78–0.93	0.001	0.84	0.74–0.95	0.004

[a] Adjusted for maternal age, BMI, smoking, education and parity

Table 4 Odds ratio of very preterm birth and extremely preterm birth in relation to NVP status

	No NVP	Mild NVP			Moderate NVP			Severe NVP		
		OR	95% CI	P value	OR	95% CI	P value	OR	95% CI	P value
Crude Odds ratio	1(reference)	0.72	0.57–0.91	0.007	0.61	0.47–0.80	< 0.001	0.44	0.30–0.66	< 0.001
Adjusted Odds ratio[a]	1(reference)	0.74	0.58–0.94	0.01	0.62	0.47–0.82	0.001	0.44	0.29–0.67	< 0.001

[a] Adjusted for maternal age, BMI, smoking, education and parity

definition/classification of NVP [16]. Various classifications of NVP were used in past studies because NVP still has no universally accepted definition/classification. Some studies classified NVP into three categories: no NVP, nausea only, and nausea/vomiting [14, 15, 19]. Other studies classified NVP into two categories, but how they assigned the categories varied [13, 16, 18]. Koren established a scoring system for NVP, classifying them into none, mild, moderate, and severe according to the number of vomiting or retching episodes and the length of nausea episodes [6, 22]. In our study, although the questionnaire about NVP had four choices, it did not collect information on duration or frequency of NVP. Therefore, we might not be able to precisely estimate the severity of NVP from our questionnaire in the manner Koren recommended. However, when we analyzed the variables of NVP by merging three choices with any symptoms of NVP into one category, the association between NVP and preterm births remained negative (data not shown).

Other possible reasons for previous inconsistent results may be the mild effect of NVP on gestational age and the difference of sample size [16]. In this study, the association between NVP and decreased risk of preterm birth was statistically significant. However, the clinical impact induced by this association is considered to be modest. Therefore, a large sample size is needed to demonstrate the association between NVP and birth outcomes. Previous studies which demonstrated an association between NVP and decreased risk of preterm birth had a large sample size. For example, Czeizel examined 38,151women and Chortatos examined 51,675 women, respectively [15, 16]. However, studies which concluded there was no association between NVP and preterm birth had smaller sample sizes [17, 18]. Our study showed the generalizability of previous findings from large cohort studies to an Asian population.

The etiopathogenesis of NVP, although unclear, is likely to be multifactorial, including placenta-mediated mechanisms [5]. Niebyl mentioned that NVP is less common in older women, multiparous women and smokers, which is attributed to the smaller placental volumes in these women [23]. In our study, NVP was less common in older women and smokers, as in Niebyl's study. Furthermore, NVP is more common in women with high BMI. This fact further supports Niebyl's speculation, because overweight and obese women generally have a heavier placenta [24]. However, multiparous women experienced NVP more often than nulliparous women in this study, which diverges from Niebyl's report. To prove the hypothesis that placental volume affects symptoms of NVP, future investigations on the association between placental characteristics and NVP status is needed.

Several limitations pertaining to this study should be considered. Information on the duration of NVP, treatment of NVP and late onset NVP could not be obtained. Therefore, we could not assess prolonged NVP and late onset NVP. The fact that information on maternal characteristics and NVP were missing in some cases was also a limitation. Some women who delivered preterm babies before 26 weeks may have failed to answer the questionnaire because they may have delivered before the questionnaire was provided. Therefore, we excluded women who had delivered before 26 weeks of gestation.

The strengths of our study are that it is a large population-based cohort study. To our knowledge, our study is the largest study to date on this topic and the first study to evaluate the association between NVP and preterm births in the Asian population. These data enabled us to analyze risks of subgroups that experienced preterm birth against a range of confounding factors, including maternal characteristics and prenatal risk factors. The fact that information on NVP were obtained before delivery is another strength of this study. Besides the adjustment for confounders, the standardized healthcare system in Japan and the relatively homogeneous Japanese pregnant population should limit possibilities of residual confounding.

Conclusion

NVP was inversely associated with preterm births, especially for very preterm births and extremely preterm births. Further investigation of the association between severity of NVP and placental characteristics or hormonal milieu is needed.

Abbreviations
aOR: Adjusted odds ratio; BMI: Body mass index; CI: Confidence interval; cOR: Crude odds ratio; JECS: The Japan Environment and Children's Study; NVP: Nausea and vomiting during pregnancy; OR: Odds ratio

Acknowledgements

We would like to express our appreciation to all participants of this study and to all individuals involved in the data collection. Members of JECS as of 2016 (principal investigator, Toshihiro Kawamoto): Hirohisa Saito (Medical Support Center for JECS, National Center for Child Health and Development, Tokyo, Japan), Reiko Kishi (Hokkaido Regional Center for JECS, Hokkaido University, Sapporo, Japan), Nobuo Yaegashi (Miyagi Regional Center for JECS, Tohoku University, Sendai, Japan), Koichi Hashimoto (Fukushima Regional Center for JECS, Fukushima Medical University, Fukushima, Japan), Chisato Mori (Chiba Regional Center for JECS, Chiba University, Chiba, Japan), Shuichi Ito (Kanagawa Regional Center for JECS, Yokohama City University, Yokohama, Japan), Zentaro Yamagata (Koshin Regional Center for JECS, University of Yamanashi, Chuo, Japan), Hidekuni Inadera (Toyama Regional Center for JECS, University of Toyama, Toyama, Japan), Michihiro Kamijima (Aichi Regional Center for JECS, Nagoya City University, Nagoya, Japan), Toshio Heike (Kyoto Regional Center for JECS, Kyoto University, Kyoto, Japan), Hiroyasu Iso (Osaka Regional Center for JECS, Osaka University, Suita, Japan), Masayuki Shima (Hyogo Regional Center for JECS, Hyogo College of Medicine, Nishinomiya, Japan), Yasuaki Kawai (Tottori Regional Center for JECS, Tottori University, Yonago, Japan), Narufumi Suganuma (Kochi Regional Center for JECS, Kochi University, Nankoku, Japan), Koichi Kusuhara (Fukuoka Regional Center for JECS, University of Occupational and Environmental Health, Kitakyushu, Japan), and Takahiko Katoh (South Kyushu/Okinawa Regional Center for JECS, Kumamoto University, Kumamoto, Japan).

Funding

The Japan Environment and Children's Study was funded by the Japanese Ministry of Environment. The findings and conclusions of this article are solely the responsibility of the authors and do not represent the official views of the above government agency.

Authors' contributions

Study Concept and design: NMi, ME, KY and MS. Analysis of data: NMi, ME and MS. Interpretation of data: NMi, ME, KY, MS, KY, NMa, MF and NS. Drafting of the manuscript: NMi. Critical revision of the manuscript: NMi, ME, KY, MS, KY, NMa, MF, NS and JECS group. All authors read and approved the final manuscript.

Competing interests

The authors declare that they have no competing interests.

Author details

[1]Department of Environmental Medicine, Kochi Medical School, Kochi University, Kohasu, Oko-cho, Nankoku, Kochi 783-8505, Japan. [2]Integrated Center for Advanced Medical Technologies, Kochi Medical School, Kochi University, Kochi, Japan. [3]Department of Obstetrics and Gynecology, Kochi Medical School, Kochi University, Kochi, Japan. [4]Department of Pediatrics, Kochi Medical School, Kochi University, Kochi, Japan. [5]Cancer Prevention and Control Division, Kanagawa Cancer Center Research Institute, Kanagawa, Japan.

References

1. Einarson TR, Piwko C, Koren G. Quantifying the global rates of nausea and vomiting of pregnancy: a meta analysis. J Popul Ther Clin Pharmacol. 2013; 20:171–83.
2. Colodro-Conde L, Cross SM, Lind PA, Painter JN, Gunst A, Jern P, Johansson A, Lund Maegbaek M, Munk-Olsen T, Nyholt DR, et al. Cohort Profile: Nausea and vomiting during pregnancy genetics consortium (NVP Genetics Consortium). Int J Epidemiol. 2017;46(2):e17.
3. Lagiou P, Tamimi R, Mucci LA, Trichopoulos D, Adami HO, Hsieh CC. Nausea and vomiting in pregnancy in relation to prolactin, estrogens, and progesterone: a prospective study. Obstet Gynecol. 2003;101:639–44.
4. Masson GM, Anthony F, Chau E. Serum chorionic gonadotrophin (hCG), schwangerschaftsprotein 1 (SP1), progesterone and oestradiol levels in patients with nausea and vomiting in early pregnancy. Br J Obstet Gynaecol. 1985;92:211–5.
5. Bustos M, Venkataramanan R, Caritis S. Nausea and vomiting of pregnancy - What's new? Auton Neurosci. 2017;202:62–72.
6. Lacasse A, Rey E, Ferreira E, Morin C, Berard A. Validity of a modified pregnancy-unique quantification of Emesis and nausea (PUQE) scoring index to assess severity of nausea and vomiting of pregnancy. Am J Obstet Gynecol. 2008;198:71–7.
7. Sherman PW, Flaxman SM. Nausea and vomiting of pregnancy in an evolutionary perspective. Am J Obstet Gynecol. 2002;186:190–7.
8. Flaxman SM, Sherman PW. Morning sickness: adaptive cause or nonadaptive consequence of embryo viability? Am Nat. 2008;172:54–62.
9. Huxley RR. Nausea and vomiting in early pregnancy: its role in placental development. Obstet Gynecol. 2000;95:779–82.
10. Koren G, Madjunkova S, Maltepe C. The protective effects of nausea and vomiting of pregnancy against adverse fetal outcome–a systematic review. Reprod Toxicol. 2014;47:77–80.
11. Hinkle SN, Mumford SL, Grantz KL, Silver RM, Mitchell EM, Sjaarda LA, Radin RG, Perkins NJ, Galai N, Schisterman EF. Association of Nausea and Vomiting during Pregnancy with Pregnancy Loss: a secondary analysis of a randomized clinical trial. JAMA Intern Med. 2016;176:1621–7.
12. Chan RL, Olshan AF, Savitz DA, Herring AH, Daniels JL, Peterson HB, Martin SL. Severity and duration of nausea and vomiting symptoms in pregnancy and spontaneous abortion. Hum Reprod. 2010;25:2907–12.
13. Klebanoff MA, Koslowe PA, Kaslow R, Rhoads GG. Epidemiology of vomiting in early pregnancy. Obstet Gynecol. 1985;66:612–6.
14. Weigel MM, Weigel RM. Nausea and vomiting of early pregnancy and pregnancy outcome. An epidemiological study. Br J Obstet Gynaecol. 1989; 96:1304–11.
15. Chortatos A, Haugen M, Iversen PO, Vikanes A, Eberhard-Gran M, Bjelland EK, Magnus P, Veierod MB. Pregnancy complications and birth outcomes among women experiencing nausea only or nausea and vomiting during pregnancy in the Norwegian mother and child cohort study. BMC Pregnancy Childbirth. 2015;15:138.
16. Czeizel AE, Puho E. Association between severe nausea and vomiting in pregnancy and lower rate of preterm births. Paediatr Perinat Epidemiol. 2004;18:253–9.
17. Temming L, Franco A, Istwan N, Rhea D, Desch C, Stanziano G, Joy S. Adverse pregnancy outcomes in women with nausea and vomiting of pregnancy. J Matern Fetal Neonatal Med. 2014;27:84–8.
18. Naumann CR, Zelig C, Napolitano PG, Ko CW. Nausea, vomiting, and heartburn in pregnancy: a prospective look at risk, treatment, and outcome. J Matern Fetal Neonatal Med. 2012;25:1488–93.
19. Weigel MM, Reyes M, Caiza ME, Tello N, Castro NP, Cespedes S, Duchicela S, Betancourt M. Is the nausea and vomiting of early pregnancy really feto-protective? J Perinat Med. 2006;34:115–22.
20. Kawamoto T, Nitta H, Murata K, Toda E, Tsukamoto N, Hasegawa M, Yamagata Z, Kayama F, Kishi R, Ohya Y, et al. Rationale and study design of the Japan environment and children's study (JECS). BMC Public Health. 2014;14:25.
21. Tucker J, McGuire W. Epidemiology of preterm birth. BMJ. 2004;329:675–8.
22. Koren G, Boskovic R, Hard M, Maltepe C, Navioz Y, Einarson A. Motherisk—PUQE (pregnancy-unique quantification of emesis and nausea) scoring system for nausea and vomiting of pregnancy. Am J Obstet Gynecol. 2002;186:228–31.

Folic acid supplementation, preconception body mass index, and preterm delivery: findings from the preconception cohort data in a Chinese rural population

Yuanyuan Wang[1,2], Zongfu Cao[1,2], Zuoqi Peng[1], Xiaona Xin[1,2], Ya Zhang[1], Ying Yang[1], Yuan He[1], Jihong Xu[1] and Xu Ma[1,2]*

Abstract

Background: Folic acid (FA) supplementation before and during the first trimester can reduce the risk of occurrence of preterm delivery (PTD). Preconception body mass index (BMI) is also associated with PTD. This study aimed to investigate the combined effect of FA supplements and preconception BMI on the risk of PTD.

Methods: The data of a cohort from 2010–2011 that was obtained through a preconception care service in China was used (including 172,206 women). A multivariable regression model was used to investigate the association between maternal preconception conditions and the risk of PTD. The interaction of preconception BMI and FA supplementation was measured by a logistic regression model.

Results: Taking FA supplements in the preconception period or in the first trimester reduced the risk of PTD (odds ratio [OR] = 0.58 and OR = 0.61, respectively). Women with an abnormal BMI had an increased risk of PTD (OR = 1.09, OR = 1.10, and OR = 1.17 for underweight, overweight, and obese, respectively). Preconception BMI showed an interaction with the protective effect of FA supplementation for PTD. With regard to the interaction of FA supplementation, the adjusted odds ratio (aOR) was 0.57 (95 % CI: 0.51, 0.64) in underweight women, 0.85 (95 % CI: 0.73, 0.98) in overweight women, and 0.77 (95 % CI, 0.65, 0.91) in obese women. Preconception BMI also showed an interaction with the time of FA supplementation. Women with a normal BMI who began to take FA supplements in the preconception period had the lowest risk of PTD (aORs: 0.58 vs. 0.65 beginning in the first trimester). The aORs at preconception and the first trimester in the underweight group were 0.56 vs. 0.60. The aORs at preconception and the first trimester were 0.94 vs. 0.65 and 1.15 vs. 0.60 in the overweight and obesity groups, respectively.

Conclusions: In our study, FA supplements reduced the risk of PTD, while abnormal BMI raised the risk of PTD, although higher BMI categories did not have this higher risk once adjusted analysis was conducted. The protective effect of FA supplementation for PTD was reduced in women with overweight or obesity. To get better protection of FA supplementation, women with normal BMI or underweight should begin to use in preconception, while women with overweight or obesity should begin to use after conception.

Keywords: Folic acid supplement, Maternal body mass index, Interaction, Preterm deivery, Preconception

* Correspondence: genetic88@126.com
[1]National Research Institute for Family Planning, No. 12, Dahuisi Road, Haidian District, Beijing 100081, China
[2]Graduate School of Peking Union Medical College, No. 9, Dongdansantiao, Dongcheng District, Beijing 100730, China

Background

Preterm delivery (PTD) is defined as neonates who are born alive before 37 weeks of pregnancy are completed. PTD is the second largest direct cause of child deaths in children younger than 5 years and causes approximately 1 million deaths annually worldwide. Additionally, PTD causes lifelong problems for many survivors [1].

The incidence of PTD was 7.1 % in a multicenter, hospital-based investigation (based on 107,905 deliveries) in China. The proportion of PTD among the causes of neonatal death has significantly increased from 33.6 % in 2003 to 40.9 % in 2008. PTD is the leading cause of neonatal death in China [2]. Because of the large population in China, China has become the second largest country with annual preterm deliveries. PTD is a serious public health problem in China.

PTD is thought to be a syndrome that is initiated by multiple mechanisms. However, the precise mechanism of PTD has not been established. Therefore, factors associated with preterm birth, but not obviously in the causal pathway, have been sought to explain preterm labor.

Folic acid (FA), an oxidized synthetic water-soluble member of the vitamin-B complex family, plays an essential role in one-carbon metabolism. The clinical application of FA supplementation to prevent neural tube defects (NTD) had been well proven in the last 20–25 years. Pregnant women are at risk of folate deficiency because pregnancy greatly increases folate requirements, especially during periods of rapid fetal growth (i.e., in the second and third trimesters). Although the relation between maternal folate status with NTD has been well established [3, 4], the association of folate status with other adverse pregnancy outcomes is still unclear [5]. Recently, some researchers have investigated maternal FA supplementation and PTD, but the findings were largely inconclusive. Some results supported protective effects [6–9] and some did not [10–14, 15]. A large population-based cohort study conducted in China showed that daily intake of 0.4 mg folic acid reduced the risk of PTD [6]. A cohort in Singapore showed that higher plasma folate concentrations were associated with a longer gestational age and tended to be associated with a lower risk of PTD [16]. Similar results were obtained in some prospective observational studies in the USA [17, 18]. Some researches have shown that maternal FA supplementation during pregnancy protects against lipopolysaccharide-induced PTD through its anti-inflammatory effects [19–21]. Researchers have hypothesized that lower maternal serum folate concentrations during pregnancy is associated with higher maternal plasma homocysteine concentrations, which cause pre-eclampsia and affect placental function, eventually leading to PTD [22, 23].

Abnormal preconception body mass index (BMI) is a risk factor for PTD [24, 25, 26]. The spontaneous PTD rate is higher in pre-pregnancy underweight women (BMI <18.5 kg/m^2) than in normal-weight women [27, 28]. Some researchers have found that indicated PTD and premature rupture of the membranes are associated with preconception obesity, especially in extremely obese groups [27, 29]. Obese women are more likely to develop pre-eclampsia and diabetes, and have indicated preterm births associated with these disorders [30]. In a Boston birth cohort, pre-pregnancy obesity was associated with a decreased odds of PTD (0.76) and underweight was nearly associated with an increased odds of PTD (1.46) for spontaneous delivery [30].

Maternal BMI and FA supplementation can affect the risk of PTD. Some studies have shown that there is an inverse interaction between BMI and serum folate levels [31, 32]. Distribution of folate in the body is significantly affected by obesity, and should pregnancy occur, it may reduce the amount of folate available to the developing embryo [33–35]. The FA supplement guideline in Canada suggests that women with a BMI >35 kg/m^2 should take 5-mg folate supplements daily to prevent a poor outcome [36].

Whether there is any interactive effect between preconception BMI and FA supplementation for PTD is unclear. These previous studies mentioned above were mostly based on Caucasians, and there is a lack of Chinese population data. In this study, we aimed to determine whether FA supplementation can reduce the risk of PTD in China. We also investigated whether there is an interaction between FA supplementation and maternal BMI for the risk of PTD in the Chinese population.

Methods

Study design

This study was designed as a retrospective cohort study. From 2010, the free National Pre-pregnancy Checkups Project (NPCP) for rural women was carried out, which collected the largest pregnancy cohort data from the preconception stage in China. The NPCP is a population-based, free, preconception medical examination and services for rural reproductive-age couples who are trying to conceive in China. The NPCP covers couples who are preparing for pregnancy, from a preconception examination to pregnancy outcome follow-up. In 2010, the NPCP was first carried out in a 100-district region in China. In this study, examination data of the 100 districts in 2010 was used. The 100 districts are distributed throughout 18 provinces, including four provinces in eastern China (Jiangsu, Zhejiang, Shandong, and Guangdong), six provinces in central China (Hebei, Jilin, Anhui, Henan, Hubei, and Hunan), and eight provinces in western China (Guangxi, Chongqing, Sichuan, Guizhou, Yunnan, Shanxi, Gansu, and Xinjiang). The total population of the research area in 2010 was 7.16 million (females, 3.49 million; males, 3.67 million, approximately 5 % of the total population of

China [37]). The rural population in the 100 districts was 4.76 million (66 % of the total population). Rural couples trying to conceive who lived in these areas could receive a free medical checkup in county-level medical institutions from January 2010 to December 2010 in the project. The clinical data were collected during the preconception medical examination. Information on socioeconomic background, reproductive history and history of illness, lifestyle behaviors, and dietary habits were carefully collected through face-to-face interviews by qualified nurses. Physical and biochemical examinations were also carried out by medical staff at the same time, including measurement of maternal height, weight, blood pressure, and hemoglobin levels.

After the examination, the couples received two follow-up interviews. The first interview was a telephone interview carried out by a trained nurse 3 months after conception. This interview was designed to obtain information of the last menstrual period and FA supplement use status (including the time when first taking FA). The second interview was carried out face-to-face or by telephone 1 month after delivery. Newborn information was collected by a trained interviewer according to the participants' answers. The current study was conducted in accordance with the Declaration of Helsinki (2000) of the World Medical Association and the protocols were approved by the Institutional Research Review Board at the National Population and Family Planning Commission. Informed consent in Chinese was obtained from all NFPC participants.

Study population

Couples who attended the preconception medical examination and obtained successful conception within 6 months in the cohort were eligible (200,165). A total of 19,398 participants were excluded because of missing data, lost to follow-up, abortion (spontaneous or induced), and stillbirth. Women with post-term pregnancy (≥42 weeks) and multiple pregnancies were not included in the study (8561). Finally, 172,206 pregnancies were selected for analysis (Fig. 1).

Definition of variables

The outcome variable in this analysis was PTD, which was defined as neonates who were born alive before 37 weeks of pregnancy were completed. Gestational age was calculated from the last menstrual period and the birth date. The independent variables were those expected to be associated with PTD based on current literature [38], including pertinent health variables (maternal preconception BMI, anemia, diabetes, and hypertension), pregnancy history, health behavior, and demographic variables. Preconception BMI (kg/m^2) was calculated using maternal weight and height during the preconception physical examination.

Because the participants in this study were all Chinese women, Chinese BMI classification standards were used in this study to classify different BMI groups. BMI <18.5 was considered underweight, BMI ≥18.5 and <24 was considered normal, BMI ≥24 and <28 was considered overweight, and BMI ≥28 was considered obese according to the Chinese population standards [39, 40].

FA supplementation was based on self-reported use in the first interview. FA supplementation was defined as women who had used supplements and had either taken FA alone or multivitamins (containing FA). FA supplement information was obtained in the first trimester follow-up. Therefore, we divided FA supplementation into three groups according to the time when the participants began to take FA: none, after conception, and preconception. Hypertension was defined as high blood pressure in the preconception examination (SBP ≥140 mmHg or DBP ≥90 mmHg) and self-reported hypertension. Diabetes was defined as self-reported diabetes or blood sugar ≥7 mmol/L. Anemia was defined as hemoglobin levels <110 g/L when the participant took the biochemical examination in the preconception service. Preconception dietary habits were defined as risk factors based on the self report, such as "dislike vegetables" and "vegetarian", which indicated "seldom eat meat and eggs". Tobacco use was defined as smoking at least one cigarette per day for at least 1 year in current smokers.

Statistical analysis

All analyses were generated using SAS software (version 8.2, SAS Institute Inc., North Carolina). The general characteristics of mothers and children based on different categories of maternal preconception BMI and FA supplementation were compared using the chi-squared test and t-test. Logistic regression was used to estimate the crude odds ratio (cOR) and the adjusted odds ratio (aOR) with 95 % confidence intervals (CIs) of PTD [41]. Covariates in the multivariable models included demographic factors (maternal age, education level, ethnic group, and career) and preconception risk factors (hypertension, anemia, alcohol use). The time of FA supplement was calculated by setting the dummy variable. The effect of FA supplementation of different weight group was calculated through the contrasts estimated in the model. A significant p value was set at 0.05.

Results

The mean age of the participants was 24.98 ± 3.87 years and the mean gestational age was 39.14 ± 1.67 weeks. The mean BMI was 21.03 ± 5.39 kg/m^2. A total of 9573 infants were born PTD. 159,635 (92.7 %) mothers were 21–35 years old, 163,767 mothers were Han ethnic (95.1 %), and 163,423 had at least a junior or higher

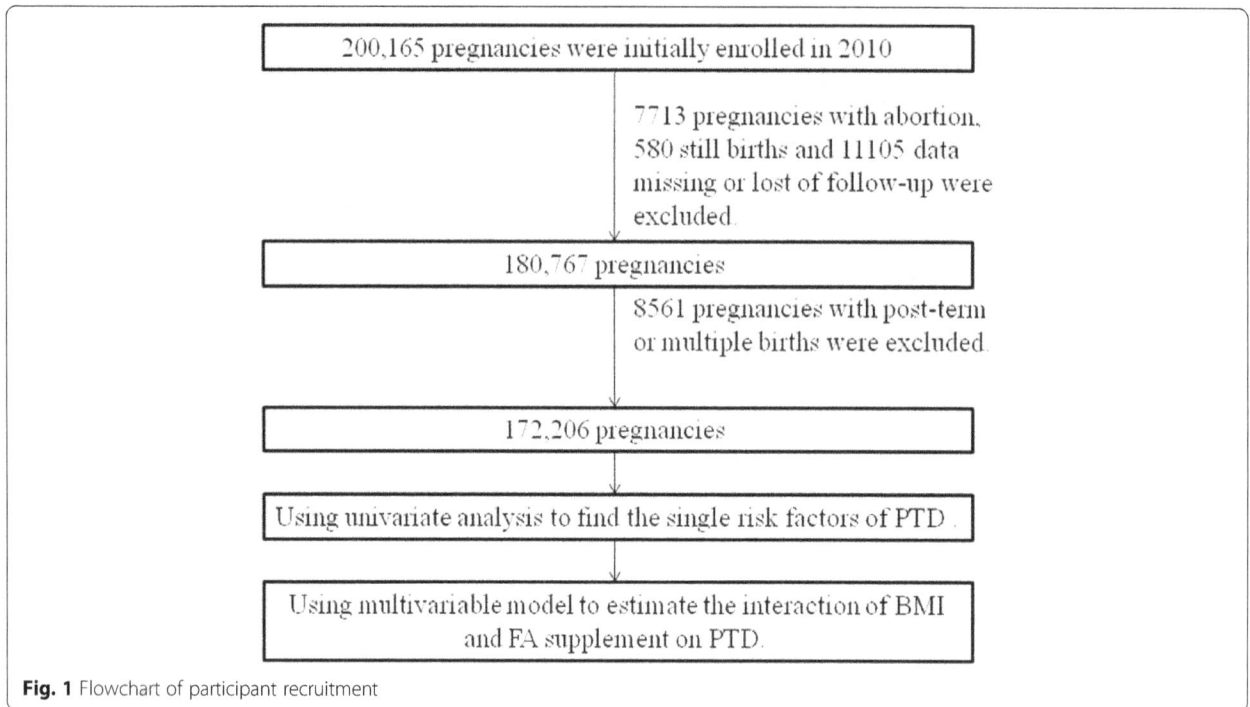

Fig. 1 Flowchart of participant recruitment

school education (94.9 %). The proportion of FA supplementation was 76.8 % and the proportion of an abnormal BMI (obese, overweight, and underweight) was 24.5 %. We compared maternal characteristics grouped by preconception BMI and FA supplementation status. Overweight or obese women were more likely to have hypertension or diabetes at preconception than women with a normal BMI or underweight women (Table 1). The proportion of women with high school or higher education experience was higher in women using FA than in nonusers. More population characteristics are shown in Table 1.

Women with an abnormal BMI had an increased risk of PTD (OR = 1.09, OR = 1.10, and OR = 1.17 for underweight, overweight, and obese, respectively). Preconception disease also raised the risk of PTD (OR = 1.49 and OR = 1.19 for hypertension and anemia, respectively). Women using alcohol had a higher risk of PTD (OR = 1.24). The risk of PTD was decreased by taking FA supplements, and this phenomenon was time-related. Taking FA supplements in the preconception period or in the first trimester reduced the risk of PTD (OR = 0.58 and OR = 0.61, respectively). The difference between the preconception period and the first trimester was not significant by transforming the first trimester as the reference group ($p = 0.053$). Details were listed in Table 2.

An interaction effect was found between preconception BMI and FA supplementation for PTD (Table 3). Taking FA supplements reduced the risk of PTD in all groups. Non-users with a normal BMI had a baseline risk of 7.95

PTD births per 100 live births, whereas mothers who took FA supplements had 4.69 PTD births per 100 live births (OR = 0.60). The OR of FA supplementation varied in different BMI groups. In underweight group, the OR of FA was 0.57 (95 % CI: 0.51, 0.64); in overweight group, the OR was 0.85 (95 % CI: 0.73,0.98); in obese group, the OR was 0.77 (95 % CI: 0.65,0.91). The interaction between maternal BMI and time of FA supplements was compared to examine why the protective effect was different among different BMI groups. We found that the protective effect of FA supplement in women with normal or underweight had similar values. The effect of FA supplement was different in overweight and obesity group, especially in preconception. Women with a BMI <24 kg/m^2 (including normal and underweight groups) who took FA supplements from preconception had a lower risk for PTD than in the first trimester (OR: 0.58 vs. 0.65 in the normal weight group, 0.56 vs. 0.60 in the underweight group). Women with a BMI ≥24 kg/m^2 (including the overweight and obese groups) who took FA supplements from the first trimester had a lower risk of PTD than at preconception (OR: 0.65 vs. 0.94 in the overweight group, 0.60 vs. 1.15 in the obesity group). Compared with no takers, obese women took FA supplement in preconception had an OR of 1.15 (not statistical significant).

Discussion

In our research population, the proportion of FA supplementation was as high as 76.8 % and more than 50 % women began to take FA supplements before conception.

Table 1 Maternal characteristics in study population grouped by preconception body mass index and folic acid supplement

	Preconception body mass index(kg^2)				P	Folic acid supplement			P
	<18.5	18.5-23.9	24-27.9	≥28		Never	1st trimester	Preconception	
Maternal characteristics									
No of subject	23429	129982	15880	2915		39871	41457	90878	
Demographic information (%)									
Maternal age (yr)	24.96(3.19)	24.18(3.82)	26.01(4.54)	26.60(4.70)	<0.001	24.85(3.94)	24.77(3.69)	25.13(3.90)	<0.001
Maternal education level									
Primary school	4.72	4.96	6.78	8.03	<0.001	5.01	4.51	5.50	<0.001
Junior school	60.56	67.38	71.79	72.42		73.50	63.63	65.57	
High school	21.82	18.81	15.29	14.68		15.35	20.68	19.51	
College and above	12.89	8.85	6.13	4.87		6.14	11.18	9.42	
House wife									
Yes	2.60	2.21	2.15	2.06	0.002	2.11	2.41	2.24	0.013
No	97.40	97.79	97.85	97.94		97.89	97.59	97.76	
Chinese Ethnic group									
Chinese Han	95.36	95.02	95.41	95.64	0.015	94.98	96.47	94.55	<0.001
Others	4.64	4.98	4.59	4.36		5.02	3.53	5.45	
Maternal risk factors (%)									
Previous preterm delivery									
No	99.75	99.83	99.62	99.59	<0.001	99.79	99.83	99.78	0.239
Yes	0.25	0.17	0.38	0.41		0.21	0.17	0.22	
Preconception hypertension									
No	98.41	97.99	95.74	90.05	<0.001	97.29	98.08	97.71	<0.001
Yes	1.59	2.01	4.26	9.95		2.71	1.92	2.29	
Anemia									
No	84.54	85.99	85.21	87.38	<0.001	83.98	83.41	87.58	<0.001
Yes	15.46	14.01	14.79	12.62		16.02	16.59	12.42	
Diabetes mellitus									
No	98.34	98.77	98.05	96.84	<0.001	98.63	98.28	98.76	<0.001
Yes	1.66	1.23	1.95	3.16		1.37	1.72	1.24	
Dislike vegetables									
No	99.24	99.37	99.17	99.11	0.004	99.27	99.34	99.34	0.286
Yes	0.76	0.63	0.83	0.89		0.73	0.66	0.66	
Preconception alcohol use									
No	96.79	97.01	97.20	97.32	0.080	97.43	96.83	96.89	<0.001
Yes	3.21	2.99	2.80	2.68		2.57	3.17	3.11	
Preconception Tobacco use									
No	99.63	99.70	99.57	99.31	<0.001	99.70	99.58	99.70	0.001
Yes	0.37	0.30	0.43	0.69		0.30	0.42	0.30	
Preterm delivery									
No	94.11	94.57	94.05	93.69	0.001	92.08	94.98	95.23	<0.001
Yes	5.89	5.43	5.95	6.31		7.92	5.02	4.77	

The reason for the high rate of supplementation in this population was based on a nation-wide free FA supplementation program, which was implemented in rural areas of China since 2009. The Chinese guideline of FA supplements is 0.4 mg/d from preconception to the end of the first trimester. Women who had rural household

Table 2 Crude odds ratio (95 % confidence intervals) of preterm delivery by maternal characteristics and single risk factor

	Number	PTD		
		%	cOR (95 % CI)	P value
Maternal characteristics				
Maternal age				
≤ 20 years	8844	5.89	1.07 (0.98,1.17)	0.14
21–35 years	159640	5.53	1	
> 35 years	3722	6.18	1.13 (0.98,1.29)	0.09
Maternal education level				
Primary school and below	8866	4.87		
Junior school	115279	6.02	1.25 (1.13,1.38)	<0.01*
High school	32418	4.42	0.90 (0.81,1.01)	0.07
College and above	15643	4.88	1 (0.89,1.13)	0.97
Maternal career				
House wife	3878	7.01	1	
Others	168328	5.53	1.29 (1.14,1.46)	<0.01*
Chinese Ethnic group				
Chinese Han	163786	5.67	1	
Others	8420	3.46	0.60 (0.53,0.67)	<0.01*
Maternal risk factors				
Previous preterm delivery				
No	171852	5.56	1	
Yes	354	6.78	1.24 (0.82,1.87)	0.32
Preconception BMI				
Underweight	23429	5.89	1.09 (1.03,1.16)	<0.01*
Normal weight	129982	5.43	1	
Overweight	15880	5.95	1.10 (1.03,1.18)	0.01*
Obese	2915	6.31	1.17 (1.01,1.36)	0.04*
Preconception hypertension				
No	168248	5.5	1	
Yes	3958	7.98	1.49 (1.33,1.67)	<0.01*
Anemia				
No	147657	5.42	1	
Yes	24549	6.37	1.19 (1.12,1.25)	<0.01*
Diabetes mellitus				
No	169819	5.55	1	
Yes	2387	6.12	1.11 (0.94,1.31)	0.23
Folic acid supplement				
Never	39871	7.92	1	
1st trimester	41457	5.02	0.61(0.58,0.65)	<0.01*
Preconception	90878	4.77	0.58(0.56,0.61)	<0.01*
Dislike vegetables				
No	171047	5.55	1	
Yes	1159	6.47	1.18(0.93,1.49)	0.17
Preconception alcohol use				

Table 2 Crude odds ratio (95 % confidence intervals) of preterm delivery by maternal characteristics and single risk factor (Continued)

No	167040	5.52	1	
Yes	5166	6.78	1.24 (1.11,1.39)	<0.01*
Preconception tobacco use				
No	171641	5.56	1	
Yes	565	6.19	0.85 (0.58,1.25)	0.42

Note: cOR = crude odds ratio

registration and planned to become pregnant were eligible to obtain FA tablets containing 0.4 mg FA for 6 months at no charge [42].

A negative association was found between FA supplementation and the risk of PTD in our population. FA supplementation showed a strong protective effect on PTD. This protective rate varied from 35 % to 40 % according to different supplementation times. Women who began to take FA supplements in the preconception period had the lowest risk of PTD (cOR = 0.58, details in Table 2). Similar results were reported in the USA, where the duration of preconceptional folate supplementation affected the protective effect for PTD. In a meta-analysis, many observational studies suggested a slight reduction in PTD, which was not consistent with the results from randomized, controlled trials [43]. The risk of spontaneous preterm birth decreased with the duration of preconceptional folate supplementation, and taking FA supplements over 1 year could reduce the risk of early spontaneous preterm birth by 50–70 %. In contrast, a cohort of Norwegians showed the opposite result, where preconceptional FA supplementation starting more than 8 weeks before conception was associated with an increased risk of PTD (hazard ratio = 1.19) [44]. Another study showed a 20 % lowered risk of PTD was found in the first trimester compared with preconception [33].

In our population, we found that women who were underweight/overweight/obese were at increased risk of PTD in single risk factor analysis (Table 2). Similar results were also reported in the USA and India [29, 45, 46]. Spontaneous preterm birth could be caused by maternal

Table 3 Effect of FA supplement in different BMI group for PTD

BMI group	FA supplement OR (95 % CI)					
	No	Yes		1st trimester		Preconception
Normal	ref	0.60	(0.57,0.63)	0.65	(0.61,0.69)	0.58 (0.55,0.62)
Underweight	ref	0.57	(0.51,0.64)	0.60	(0.52,0.69)	0.56 (0.49,0.63)
Overweight	ref	0.85	(0.73,0.98)	0.65	(0.53,0.79)	0.94 (0.80,1.10)
Obesity	ref	0.77	(0.65,0.91)	0.60	(0.37,0.97)	1.15 (0.81,1.64)

Note: Adjusted for maternal education, career, ethnic, hypertension, anemia, alcohol use thinness associated with decreased blood volume and fewer vitamins and minerals, which are associated with increased maternal infections. Serum folate levels are lower in obese women than in normal or underweight women [32]. Obese women are more likely to develop pre-eclampsia and diabetes, and indicated preterm births are associated with these disorders [42]. In this study, we could only compare the interaction between FA supplementation and maternal BMI. The direct factor (folate levels) in the population was not compared (without original data). FA supplementation can reduce homocysteine, which causes pre-eclampsia and affects placental function and fetal maturity, eventually leading to PTD. Therefore, analyzing the interaction of FA and BMI for prevention of PTD is important.

An interaction between FA supplements and maternal BMI was found in our population, and the protective effect of FA varied in different BMI groups. Taking FA supplements of 0.4 mg/d (regardless of when they started) reduced the risk of PTD in all of the BMI groups. The time of taking FA supplement was very important in women with abnormal BMI. In the underweight group, there was very little difference between 1st trimester and preconception. But in overweight and obesity group, the difference was very large. We hypothesize that maternal body size is associated with folate metabolism, which can influence maternal homocysteine levels and affect embryonic development and gestational weeks [23, 47]. Distribution of folate in the body is significantly affected by BMI, and obesity might reduce the amount of folate available to the developing embryo [35, 36]. Obesity-associated metabolic alterations could have an effect on folate use or increase folate requirements [48, 49]. RBC folate increased incrementally with BMI, while serum folate concentrations were lower in obese groups [50]. We conclude that FA supplementation and maternal obesity can influence homocysteine levels, which might affect placental function and eventually lead to PTD. The distribution of folate might be changed in pregnancy period. We also compared the interaction between the time of FA supplements and maternal BMI. Women with a BMI <24 kg/m^2 (including the normal and underweight groups) who took FA supplements from preconception had a lower risk for PTD than in the first trimester. Women with a BMI ≥24 kg/m^2 (including the overweight and obese groups) who took FA supplements from the first trimester had a lower risk of PTD than at preconception. Several studies have shown that different supplementation times can change the protective effect of FA [9, 51]. In a similar study on NTD, the protective of FA was also weaker in the overweight and obesity population than in the normal and underweight population [52]. We suggest that a diverse plan of FA supplementation should be carried out according to women's BMI category. The time and dose of FA supplement for obesity should be taken into account.

Limitations

The primary limitation in the present study was misclassification of FA supplemental status. We relied on the self-reported use of FA supplements, which could lead to misclassification of FA supplemental status. We compared the proportion of FA supplements in our study with other studies (77 % vs. 68–92 % [47, 53]). The name and content of the FA supplement was not investigated in the first trimester interview. Therefore, we could not separate FA supplements and multiple vitamin supplements, including FA. Dietary folate was also not estimated in this cohort. We could not calculate the exact folate level. Further research should be carried out to verify the results of this study.

The second limitation of this study was that PTD could not be divided into indicated and spontaneous PTD. Pre-pregnancy obesity is associated with a higher risk of indicated, but not spontaneous, PTD [30]. This study was a retrospective cohort study. We could not analyze the risk of iatrogenic PTD because this type of PTD was not classified in the follow-up records. Detailed data should be collected to estimate the protective effect of FA between indicated PTD and spontaneous PTD in the future.

Because of the uncertainty of natural conception, we selected women who became pregnant in the following 6 months after the preconception medical examination as our research population. All statistical research was carried out in this population, which could also have reduced the effect of a change in maternal medical status on the results. Reported supplementation of FA for 1 year prior to conception has been linked with a decreased risk of preterm birth [54]. In our cohort, we did not test the protective effect of FA from 1 year before conception in our population. Because our study design only included 6 months of FA supplements in the pregnant population, the results may not apply to the whole population.

Conclusions

In our study, FA supplements reduced the risk of PTD, while abnormal BMI raised the risk of PTD, although higher BMI categories did not have this higher risk once adjusted analysis was conducted. The protective effect of FA supplementation for PTD is reduced in women whose BMI was equal or greater than 24 kg/m^2. To get better protection of FA supplementation, women with BMI < 24 kg/m^2 should begin to use in preconception, while women with BMI ≥24 kg/m^2 should begin to use after conception.

Abbreviations

FA: Folic acid; BMI: Body mass index; PTD: Preterm delivery; cOR: Crude odds ratio; aOR: Adjusted odds ratio; CIs: Confidence intervals.

Competing interests

The authors declare that they have no competing interests.

Authors' contributions

YY Wang: Study design and paper writing. ZF Cao: Statistical anlysis. ZQ Peng: Data collection. XN Xin: Data collection. Y Zhang: Data collection.Y Yang: Paper review. Y He: Paper review. JH Xu: Paper review. X Ma: Study design. All authors read and approved the final manuscript.

Acknowledgements

We thank all the participants in this research and all the medical staffs in the 100 counties for their hard work in NFPC.

Financial support

This study was supported by the "Five-twelfth" National Science and Technology Support Program (No.2012BAI41B08, No.2013BAI12B01) and the National Natural Science Foundation(No.41401469),People's Republic of China.

References

1. Gravett MG, Rubens CE. Global Alliance to Prevent Prematurity and Stillbirth Technical Team: A framework for strategic investments in research to reduce the global burden of preterm birth. Am J Obstet Gynecol. 2012;207: 368–73.

2. Liang J, Mao M, Dai L, Li X, Miao L, Li Q, et al. Neonatal mortality due to preterm birth at 28–36 weeks' gestation in China, 2003–2008. Paediatr Perinat Epidemiol. 2011;25:593–600.

3. Werler MM, Shapiro S, Mitchell AA. Mitchell, Periconceptional folic acid exposure and risk of occurrent neural tube defects. Jama. 1993;269:1257–61.

4. Shaw GM, Schaffer D, Velie EM, Morland K, Harris JA. Periconceptional vitamin use, dietary folate, and the occurrence of neural tube defects. Epidemiology. 1995;6:219–26.

5. Rozendaal AM, van Essen AJ, te Meerman GJ, Bakker MK, van der Biezen JJ, Goorhuis-Brouwer SM, et al. Periconceptional folic acid associated with an increased risk of oral clefts relative to non-folate related malformations in the Northern Netherlands: a population based case–control study. Eur J Epidemiol. 2013;28:875–87.

6. Li Z, Ye R, Zhang L, Li H, Liu J, Ren A. Periconceptional folic acid supplementation and the risk of preterm births in China: a large prospective cohort study. Int J Epidemiol. 2014;43:1132–9.

7. Czeizel AE, Puhó EH, Langmar Z, Acs N, Bánhidy F. Possible association of folic acid supplementation during pregnancy with reduction of preterm birth: a population-based study. Eur J Obstet Gynecol Reprod Biol. 2010;148:135–40.

8. Naimi AI, Auger N. Population-wide folic acid fortification and preterm birth: testing the folate depletion hypothesis. Am J Public Health. 2015;105(4): 793–5.

9. Papadopoulou E, Stratakis N, Roumeliotaki T, Sarri K, Merlo DF, Kogevinas M, et al. The effect of high doses of folic acid and iron supplementation in early-to-mid pregnancy on prematurity and fetal growth retardation: the mother-child cohort study in Crete, Greece (Rhea study). Eur J Nutr. 2013;52:327–36.

10. Dunlop AL, Taylor RN, Tangpricha V, Fortunato S, Menon R. Maternal micronutrient status and preterm versus term birth for black and white US women. Reprod Sci. 2012;19:939–48.

11. Yamada T, Morikawa M, Yamada T, Kishi R, Sengoku K, Endo T, et al. First-trimester serum folate levels and subsequent risk of abortion and preterm birth among Japanese women with singleton pregnancies. Arch Gynecol Obstet. 2013;287:9–14.

12. Naimi AI, Auger N. Population-wide folic acid fortification and preterm birth: testing the folate depletion hypothesis. Am J Public Health. 2015;105:793–5.

13. Lassi ZS, Salam RA, Haider BA, Bhutta ZA. Folic acid supplementation during pregnancy for maternal health and pregnancy outcomes. Cochrane Database Syst Rev. 2013;3:CD006896.

14. Bakker R, Timmermans S, Steegers EA, Hofman A, Jaddoe VW. Folic acid supplements modify the adverse effects of maternal smoking on fetal growth and neonatal complications. J Nutr. 2011;141:2172–9.

15. Shah R, Mullany LC, Darmstadt GL, Mannan I, Rahman SM, Talukder RR, et al. Incidence and risk factors of preterm birth in a rural Bangladeshi cohort. BMC Pediatr. 2014;14:112.

16. Chen LW, Lim AL, Colega M, Tint MT, Aris IM, Tan CS, et al. Maternal folate status, but not that of vitamins B-12 or B-6, is associated with gestational age and preterm birth risk in a multiethnic Asian population. J Nutr. 2015;145:113–20.

17. Scholl TO, Hediger ML, Schall JI, Khoo CS, Fischer RL. Dietary and serum folate: their influence on the outcome of pregnancy. Am J Clin Nutr. 1996;63:520–5.

18. Siega-Riz AM, Savitz DA, Zeisel SH, Thorp JM, Herring A. Second trimester folate status and preterm birth. Am J Obstet Gynecol. 2004;191:1851–7.

19. Zhao M, Chen YH, Dong XT, Zhou J, Chen X, Wang H, et al. Xu DX Folic acid protects against lipopolysaccharide-induced preterm delivery and intrauterine growth restriction through its anti-inflammatory effect in mice. PLoS One. 2013;8:e82713.

20. Kim H, Hwang JY, Ha EH, Park H, Ha M, Lee SJ, et al. Association of maternal folate nutrition and serum C-reactive protein concentrations with gestational age at delivery. Eur J Clin Nutr. 2011;65:350–6.

21. Simhan HN, Himes KP, Venkataramanan R, Bodnar LM. Maternal serum folate species in early pregnancy and lower genital tract inflammatory milieu. Am J Obstet Gynecol. 2011;205(61):e1–7.

22. Dhobale M, Chavan P, Kulkarni A, Mehendale S, Pisal H, Joshi S. Reduced folate, increased vitamin B(12) and homocysteine concentrations in women delivering preterm. Ann Nutr Metab. 2012;61:7–14.

23. Kim MW, Hong SC, Choi JS, Han JY, Oh MJ, Kim HJ, et al. folate and pregnancy outcomes. J Obstet Gynaecol. 2012;32:520–4.

24. Papachatzi E, Dimitriou G, Dimitropoulos K, Vantarakis A. Pre-pregnancy obesity: maternal, neonatal and childhood outcomes. J Neonatal Perinatal Med. 2013;6:203–16.

25. Lynch AM, Hart JE, Agwu OC, Fisher BM, West NA, Gibbs RS. Association of extremes of prepregnancy BMI with the clinical presentations of preterm birth. Am J Obstet Gynecol. 2014;210(428):e1–9.

26. Dean SV, Lassi ZS, Imam AM, Bhutta ZA. Preconception care: nutritional risks and interventions. Reprod Health. 2014;11 Suppl 3:S3.

27. Fujiwara K, Aoki S, Kurasawa K, Okuda M, Takahashi T, Hirahara F. Associations of maternal pre-pregnancy underweight with small-for-gestational-age and spontaneous preterm birth, and optimal gestational weight gain in Japanese women. J Obstet Gynaecol Res. 2014;40:988–94.

28. Shin D, Song WO. Prepregnancy body mass index is an independent risk factor for gestational hypertension, gestational diabetes, preterm labor, and small- and large-for-gestational-age infants. J Matern Fetal Neonatal Med. 2015;28:1679–86.

29. Parker MG, Ouyang F, Pearson C, Gillman MW, Belfort MB, Hong X, et al. Prepregnancy body mass index and risk of preterm birth: association heterogeneity by preterm subgroups. BMC Pregnancy Childbirth. 2014;14:153.

30. Shaw GM, Carmichael SL, Yang W. Siega-Riz AM; National Birth Defects Prevention Study: Periconceptional intake of folic acid and food folate and risks of preterm delivery. Am J Perinatol. 2011;28:747–52.

31. Tinker SC, Hamner HC, Berry RJ, Bailey LB, Pfeiffer CM. Does obesity modify the association of supplemental folic acid with folate status among nonpregnant women of childbearing age in the United States? Birth Defects Res A Clin Mol Teratol. 2012;94:749–55.

32. Mojtabai R. Body mass index and serum folate in childbearing age women. Eur J Epidemiol. 2004;19(11):1029–36.

33. da Silva VR, Hausman DB, Kauwell GP, Sokolow A, Tackett RL, Rathbun SL, et al. Obesity affects short-term folate pharmacokinetics in women of childbearing age. Int J Obes (Lond). 2013;37:1608–10.

34. Kim H, Hwang JY, Kim KN, Ha EH, Park H, Ha M, et al. Relationship between body-mass index and serum folate concentrations in pregnant women. Eur J Clin Nutr. 2012;66:136–8.

35. Stern SJ, Matok I, Kapur B, Koren G. Dosage requirements for periconceptional folic acid supplementation: accounting for BMI and lean body weight. J Obstet Gynaecol Can. 2012;34:374–8.

36. Wilson RD, Johnson JA, Wyatt P, Allen V, Gagnon A, Langlois S, et al. Genetics Committee of the Society of Obstetricians and Gynaecologists of Canada and The Motherrisk Program: Pre-conceptional vitamin/folic acid supplementation 2007: the use of folic acid in combination with a multivitamin supplement for the prevention of neural tube defects and other congenital anomalies. J Obstet Gynaecol Can. 2007;29:1003–26.

37. National Bureau of Statistics of China. China Statistical Yearbook 2011. http://www.stats.gov.cn/tjsj/ndsj/2011/indexeh.htm. Accessed date 2011.
38. Goldenberg RL, Culhane JF, Iams JD, Romero R. Epidemiology and causes of preterm birth. Lancet. 2008;371:75–84.
39. National Health and Family Planning Commission of the People's Republic of China. Criteria of weight for adults. http://www.moh.gov.cn/ewebeditor/uploadfile/2013/08/20130808135715967.pdf. Accessed date 2013.
40. Chen C, Lu FC, Department of Disease Control Ministry of Health, PR China. The guidelines for prevention and control of overweight and obesity in Chinese adults. Biomed Environ Sci. 2004;17(Suppl):1–36.
41. Rothman K, Greenland S, Lash T, editors. Modern Epidemiology. Philadelphia: Lippincott Williams & Wilkins; 2008.
42. Liu J, Jin L, Meng Q, Gao L, Zhang L, Li Z, et al. Changes in folic acid supplementation behaviour among women of reproductive age after the implementation of a massive supplementation programme in China. Public Health Nutr. 2015;18:582–8.
43. Mantovani E, Filippini F, Bortolus R, Franchi M. Folic acid supplementation and preterm birth: results from observational studies. Biomed Res Int. 2014; 2014:481914.
44. Sengpiel V, Bacelis J, Myhre R, Myking S, Devold Pay AS, Haugen M, et al. Folic acid supplementation, dietary folate intake during pregnancy and risk for spontaneous preterm delivery: a prospective observational cohort study. BMC Pregnancy Childbirth. 2014;14:375.
45. Johnson TS, Rottier KJ, Luellwitz A, Kirby RS. Maternal prepregnancy body mass index and delivery of a preterm infant in Missouri 1998–2000. Public Health Nurs. 2009;26:3–13.
46. Mandal D, Manda S, Rakshi A, Dey RP, Biswas SC, Banerjee A. Maternal obesity and pregnancy outcome: a prospective analysis. J Assoc Physicians India. 2011;59:486–9.
47. Sukla KK, Tiwari PK, Kumar A, Raman R. Low birthweight (LBW) and neonatal hyperbilirubinemia (NNH) in an Indian cohort: association of homocysteine, its metabolic pathway genes and micronutrients as risk factors. PLoS One. 2013;8:e71587.
48. Goldberg BB, Alvarado S, Chavez C, Chen BH, Dick LM, Felix RJ, et al. Teratogen Information Service: Prevalence of periconceptional folic acid use and perceived barriers to the postgestation continuance of supplemental folic acid: survey results from a Teratogen Information Service. Birth Defects Res A Clin Mol Teratol. 2006;76:193–9.
49. Watkins ML, Scanlon KS, Mulinare J, Khoury MJ. Is maternal obesity a risk factor for anencephaly and spina bifida? Epidemiology. 1996;7:507–12.
50. Bird JK, Ronnenberg AG, Choi SW, Du F, Mason JB, Liu Z. Obesity is associated with increased red blood cell folate despite lower dietary intakes and serum concentrations. J Nutr. 2015;145(1):79–86.
51. Bergen NE, Jaddoe VW, Timmermans S, Hofman A, Lindemans J, Russcher H, et al. Homocysteine and folate concentrations in early pregnancy and the risk of adverse pregnancy outcomes: the Generation R Study. BJOG. 2012;119:739–51.
52. Wang M, Wang ZP, Gao LJ, Gong R, Sun XH, Zhao ZT. Maternal body mass index and the association between folic acid supplements and neural tube defects. Acta Paediatr. 2013;102:908–13.
53. Xing XY, Tao FB, Hao JH, Huang K, Huang ZH, Zhu XM, et al. Periconceptional folic acid supplementation among women attending antenatal clinic in Anhui, China: data from a population-based cohort study. Midwifery. 2012;28:291–7.
54. Bukowski R, Malone FD, Porter FT, Nyberg DA, Comstock CH, Hankins GD, et al. Preconceptional folate supplementation and the risk of spontaneous preterm birth: a cohort study. PLoS Med. 2009;6:e1000061.

The association between fine particulate matter exposure during pregnancy and preterm birth

Xiaoli Sun[1], Xiping Luo[1*], Chunmei Zhao[1], Rachel Wai Chung Ng[2], Chi Eung Danforn Lim[2,3], Bo Zhang[4] and Tao Liu[5,6*]

Abstract

Background: Although several previous studies have assessed the association of fine particulate matter ($PM_{2.5}$) exposure during pregnancy with preterm birth, the results have been inconsistent and remain controversial. This meta-analysis aims to quantitatively summarize the association between maternal $PM_{2.5}$ exposure and preterm birth and to further explore the sources of heterogeneity in findings on this association.

Methods: We searched for all studies published before December 2014 on the association between $PM_{2.5}$ exposure during pregnancy and preterm birth in the MEDLINE, PUBMED and Embase databases as well as the China Biological Medicine and Wanfang databases. A pooled OR for preterm birth in association with each 10 $\mu g/m^3$ increase in $PM_{2.5}$ exposure was calculated by a random-effects model (for studies with significant heterogeneity) or a fixed-effects model (for studies without significant heterogeneity).

Results: A total of 18 studies were included in this analysis. The pooled OR for $PM_{2.5}$ exposure (per 10 $\mu g/m^3$ increment) during the entire pregnancy on preterm birth was 1.13 (95 % CI = 1.03–1.24) in 13 studies with a significant heterogeneity (Q = 80.51, $p < 0.001$). The pooled ORs of $PM_{2.5}$ exposure in the first, second and third trimester were 1.08 (95 % CI = 0.92–1.26), 1.09 (95 % CI = 0.82–1.44) and 1.08 (95 % CI = 0.99–1.17), respectively. The corresponding meta-estimates of $PM_{2.5}$ effects in studies assessing $PM_{2.5}$ exposure at individual, semi-individual and regional level were 1.11 (95 % CI = 0.89–1.37), 1.14 (95 % CI = 0.97–1.35) and 1.07 (95 % CI = 0.94–1.23). In addition, significant meta-estimates of $PM_{2.5}$ exposures were found in retrospective studies (OR = 1.10, 95 % CI = 1.01–1.21), prospective studies (OR = 1.42, 95 % CI = 1.08–1.85), and studies conducted in the USA (OR = 1.16, 95 % CI = 1.05–1.29).

Conclusions: Maternal $PM_{2.5}$ exposure during pregnancy may increase the risk of preterm birth,but significant heterogeneity was found between studies. Exposure assessment methods, study designs and study settings might be important sources of heterogeneity, and should be taken into account in future meta-analyses.

Keywords: Fine particulate matter, Preterm birth, Meta-analysis, Adverse pregnancy outcome

Background

Preterm birth (before 37 weeks of gestation) is the leading cause of newborn deaths and the second-leading cause of death (after pneumonia) in children less than 5 years old [1]. More than 1 million children die each year worldwide due to complications of preterm birth. Many survivors face lifelong disabilities and chronic diseases, including learning disabilities, adult hypertension, diabetes, coronary heart disease, and visual and hearing problems [1, 2]. An emerging body of evidence indicates that ambient air pollution may play an important role in the incidence of preterm birth [3, 4]. As a prominent component of the ambient air pollution mixture, fine particulate matter ($PM_{2.5}$, aerodynamic diameter <2.5 μm) may cause greater harm to human health due to its specific characteristics such as smaller diameter, larger surface

* Correspondence: luoxiping07@aliyun.com; gztt_2002@163.com
[1]Gynecology Department, Guangdong Women and Children Hospital, No. 521, Xingnan Road, Panyu District, Guangzhou 511442, China
[5]Guangdong Provincial Institute of Public Health, Guangdong Provincial Center for Disease Control and Prevention, No. 160, Qunxian Road, Panyu District, Guangzhou 511430, China
Full list of author information is available at the end of the article

area, and longer suspension time in air [5, 6]. Although previous studies have estimated the association between $PM_{2.5}$ exposure during pregnancy and preterm birth, the results have been inconsistent and remain controversial [7–10].

To quantitatively summarize the association between $PM_{2.5}$ exposure and preterm birth risk, a few meta-analyses have been conducted during the past several years [11–13]. However, due to some methodological issues in previous studies, further research is needed. For example, all three meta-analyses found a significant heterogeneity between included studies [11–13]. According to the Cochrane guide, it is not appropriate to simply combine the results of articles with significant heterogeneity [14]. Although some authors have recognized this issue in their studies, the limited number of included studies prevented them from quantitatively testing the sources of heterogeneity [11, 12]. In the past several years, more studies have been conducted to estimate the association between maternal $PM_{2.5}$ exposure and preterm birth, which provides an opportunity to quantitatively explore the sources of heterogeneity between previous studies and meta-analyses.

In this study, we collected previously published studies that assessed the association between $PM_{2.5}$ exposure during pregnancy and preterm birth, and employed a meta-analysis model to quantitatively evaluate the effects of $PM_{2.5}$ exposure during different phases of pregnancy on preterm birth. We further explored the modification of exposure measurement methods, study settings and study designs on the meta-estimates of $PM_{2.5}$.

Methods

The methods for the analysis and inclusion criteria were specified in advance and documented in a protocol.

Literature search

We searched for all publications indexed in the MEDLINE, PUBMED and EMBASE databases as well as the China Biological Medicine and Wanfang databases during November and December 2014. The search strategies used combinations of the following key words: "air pollution", "particulate matter", "fine particulate matter", "fine particles", "PM", "$PM_{2.5}$", "PM $_{2.5}$", "premature birth", "preterm birth", "PTB", "preterm delivery", "PTD" and "prematurity". We also manually searched the references of every primary study for additional publications. Further publications were also identified from review articles. Only publications in English or Chinese were considered.

Inclusion and exclusion criteria

We initially screened the titles and abstracts of all studies. Studies were excluded if they were not related to fine particulate matter and preterm birth. The remaining studies

were noted as potentially eligible studies and were further viewed by two independent authors. The studies were included in this meta-analysis if they met the following criteria: (a) studies included $PM_{2.5}$ exposure during pregnancy and preterm birth that was defined as a live birth before gestational week 37; (b) studies presented sample sizes and odds ratios (OR) with 95 % confidence intervals (CI) or information that could be used to infer these results; (c) if more than one study was identified for the same population, only the study that included the most recent population or the most information was selected. Studies that did not meet the above criteria were excluded. The process of study selection is presented in detail in Fig. 1.

Data extraction

The following information was extracted from each study: authors, year and source of publication, study period, study setting, study design, $PM_{2.5}$ exposure assessment methods, data sources, sample size, $PM_{2.5}$ exposure windows, exposure range, and ORs and 95 % CIs. If a study provided associations between preterm birth and $PM_{2.5}$ exposure during the entire pregnancy and trimester-specific periods, all estimates were extracted. Several studies assessed $PM_{2.5}$ exposure based on monitoring network data and remote sensing data; we preferentially chose estimates based on monitoring network data because this assessment method was more common across all studies, which could potentially reduce the heterogeneity between studies in this meta-analysis. In addition, because there is considerable co-linearity between pollutants originating from the same sources and not all studies adjusted for air pollutants other than $PM_{2.5}$, we extracted estimates only from single pollutant models fully adjusted for other covariates. Eligibility assessment and all data extraction were conducted by two authors using a standard form, and discrepancies were resolved by discussion between authors. The authors adhered to PRISMA guidelines for meta syntheses. Ethical approval was not required for this meta analysis. We employed the New Castle Ottawa scale to assess the quality of all included studies [15]. For the retrospective studies, the quality assessment was based on participant selection, comparability and exposure assessment; For the prospective studies, the quality assessment was based on participant selection, comparability and outcome.

Meta-analysis and statistical analysis

Prior to performing the meta-analysis, we converted all ORs to a common exposure unit of 10 μg/m³ increase in $PM_{2.5}$ exposure, which allowed us to quantitatively pool estimates from different studies. Firstly, all ORs and their 95%CIs were converted by logarithms (ln), which

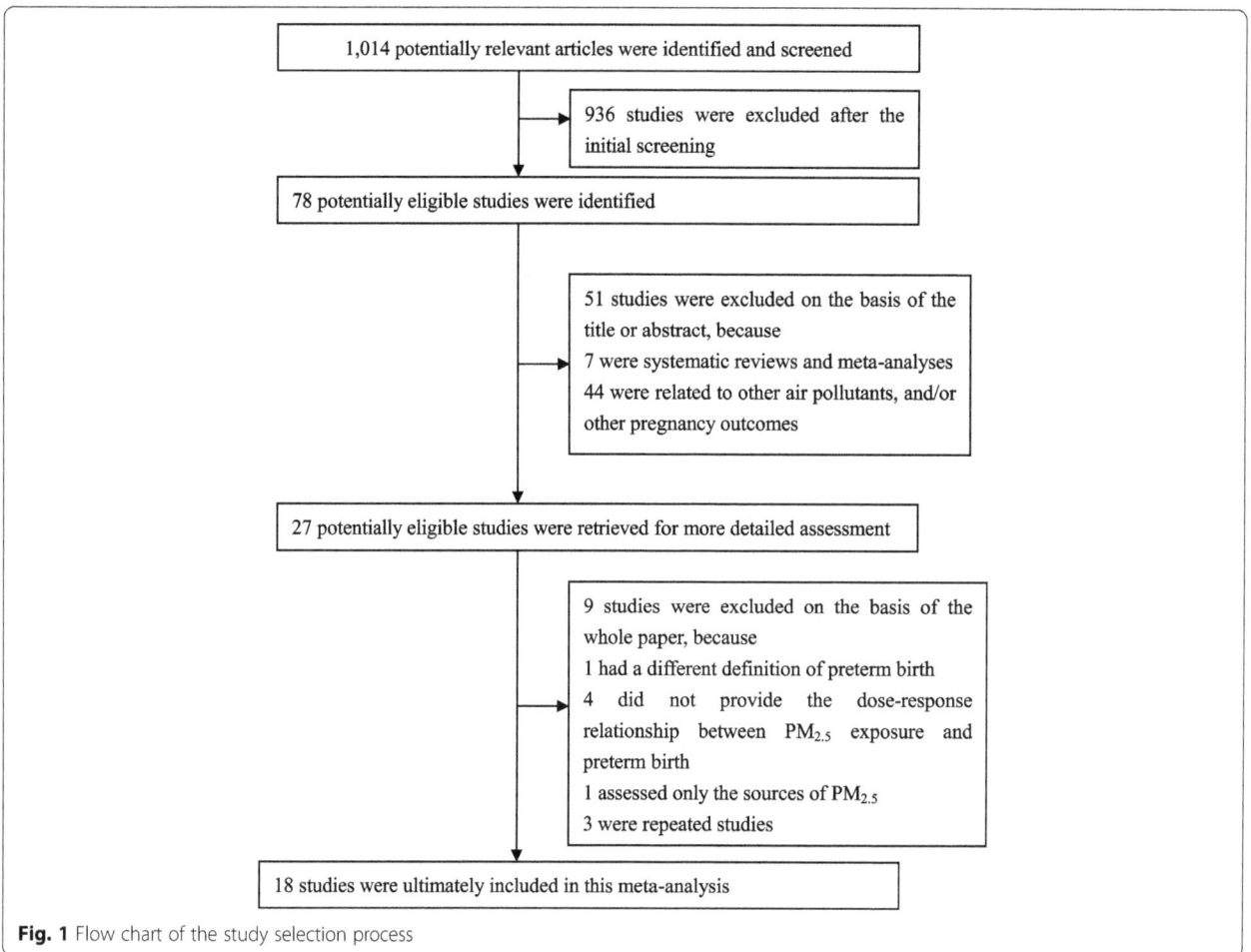

Fig. 1 Flow chart of the study selection process

were used to calculate the partial regression coefficients (β) and their standard errors (se). Then the OR_a (adjusted OR) for each 10 $\mu g/m^3$ increase in $PM_{2.5}$ exposure can be computed by the following formula:

$$OR_a = EXP(\beta \times 10/x)$$

Where x ($\mu g/m^3$) is the exposure dose for OR reported in each included study. Similarly, the 95%CI of OR_a could also be calculated. We then conducted several meta-analyses of the identified studies to quantitatively estimate the associations of $PM_{2.5}$ exposure during the entire pregnancy and trimester-specific exposure durations with preterm birth risks. Several secondary analyses were also conducted to estimate the pooled-effects of $PM_{2.5}$ exposure during the entire pregnancy on preterm birth in subgroups with different exposure measurement methods, study designs, and study settings. These subgroup analyses aimed to explore the modification effects of these characteristics on the estimates of $PM_{2.5}$ exposure on preterm birth and to further test their impacts on the heterogeneity in the reported associations.

Three exposure measurement methods were identified in the included studies: individual-level, semi-individual-level, and regional-level exposure assessment. All these three assessment methods were based on residential level. Individual-level exposure was assessed using complicated dispersion models based on traffic, meteorology, roadway geometry, vehicle emission, air quality monitoring, and land use databases [16, 17]. These models could estimate each subject's daily $PM_{2.5}$ exposure level with high accuracy. Semi-individual exposure was estimated using the daily $PM_{2.5}$ concentration from the monitoring station nearest to the individual's residence [7, 8]. Regional-level exposure was calculated using the average $PM_{2.5}$ concentration in a region or a grid with low resolution. This method did not consider the variation in $PM_{2.5}$ concentration within a region, and assumed that all subjects in this region had the same $PM_{2.5}$ exposure concentration. The $PM_{2.5}$ data usually had been obtained from monitoring networks and remote sensing [18]. The study designs of all of the included studies were divided into two categories: retrospective and prospective. In addition, several meta regression analyses were further employed to assess the impacts of study characteristics on the associations between $PM_{2.5}$ exposure and preterm birth risks.

To explore the possible heterogeneity of study results, we hypothesized that effect size may differ according to the methodological quality of the studies. The heterogeneity of the included studies was assessed using the Q statistic and I^2 statistic. Cochran's Q statistic was calculated by summing the squared deviations of each study's estimate from the overall meta-analysis estimate weighted by each study's contribution. A p-value was obtained by comparing the Q statistic with a chi-square distribution with k-1° of freedom, where k is the number of included studies [19]. If the p-value was <0.05, then a random-effects model would be selected, otherwise a fixed-effects model would be selected [20, 21]. The I^2 statistic $[I^2 = (Q - df)/Q \times 100]$ describes the percentage of variation across studies that is due to heterogeneity rather than chance. $I^2 > 50$ % demonstrated that there is a statistically significant heterogeneity [19]. We also used funnel plot asymmetry to detect potential publication bias. Egger's regression was applied to test the funnel plot symmetry, with the inverse of the standard error as the independent variable and the standardized estimate of size effect as the dependent variable [22].

Finally, a series of sensitivity analyses was performed to test the robustness of our results. Because some subgroup analyses included very few studies, we conducted sensitivity analyses only overall and in sub-groups analyses that included more than five studies. For each sensitivity analysis, we individually removed a single study with the largest OR, the smallest OR, the largest standard error, and the smallest standard error from the meta-analyses.

All statistical tests were two-sided, and P <0.05 was considered statistically significant. We used R software (version 2.15.2; R Development Core Team 2012, www.R-project.org) to analyze the data.

Results

Search results and study characteristics

Twenty-seven potentially eligible studies were identified and assessed for full text. A total of nine studies were excluded for the following reasons: having a different definition of preterm birth ($n = 1$) [23], not providing the dose–response relationship between $PM_{2.5}$ exposure and preterm birth ($n = 4$) [24–27], only assessing the sources of $PM_{2.5}$ ($n = 1$) [28], and duplication of studies whose primary results had already been included in other studies ($n = 3$) [29–31]. Eighteen studies were ultimately included in this meta-analysis, containing a total of more than 3,000 000 subjects with more than 299,000 preterm births [7–10, 16–18, 32–42]. Most studies (12/18) were conducted in the USA [7, 16, 18, 32, 34–40, 42]. There were 12 retrospective and six prospective studies. There were two studies assessing maternal $PM_{2.5}$ exposure at

individual, ten at semi-individual, and two at regional levels. The other four studies used two methods to assess $PM_{2.5}$ exposure. The average Newcastle-Ottawa quality score is 8. Detailed information about the included studies is presented in Table 1.

The pooled effects of $PM_{2.5}$ exposure in different trimesters of pregnancy on preterm birth

We estimated a significant increase of preterm birth risk associated with overall $PM_{2.5}$ exposure (per 10 µg/m³ increment) during pregnancy across all 13 included studies (OR = 1.13, 95 % CI = 1.03–1.24) (Table 2 and Fig. 2). The pooled OR values of $PM_{2.5}$ exposure in the first, second and third trimester were 1.08 (95 % CI = 0.92–1.26), 1.09 (95 % CI = 0.82–1.44) and 1.08 (95 % CI = 0.99–1.17), respectively. We did not find any significant effects of $PM_{2.5}$ exposure in either the first month (OR = 1.10, 95 % CI = 0.92–1.30) or the last month of gestation (OR = 1.05, 95 % CI = 0.97–1.13) (Table 2 and Fig. 2).

Subgroup analyses on the effects of exposure assessment methods, study designs and study settings on the associations between $PM_{2.5}$ exposure during the entire pregnancy and preterm birth

We found numerically similar pooled associations between preterm birth risk and $PM_{2.5}$ exposure in studies using different exposure assessment methods. The pooled ORs in the studies that assessed $PM_{2.5}$ exposure at individual, semi-individual and regional levels were 1.11 (95 % CI = 0.89–1.37), 1.14 (95 % CI = 0.97–1.35) and 1.07 (95 % CI = 0.94–1.23), respectively (Table 2 and Fig. 2).

We observed significant pooled estimates of $PM_{2.5}$ on preterm in studies that used a retrospective (OR = 1.10, 95 % CI = 1.01–1.21) or prospective study design (OR = 1.42, 95 % CI = 1.08–1.85). Furthermore, the latter meta-estimate of $PM_{2.5}$ was larger than the former (Table 2 and Fig. 2).

The pooled estimate of the association between $PM_{2.5}$ exposure and preterm birth was statistically significant for studies that were conducted in the USA (OR = 1.16, 95 % CI = 1.05–1.29), but the pooled estimate was not significant for studies that were conducted in other countries (OR = 0.98, 95 % CI = 0.95–1.01) (Table 2 and Fig. 2).

In addition, several meta regression analyses were employed to further evaluate the impacts of study characteristics on the associations between $PM_{2.5}$ exposure and preterm birth risks (Additional file 1: Figure S1). We observed similar results with the subgroup analyses. For instance, the combined estimate of $PM_{2.5}$ exposure during the entire pregnancy were higher in prospective studies than in retrospective studies ($\beta = 0.25$, $P = 0.120$).

Table 1 Characteristics of the studies included in the meta-analysis

Authors	Study setting	Study period	Study design	Exposure assessment level	Data source	No. of participants	No. of cases	Exposure period	Exposure range (mean (IQR) μg/m³)	Quality score[a]
Wilhelm et al. [39]	California, USA	1999–2000	Retrospective	Semi-individual level	Monitoring network data	106,483	92,68	TS	21.0 (NA)	8
Huynh et al. [7]	California, USA	1999–2000	Retrospective	Semi-individual level	Monitoring network data	42,692	10,673	WP and TS	18.0 (8.7)	8
Jalaludin et al. [33]	Sydney, Australia	1998–2000	Retrospective	Regional level and semi-individual level	Monitoring network data	123,840	6011	TS	9.0 (4.5)	8
Ritz et al. [37]	California, USA	2003	Prospective	Semi-individual level	Monitoring network data	58,316	5924	TS	20.0 (NA)	7
Brauer et al. [8]	Vancouver, Canada	1999–2002	Prospective	Semi-individual level	Monitoring network data	70,249	3748	WP	5.1 (1.1)	7
Wu et al. [16]	California, USA	1997–2006	Retrospective	Individual level	Monitoring network data	81,186	6712	WP	1.8 (1.4)	9
Gehring et al. [17]	North, west, and center of the Netherlands	1996–1997	Prospective	Individual level	Monitoring network data and land use regression model	3853	165	WP and TS	20.1 (4.6)	7
Rudra et al. [38]	Washington, USA	1996–2006	Retrospective	Semi-individual level	Monitoring network data	3509	369	TS	10.1 (NA)	9
Kloog et al. [34]	Massachusetts, USA	2000–2008	Retrospective	Semi-individual level	Remote sensing data	634,244	61,972	WP	9.6 (5.3)	9
Lee et al. [35]	Pittsburgh, USA	1997–2002	Prospective	Semi-individual level	Monitoring network data	34,705	1940	TS	15.6 (4.0)	7
Chang et al. 2015	Atlanta, USA	1999–2005	Retrospective	Semi-individual level	Monitoring network data	175,891	18,648	WP and TS	17.3 (3.1)	8
Fleischer et al. [10]	22 countries	2004–2008	Retrospective	Regional level	Remote sensing data	192,900	13,379	WP	1.4–98.1 (NA)	7
Nannam et al. 2014 [41]	Northwest England	2004–2008	Retrospective	Semi-individual level and individual level	Monitoring network data	265,613	38,608	WP and TS	22.1 (4.6)	9
Ha et al. [42]	Florida, USA	2004–2005	Retrospective	Regional level and semi-individual level	Monitoring network data	423,719	39,082	WP and TS	9.9 (2.0)	8
Hyder et al. [18]	Connecticut and Massachusetts, USA	2000–2006	Retrospective	Regional level and semi-individual level	Monitoring network data and remote sensing data	647,942	41,868	WP and TS	11.9 (2.4)	8
Gray et al. [32]	North Carolina, USA	2002–2006	Retrospective	Regional level	Monitoring network data	457,642	40,746	WP	13.6 (2.0)	8
Pereira et al. [9]	Connecticut, USA	2000–2006	Prospective	Semi-individual level	Monitoring network data	61,688	-	WP and TS	12.4 (2.3)	9
Pereira et al. [56]	Perth, Australia	1997–2007	Prospective	Semi-individual level	Monitoring network data	31,567	-	WP and TS	8.6 (2.2)	9

NA: Data not available
[a]: Newcastle-Ottawa quality score
-: The number of cases was not available because these studies were longitudinal studies that assessed the effects of PM$_{2.5}$ on preterm birth across successive pregnancies. NA: Data not available

Table 2 Pooled associations between PM$_{2.5}$ exposure (per 10 µg/m^3 increment) during pregnancy and preterm birth risks in different subgroups

Subgroups	No. of studies	Heterogeneity test Q	Heterogeneity test P	Summary OR (95 % CI)	Hypothesis test Z	Hypothesis test P	I^2 (%)	Egger's test t	Egger's test P
Exposure during the entire pregnancy	13	80.51	<0.001	1.13* (1.03–1.24)	2.59	0.010	91.4	2.20	0.051
Specific trimester									
First trimester exposure	10	89.14	<0.001	1.08 (0.92–1.26)	0.96	0.334	91.3	0.68	0.517
Second trimester exposure	5	138.69	<0.001	1.09 (0.82–1.44)	0.60	0.548	98.7	0.311	0.776
Third trimester exposure	9	44.83	<0.001	1.08** (0.99–1.17)	1.70	0.089	92.1	1.58	0.157
First month of gestation	3	22.03	<0.001	1.10 (0.92–1.30)	1.03	0.301	91.0	0.58	0.666
Within one month before birth	6	51.49	<0.001	1.01 (0.86–1.19)	0.09	0.926	96.8	0.03	0.980
Exposure assessment method[a]									
Individual exposure	3	4.94	0.085	1.11 (0.89–1.37)	0.93	0.352	61.3	1.74	0.332
Semi-individual exposure	9	55.86	<0.001	1.14 (0.97–1.35)	1.56	0.119	93.0	0.35	0.737
Regional level	4	46.19	<0.001	1.07 (0.94–1.23)	1.00	0.319	93.8	0.11	0.921
Study design[a]									
Retrospective studies	9	70.98	<0.001	1.10* (1.01–1.21)	2.12	0.034	93.3	2.31	0.055
Prospective studies	4	4.64	0.201	1.42* (1.08–1.85)	2.52	0.012	39.5	0.10	0.927
Study setting[a]									
USA	8	50.49	<0.001	1.16* (1.05–1.29)	2.73	0.006	90.6	1.80	0.121
Others	5	7.90	0.095	0.98 (0.95–1.01)	1.11	0.268	0.1	1.62	0.205

[a]: All of these subgroup analyses were conducted for the studies that assessed the association between PM$_{2.5}$ exposure during the entire pregnancy and preterm birth. All of these estimates were ORs for each 10 µg/m^3 increment of PM$_{2.5}$ exposure during the entire pregnancy

*: $p < 0.05$

**: $0.05 < p < 0.10$

Sensitivity analyses on the associations between PM$_{2.5}$ exposure and preterm birth

In the meta-analysis that included studies assessing PM$_{2.5}$ exposure at the semi-individual level, the PM$_{2.5}$ meta-estimate became significant after excluding a single study with the smallest effect size. Beyond that, we did not find any significant change in the PM$_{2.5}$ meta-estimates in other meta-analyses after excluding a single study with the largest effect size, the smallest effect size, the largest standard error, or the smallest standard error (Fig. 3).

Heterogeneity and publication bias

We observed significant heterogeneities in most of the meta-analyses. However, in some subgroup analyses, such as the subgroup of prospective studies, there were no significant heterogeneities between studies. These findings indicate that the three characteristics that we took into account in this study were important sources of heterogeneities between studies. We did not find any statistically significant publication bias in any of the meta-analyses (Table 2 and Fig. 4).

Discussion

In this meta-analysis, we quantitatively assessed the association between maternal PM$_{2.5}$ exposure during pregnancy and preterm birth risk. We observed a clearly significant association between PM$_{2.5}$ exposure during pregnancy and preterm birth risk, which is consistent with the results of previous meta-analyses [11, 13]. Sapkota et al. estimated a pooled OR of 1.15 (95 % CI = 1.14–1.16) for preterm birth per 10 µg/m^3 increment in PM$_{2.5}$ exposure during the entire pregnancy [11]. Zhu et al. reported that a 10 µg/m^3 increase in PM$_{2.5}$ exposure over the entire pregnancy was positively associated with a 10 % (95 CI % = 3.0–18 %) increase in preterm birth risk [11] Stieb et al.'s meta-analysis also found a positive but non-significant association between PM$_{2.5}$ exposure and preterm birth (OR = 1.05, 95 CI % = 0.98–1.13). The lack of statistical significance may be due to the small quantity of included studies ($n = 4$) [12]. These results further demonstrate the adverse effect of PM$_{2.5}$ exposure during pregnancy on preterm birth. Air pollution is ubiquitous, and all populations are exposed to it at some level. Immature fetuses are more susceptible to air pollution [43]. Therefore, these results are important for policy makers and public health practitioners worldwide.

Although the mechanisms of PM$_{2.5}$ leading to preterm birth are not well understood, inhaled PM$_{2.5}$ can penetrate the gas exchange region of the lungs and enter the bloodstream. Toxic chemicals such as carcinogenic polycyclic aromatic hydrocarbons and harmful metals could cause systemic oxidative stress, oxidative stress-induced DNA

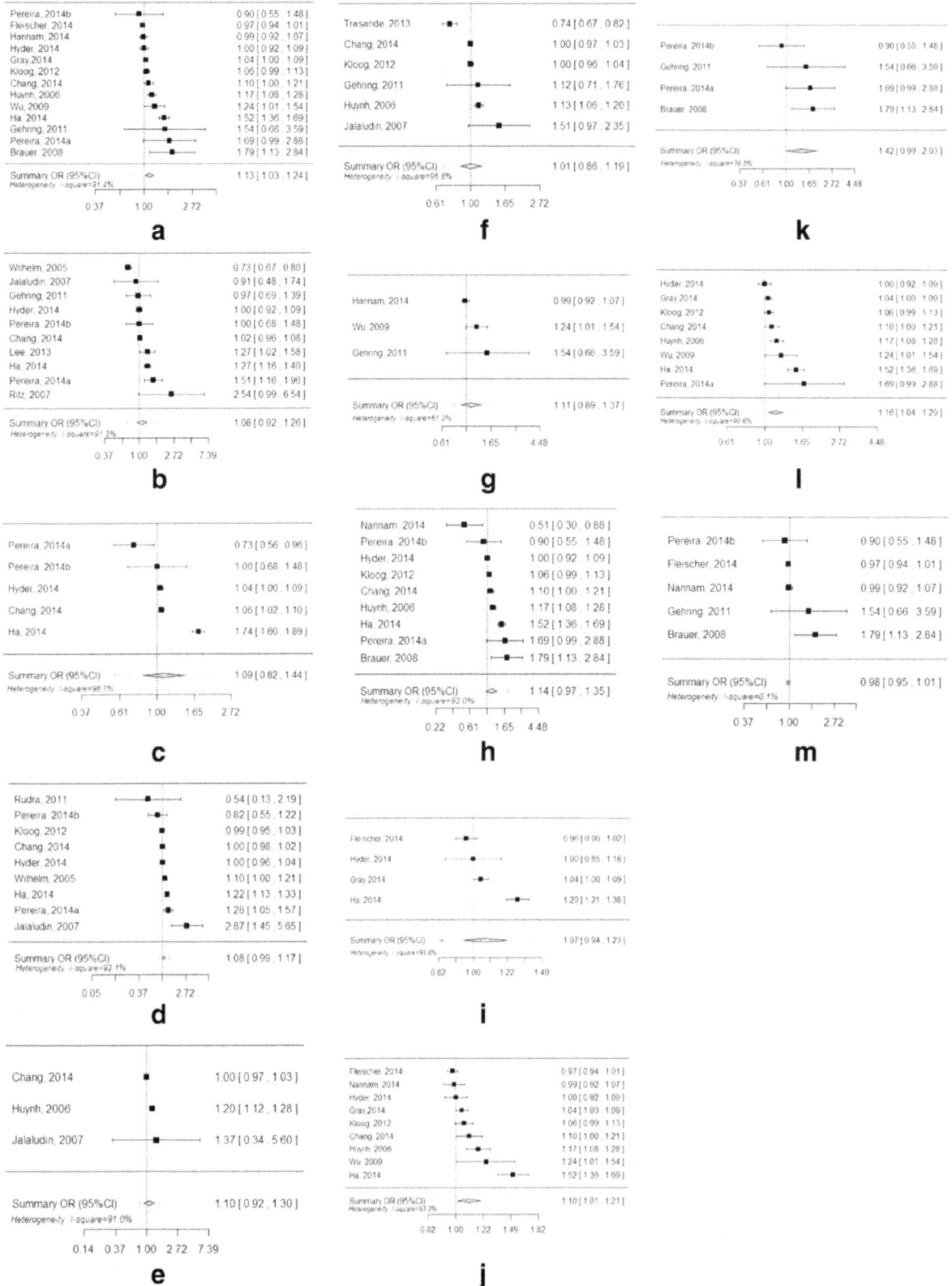

Fig. 2 (See legend on next page.)

(See figure on previous page.)
Fig. 2 Forest plots for the pooled ORs for the association between PM$_{2.5}$ exposure (per 10 µg/m^3 increment) during the pregnancy and preterm birth. **a**: In studies that assessed PM$_{2.5}$ exposure during the entire pregnancy. **b**: In studies that assessed PM$_{2.5}$ exposure in the first trimester. **c**: In studies that assessed PM$_{2.5}$ exposure in the second trimester. **d**: In studies that assessed PM$_{2.5}$ exposure in the third trimester. **e**: In studies that assessed PM$_{2.5}$ exposure in the first month of gestation. **f**: In studies that assessed PM$_{2.5}$ exposure within one month before birth. **g**: In studies that assessed PM$_{2.5}$ exposure at individual level. **h**: In studies that assessed PM$_{2.5}$ exposure at semi-individual level. **i**: In studies that assessed PM$_{2.5}$ exposure at regional level. **j**: In retrospective studies. **k**: In prospective studies. **l**: In studies conducted in the USA. **m**: In studies conducted in other countries

damage, pulmonary and placental inflammation, blood coagulation, endothelial dis-function, and hemodynamic changes [44]. These responses could interfere with the transplacental oxygen and nutrient transport from mothers to fetuses, and has the potential to negatively impact fetal growth and development, particularly during critical periods of organogenesis [43, 45, 46]. In addition, The early activation of cytokines favoring inflammation may play an important role in the PM$_{2.5}$-preterm link, because inflammatory mediators such as interleukin 1-β (IL-1β) and tumor necrosis factor-α (TNF-α) can trigger the premature onset of labor [46].

The question of which gestational windows are more susceptible to air pollution has been explored in several previous studies. Although some studies supported early pregnancy (the first month or first trimester) [7, 35, 37], other studies supported later pregnancy (the third trimester, the last month, or the last week) [33, 39] as the window of susceptibility. A meta-analysis also observed a pronounced association between PM$_{2.5}$ exposure during the third trimester and preterm risk [11]. It was debated that PM$_{2.5}$ exposure during the later pregnancy might induce early activation of cytokines favoring inflammation, and trigger the premature onset of labor [46]. By contrast, the implantation of the fetus and the formation of the placenta occur during the first trimester, and higher PM$_{2.5}$ exposure during this time period might cause genetic mutations, and hence increase the risks of fetal malformation, miscarriage and even death [47]. These serious harmful effects might attenuate the association between PM$_{2.5}$ exposure in early pregnancy and preterm outcome. However, in this study we observed nearly identical pooled estimates of PM$_{2.5}$ exposure during the first, second and third trimester, which indicates that more studies are needed in the future to explore which gestational windows are more susceptible to air pollution.

Exposure assessment is an important issue in studies estimating the effects of ambient air pollution on health. In this meta-analysis, we selected studies that assessed PM$_{2.5}$ exposure at the individual, semi-individual or regional level. Using monitoring data for nearby areas or regional average PM$_{2.5}$ concentrations measured at monitoring stations may provide a misrepresentation of exposure because this method does not take into account the spatial misalignment between an individual's

residence and monitoring sites, and ignores the fact that individuals have different activity models (indoor and outdoor activity time) and could have changed their residential address during pregnancy [8, 48, 49]. Some recent studies used complicated dispersion models to quantitatively assess individual PM$_{2.5}$ exposure [16, 17]. These models included data on several variables including traffic, meteorology, roadway geometry, vehicle emission, air quality, and land use. However, the accessibility of these datasets usually limits the wide employment of these dispersion models, particularly in some developing countries where the information on land use, traffic and vehicle emission is limited. In recent years, some studies used personal monitors to assess maternal exposure to air pollutants in different trimesters [50, 51]. These methods could theoretically reduce the bias in exposure assessment. In this study, although we observed stronger pooled associations between PM$_{2.5}$ exposure and preterm birth in studies that assessed PM$_{2.5}$ exposure at the individual and semi-individual levels than for studies that used regional-level methods, the lack of significant associations indicate that more studies are needed in the future, especially studies assessing PM$_{2.5}$ exposure at the individual level. For example, we only included three studies that used the individual-level assessment method, and their pooled estimate was dominated by a single study.

It is well known that the toxicity and health impacts of PM$_{2.5}$ may vary by geographic area [52]. Therefore, it is reasonable to conduct subgroup meta-analyses to test the variation in PM$_{2.5}$ estimates between regions. In this study, because most of the included studies were conducted in the USA, we divided all studies into two groups (USA and other countries). However, we found a significant meta-estimate of PM$_{2.5}$ exposure only for the US studies. This discrepancy may be partially related to the small number ($n = 5$) of studies in the second group, which indicates that more studies in countries other than the USA are needed, especially in middle or low income countries with higher levels of air pollution. For example, only one study has been found that assessed the association between PM$_{2.5}$ exposure and preterm birth in China and India. These two countries have the most severe PM$_{2.5}$ pollution [53], and the largest number of preterm births worldwide [1]. Studies in these countries could provide important information for policy

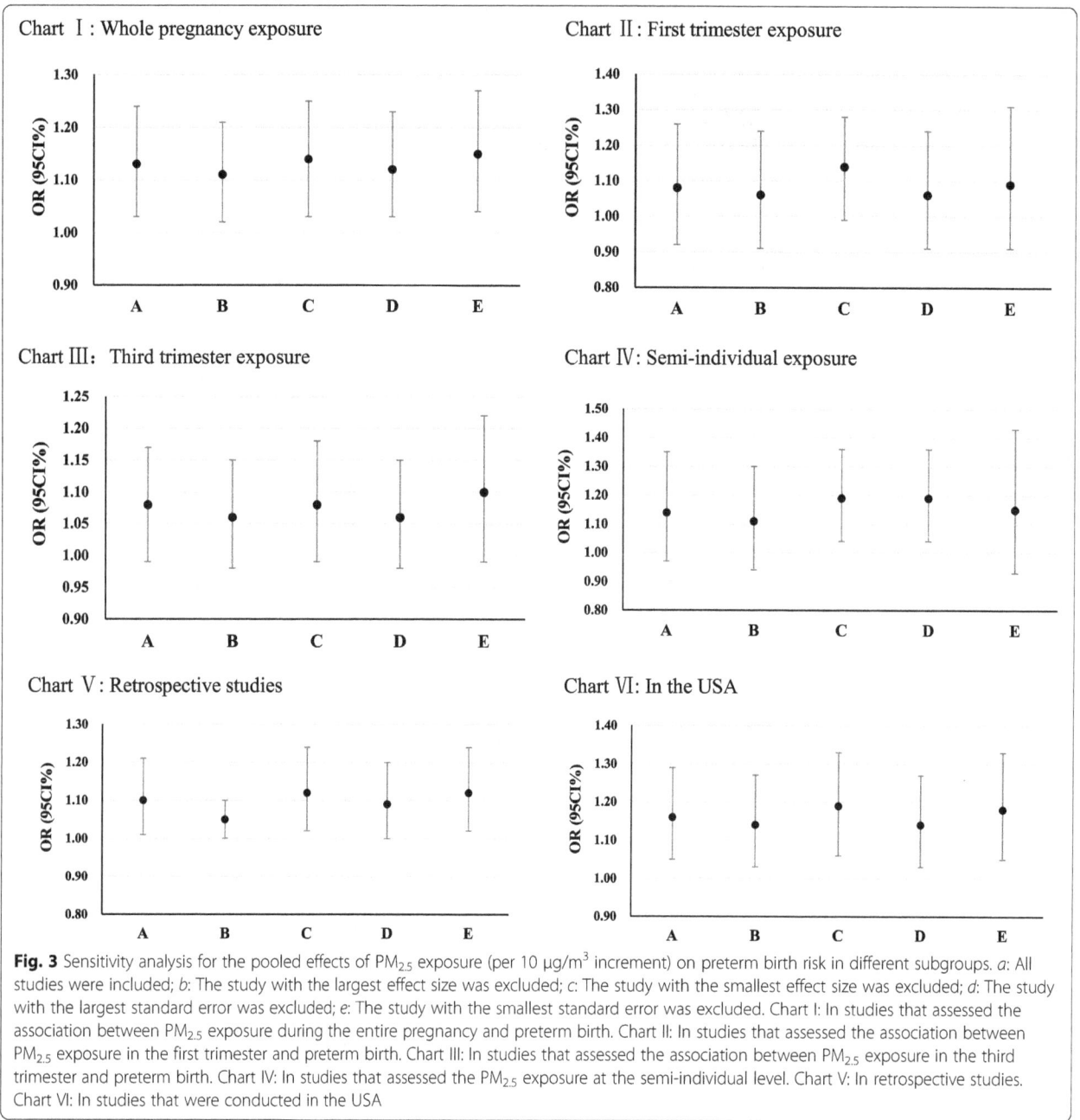

Fig. 3 Sensitivity analysis for the pooled effects of PM$_{2.5}$ exposure (per 10 µg/m^3 increment) on preterm birth risk in different subgroups. *a*: All studies were included; *b*: The study with the largest effect size was excluded; *c*: The study with the smallest effect size was excluded; *d*: The study with the largest standard error was excluded; *e*: The study with the smallest standard error was excluded. Chart I: In studies that assessed the association between PM$_{2.5}$ exposure during the entire pregnancy and preterm birth. Chart II: In studies that assessed the association between PM$_{2.5}$ exposure in the first trimester and preterm birth. Chart III: In studies that assessed the association between PM$_{2.5}$ exposure in the third trimester and preterm birth. Chart IV: In studies that assessed the PM$_{2.5}$ exposure at the semi-individual level. Chart V: In retrospective studies. Chart VI: In studies that were conducted in the USA

makers and public health practitioners to reduce the health impacts of air pollution.

Although this meta-analysis estimated the pooled effects of PM$_{2.5}$ concentrations on preterm birth risks, the limited number of studies restricted us from further exploring the effects of the chemical components of PM$_{2.5}$ on preterm birth. PM$_{2.5}$ is a mixture of multiple inorganic and organic components, and its health effects can vary based on components and origins [54, 55]. Only two of the included studies assessed the association between the components and sources of PM$_{2.5}$ and preterm birth. Pereira et al.

observed that preterm birth in Connecticut, USA was associated with increased exposure to dust, motor vehicle emissions, oil combustion and regional sulfur PM$_{2.5}$ sources during the entire pregnancy [56]. Darrow et al.'s study in Atlanta, USA found that preterm birth was significantly associated with sulfates and water-soluble metals in PM$_{2.5}$, but not associated with other components [30]. These results demonstrate that studies on the association between PM$_{2.5}$ components and sources and preterm birth are still limited, and more studies are needed in the future.

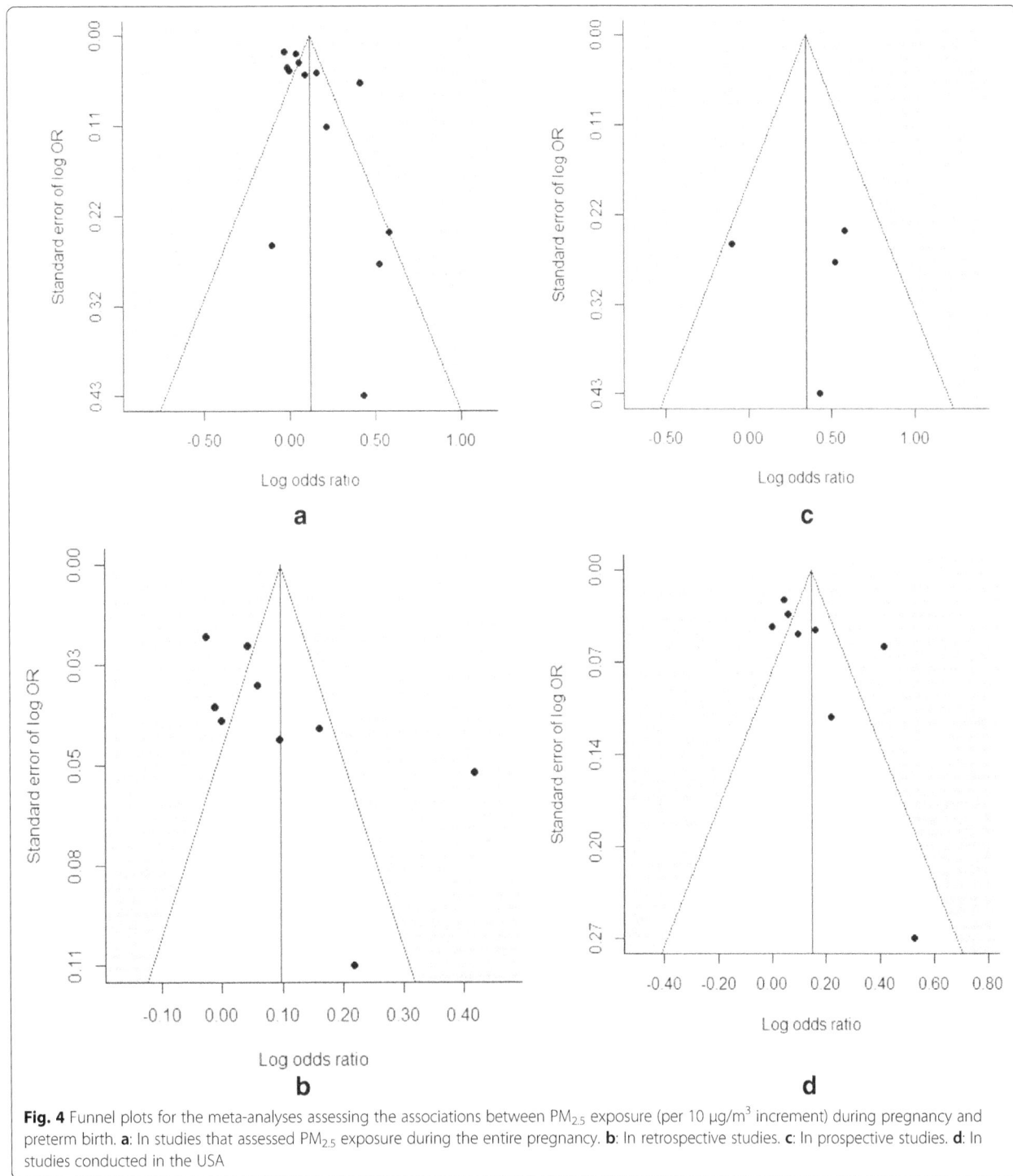

Fig. 4 Funnel plots for the meta-analyses assessing the associations between PM$_{2.5}$ exposure (per 10 μg/m^3 increment) during pregnancy and preterm birth. **a**: In studies that assessed PM$_{2.5}$ exposure during the entire pregnancy. **b**: In retrospective studies. **c**: In prospective studies. **d**: In studies conducted in the USA

Another factor affecting the heterogeneity between studies is the way that the studies controlled for confounders [57]. All of the studies included in this meta-analysis provided adjusted estimates of PM$_{2.5}$ exposure. Some common confounders, such as maternal age, race/ethnicity, income, education, smoking status during pregnancy, infant sex, parity, and birth season, were adjusted

for in most studies. However, almost all of the maternal and infant information was from public records, such as birth certificates, which limited the ability to control for other important confounders, such as maternal stress, activity level, nutrition, indoor pollution, and factors that varied spatially [36, 50, 51]. Therefore, improving the data quality of public records is one way to improve related studies. Future longitudinal studies that collect more detailed information at the individual level would be beneficial.

With reference to the limitations of this meta-analysis, we found high heterogeneity between included studies. Therefore, we used a random-effects model to quantitatively combine the individual estimate in studies with high heterogeneities. We also employed sub-group analyses and meta-regression analyses to explore the sources of heterogeneity. The results showed that although exposure assessment methods, study designs and study settings partially explained the heterogeneity, significant heterogeneities were still found in most sub-group analyses. These findings indicate that the heterogeneity across the included studies may also have been affected by other factors that we did not consider in this study, such as socioeconomic status and chemical constituents of $PM_{2.5}$, due to the limited quantity of related studies. Therefore, further studies are needed to explore the sources of heterogeneity in the future.

Conclusions

In summary, this meta-analysis observed a clear association between $PM_{2.5}$ exposure during pregnancy and preterm birth risk. However, a significant heterogeneity was found between included studies. The exposure assessment method, study design and study setting might be important sources of the heterogeneity, and should be taken into account in future meta-analyses. This study extends our understanding of the effects of maternal $PM_{2.5}$ exposure on preterm birth, and highlights that it is crucial to reduce ambient $PM_{2.5}$ pollution and reduce maternal $PM_{2.5}$ exposure during pregnancy to improve birth outcomes.

Additional file

Additional file 1: Figure S1. Meta regression analyses on the effects of study characteristics on the associations between $PM_{2.5}$ exposure and preterm birth risks. Chart A: The effects of $PM_{2.5}$ exposure during different trimester (the first, second and third trimester) of pregnancy on the pooled estimate of $PM_{2.5}$. Chart B: The effects of $PM_{2.5}$ exposure assessed by different methods (regional, semi-individual and individual level) on the pooled estimate of $PM_{2.5}$. Chart C: The effects of study designs (retrospective and prospective studies) on the pooled estimate of $PM_{2.5}$. Chart D: The effects of study settings (the USA and other countries) on the pooled estimate of $PM_{2.5}$

Abbreviations
$PM_{2.5}$: Fine particulate matter with aerodynamic diameter <2.5 μm; OR: Odds ratio; CI: Confidence interval; USA: The United States of America; PTB: Preterm birth; PTD: Preterm delivery; NA: Data not available.

Competing interests
The authors declare that they have no competing interests.

Authors' contributions
XS participated in the design and coordination of the study, and drafting the manuscript. XL conceived the study. CZ searched for the studies, collected and analyzed the data. RC participated in the design of this study and edited

the manuscript. CD participated in the design of this study and edited the manuscript. BZ did the data management and analyzed the data. TL conceived the study. All authors read and approved the final manuscript.

Acknowledgments and funding
This work was supported by the, Natural Science Foundation of Guangdong Province (2015A030310220) National Natural Science Foundation of China (81502819) , Fundamental Research Funds for the Central Universities (12ykpy13) and Postdoctoral Science Foundation of China (2013 M542230)

Author details
[1]Gynecology Department, Guangdong Women and Children Hospital, No. 521, Xingnan Road, Panyu District, Guangzhou 511442, China. [2]Sydney South West Clinical School, Faculty of Medicine, University of New South Wales, Sydney, Australia. [3]Faculty of Science, University of Technology Sydney, Ultimo, Australia. [4]Department of Preventive Medicine, School of Public Health, Sun Yat-sen University, Guangzhou 510080, China. [5]Guangdong Provincial Institute of Public Health, Guangdong Provincial Center for Disease Control and Prevention, No. 160, Qunxian Road, Panyu District, Guangzhou 511430, China. [6]Environment and Health, Guangdong Provincial Key Medical Discipline of Twelfth Five-Year Plan, Guangzhou 511430, China.

References
1. March of Dimes, PMNCH, Save the Children, WHO. Born Too Soon: The Global Action Report on Preterm Birth. CP Howson, MV Kinney, JE Lawn, editors. Geneva; World Health Organization. 2012.
2. Saigal S, Doyle LW. An overview of mortality and sequelae of preterm birth from infancy to adulthood. Lancet. 2008;371(9608):261–9.
3. Shah PS, Balkhair T, Knowledge Synthesis Group on Determinants of Preterm LBWb. Air pollution and birth outcomes: a systematic review. Environ Int. 2011;37(2):498–516.
4. Nieuwenhuijsen MJ, Dadvand P, Grellier J, Martinez D, Vrijheid M. Environmental risk factors of pregnancy outcomes: a summary of recent meta-analyses of epidemiological studies. Environ Health. 2013;12:6.
5. Englert N. Fine particles and human health—a review of epidemiological studies. Toxicol Lett. 2004;149(1):235–42.
6. Parker JD, Woodruff TJ, Basu R, Schoendorf KC. Air pollution and birth weight among term infants in California. Pediatrics. 2005;115(1):121–8.
7. Huynh M, Woodruff TJ, Parker JD, Schoendorf KC. Relationships between air pollution and preterm birth in California. Paediatr Perinat Ep. 2006;20(6):454–61.
8. Brauer M, Lencar C, Tamburic L, Koehoorn M, Demers P, Karr C. A cohort study of traffic-related air pollution impacts on birth outcomes. Environ Health Perspect. 2008;116(5):680–6.
9. Pereira G, Bell ML, Belanger K, de Klerk N. Fine particulate matter and risk of preterm birth and pre-labor rupture of membranes in Perth, Western Australia 1997–2007: A longitudinal study. Environ Int. 2014;73C:143–9.
10. Fleischer NL, Merialdi M, van Donkelaar A, Vadillo-Ortega F, Martin RV, Betran AP, et al. Outdoor air pollution, preterm birth, and low birth weight: analysis of the world health organization global survey on maternal and perinatal health. Environ Health Perspect. 2014;122(4):425–30.
11. Sapkota A, Chelikowsky AP, Nachman KE, Cohen AJ, Ritz B. Exposure to particulate matter and adverse birth outcomes: a comprehensive review and meta-analysis. Air Qual, Atmos Hlth. 2012;5(4):369–81.
12. Stieb DM, Chen L, Eshoul M, Judek S. Ambient air pollution, birth weight and preterm birth: a systematic review and meta-analysis. Environ Res. 2012;117:100–11.
13. Zhu X, Liu Y, Chen Y, Yao C, Che Z, Cao J. Maternal exposure to fine particulate matter (PM) and pregnancy outcomes: a meta-analysis. Environ Sci Pollut Res Int. 2015; DOI 10.1007/s11356-014-3458-7.
14. Higgins JP, Green S. Cochrane handbook for systematic reviews of interventions, vol. 5. Chichester: John Wiley & Sons, Ltd; 2008.
15. Wells G, Shea B, O'connell D, Peterson J, Welch V, Losos M, et al. The Newcastle-Ottawa Scale (NOS) for assessing the quality of nonrandomised studies in meta-analyses. http://www.medicine.mcgill.ca/rtamblyn/Readings/The%20Newcastle%20-%20Scale%20for%20assessing%20the%20quality%20of%20nonrandomised%20studies%20in%20meta-analyses.pdf. [Accessed January 3, 2015]

16. Wu J, Ren C, Delfino RJ, Chung J, Wilhelm M, Ritz B. Association between local traffic-generated air pollution and preeclampsia and preterm delivery in the south coast air basin of California. Environ Health Perspect. 2009;117(11):1773–9.

17. Gehring U, Wijga AH, Fischer P, de Jongste JC, Kerkhof M, Koppelman GH, et al. Traffic-related air pollution, preterm birth and term birth weight in the PIAMA birth cohort study. Environ Res. 2011;111(1):125–35.

18. Hyder A, Lee HJ, Ebisu K, Koutrakis P, Belanger K, Bell ML. PM2.5 exposure and birth outcomes: use of satellite- and monitor-based data. Epidemiology. 2014;25(1):58–67.

19. Higgins JP, Thompson SG, Deeks JJ, Altman DG. Measuring inconsistency in meta-analyses. BMJ. 2003;327(7414):557–60.

20. Hamra GB, Guha N, Cohen A, Laden F, Raaschou-Nielsen O, Samet JM, et al. Outdoor Particulate Matter Exposure and Lung Cancer: A Systematic Review and Meta-Analysis. Environ Health Perspect. 2014;122(9):906–11.

21. DerSimonian R, Laird N. Meta-analysis in clinical trials. Control Clin Trials. 1986;7(3):177–88.

22. Egger M, Davey Smith G, Schneider M, Minder C. Bias in meta-analysis detected by a simple, graphical test. BMJ. 1997;315(7109):629–34.

23. Rappazzo KM, Daniels JL, Messer LC, Poole C, Lobdell DT. Exposure to fine particulate matter during pregnancy and risk of preterm birth among women in New Jersey, Ohio, and Pennsylvania, 2000–2005. Environ Health Perspect. 2014;122(9):992.

24. Chang HH, Reich BJ, Miranda ML. A spatial time-to-event approach for estimating associations between air pollution and preterm birth. J R Stat Soc: Ser C: Appl Stat. 2013;62(2):167–79.

25. Chang HH, Reich BJ, Miranda ML. Time-to-event analysis of fine particle air pollution and preterm birth: results from North Carolina, 2001–2005. Am J Epidemiol. 2012;175(2):91–8.

26. Warren J, Fuentes M, Herring A, Langlois P. Spatial-Temporal Modeling of the Association between Air Pollution Exposure and Preterm Birth: Identifying Critical Windows of Exposure. Biometrics. 2012;68(4):1157–67.

27. Symanski E, Davila M, McHugh MK, Waller DK, Zhang X, Lai D. Maternal Exposure to Fine Particulate Pollution During Narrow Gestational Periods and Newborn Health in Harris County, Texas. Matern Child Health J. 2014;18(8):2003–12.

28. Sram RJ, Benes I, Binkova B, Dejmek J, Horstman D, Kotesovec F, et al. Teplice program–the impact of air pollution on human health. Environ Health Perspect. 1996;104 Suppl 4:699–714.

29. Wu J, Wilhelm M, Chung J, Ritz B. Comparing exposure assessment methods for traffic-related air pollution in an adverse pregnancy outcome study. Environ Res. 2011;111(5):685–92.

30. Darrow LA, Klein M, Flanders WD, Waller LA, Correa A, Marcus M, et al. Ambient air pollution and preterm birth: a time-series analysis. Epidemiology. 2009;20(5):689–98.

31. Wilhelm M, Ghosh JK, Su J, Cockburn M, Jerrett M, Ritz B. Traffic-related air toxics and preterm birth: a population-based case–control study in Los Angeles County, California. Environ Health. 2011;10:89.

32. Gray SC, Edwards SE, Schultz BD, Miranda ML. Assessing the impact of race, social factors and air pollution on birth outcomes: a population-based study. Environ Health. 2014;13(4):1–8.

33. Jalaludin B, Mannes T, Morgan G, Lincoln D, Sheppeard V, Corbett S. Impact of ambient air pollution on gestational age is modified by season in Sydney, Australia. Environ Health. 2007;6(16):1–9.

34. Kloog I, Melly SJ, Ridgway WL, Coull BA, Schwartz J. Using new satellite based exposure methods to study the association between pregnancy PM2.5 exposure, premature birth and birth weight in Massachusetts. Environ Health. 2012;11(1):1–8.

35. Lee PC, Roberts JM, Catov JM, Talbott EO, Ritz B. First trimester exposure to ambient air pollution, pregnancy complications and adverse birth outcomes in Allegheny County, PA. Matern Child Health J. 2013;17(3):545–55.

36. Pereira G, Belanger K, Ebisu K, Bell ML. Fine particulate matter and risk of preterm birth in connecticut in 2000–2006: a longitudinal study. Am J Epidemiol. 2014;179(1):67–74.

37. Ritz B, Wilhelm M, Hoggatt KJ, Ghosh JKC. Ambient air pollution and preterm birth in the environment and pregnancy outcomes study at the University of California, Los Angeles. Am J Epidemiol. 2007;166(9):1045–52.

38. Rudra CB, Williams MA, Sheppard L, Koenig JQ, Schiff MA. Ambient carbon monoxide and fine particulate matter in relation to preeclampsia and preterm delivery in western Washington State. Environ Health Perspect. 2011;119(6):886–92.

39. Wilhelm M, Ritz B. Local variations in CO and particulate air pollution and adverse birth outcomes in Los Angeles County, California, USA. Environ Health Perspect. 2005;113(9):1212–21.

40. Chang HH, Warren JL, Darrow LA, Reich BJ, Waller LA. Assessment of critical exposure and outcome windows in time-to-event analysis with application to air pollution and preterm birth study. Biostatistics. 2015;16(3):509–21. kxu060.

41. Hannam K, McNamee R, Baker P, Sibley C, Agius R. Air pollution exposure and adverse pregnancy outcomes in a large UK birth cohort: use of a novel spatio-temporal modelling technique. Scand J Work Environ Health. 2014;40(5):518–30.

42. Ha S, Hu H, Roussos-Ross D, Haidong K, Roth J, Xu X. The effects of air pollution on adverse birth outcomes. Environ Res. 2014;134:198–204.

43. Backes CH, Nelin T, Gorr MW, Wold LE. Early life exposure to air pollution: how bad is it? Toxicol Lett. 2013;216(1):47–53.

44. Parker JD, Woodruff TJ. Influences of study design and location on the relationship between particulate matter air pollution and birthweight. Paediatr Perinat Ep. 2008;22(3):214–27.

45. Kannan S, Misra DP, Dvonch JT, Krishnakumar A. Exposures to airborne particulate matter and adverse perinatal outcomes: a biologically plausible mechanistic framework for exploring potential effect modification by nutrition. Environ Health Perspect. 2006;114(11):1636–42.

46. Vadillo-Ortega F, Osornio-Vargas A, Buxton MA, Sánchez BN, Rojas-Bracho L, Viveros-Alcaráz M, et al. Air pollution, inflammation and preterm birth: A potential mechanistic link. Med Hypotheses. 2014;82(2):219–24.

47. Lin C-C, Santolaya-Forgas J. Current concepts of fetal growth restriction: part I. Causes, classification, and pathophysiology. Obstet Gynecol. 1998; 92(6):1044–55.

48. Zeger SL, Thomas D, Dominici F, Samet JM, Schwartz J, Dockery D, et al. Exposure measurement error in time-series studies of air pollution: concepts and consequences. Environ Health Perspect. 2000;108(5):419–26.

49. Berrocal VJ, Gelfand AE, Holland DM, Burke J, Miranda ML. On the use of a PM2.5 exposure simulator to explain birthweight. Environmetrics. 2011;22(4):553–71.

50. Jedrychowski W, Perera F, Mrozek-Budzyn D, Mroz E, Flak E, Spengler JD, et al. Gender differences in fetal growth of newborns exposed prenatally to airborne fine particulate matter. Environ Res. 2009;109(4):447–56.

51. Jedrychowski W, Bendkowska I, Flak E, Penar A, Jacek R, Kaim I, et al. Estimated risk for altered fetal growth resulting from exposure to fine particles during pregnancy: an epidemiologic prospective cohort study in Poland. Environ Health Perspect. 2004;112(14):1398–402.

52. Laden F, Neas LM, Dockery DW, Schwartz J. Association of fine particulate matter from different sources with daily mortality in six US cities. Environ Health Perspect. 2000;108(10):941–7.

53. Van Donkelaar A, Martin RV, Brauer M, Kahn R, Levy R, Verduzco C, et al. Global estimates of ambient fine particulate matter concentrations from satellite-based aerosol optical depth: development and application. Environ Health Perspect. 2010;118(6):847–55.

54. Habre R, Moshier E, Castro W, Nath A, Grunin A, Rohr A, et al. The effects of PM2.5 and its components from indoor and outdoor sources on cough and wheeze symptoms in asthmatic children. J Expo Sci Env Epid. 2014;24:380–7.

55. Kelly FJ, Fussell JC. Size, source and chemical composition as determinants of toxicity attributable to ambient particulate matter. Atmos Environ. 2012; 60:504–26.

56. Pereira G, Bell ML, Lee HJ, Koutrakis P, Belanger K. Sources of Fine Particulate Matter and Risk of Preterm Birth in Connecticut, 2000–2006: A Longitudinal Study. Environ Health Perspect. 2014;122(10):1117–22.

57. Morello-Frosch R, Jesdale BM, Sadd JL, Pastor M. Ambient air pollution exposure and full-term birth weight in California. Environ Health. 2010;9(44):1–13.

19

Serum screening in first trimester to predict pre-eclampsia, small for gestational age and preterm delivery

Yan Zhong, Fufan Zhu and Yiling Ding[*]

Abstract

Background: Early assessment before the establishment of placental dysfunction has the potential to improve treatment and prognosis for clinical practice. The objective of the study is to investigate the accuracy of serum biochemical markers(Pregnancy- Associated Plasma Protein-A (PAPP-A), human Chorionic Gonadotropin (hCG), Placental Growth Factor (PlGF), Placental Protein 13 (PP13) used in first trimester serum screening in predicting preelampsia, small for gestational age (SGA) and preterm delivery.

Methods: The data sources included Medline, Embase, Cochrane library, Medion, hand searching of relevant journals, reference list checking of included articles and contact with experts. Two reviewers independently selected the articles. Two authors independently extracted data on study characteristics, quality and results.

Results: The results showed low predictive accuracy overall. For preeclampsia, the best predictor was PlGF; LR + 4.01 (3.74, 4.28), LR-(0.67, 0.64, 0.69). The predictive value of serum markers for early preeclampsia was better than that of late preeclampsia. For SGA the best predictor was PP13; LR+ 3.70 (3.39, 4.03), LR- 0.70 (0.67, 0.73). For preterm delivery, the best predictor was PP13; LR+ 4.16 (2.72, 5.61), LR- 0.56 (0.45, 0.67).

Conclusion: First trimester screening analytes have low predictive accuracy for pre-eclampsia, small for gestational age and preterm delivery. However, the predict value of first trimester analytes is not worse than that of the second trimester markers.

Background

Preeclampsia, fetal growth restriction (FGR) and preterm delivery are major contributors to perinatal mortality and morbidity. They not only alter the immediate outcomes of pregnancy at the time of delivery but also the long-term cardiovascular health of the affected women and children. For example, a history of preeclampsia increases a female's risk of myocardial infarction, stroke or diabetes mellitus by two to eight fold over the next two decades [1]. Moreover, newborns diagnosed with FGR at birth have a two to eight fold increased risk for hypertension, cardiovascular disease, diabetes mellitus or renal disease as adults [2, 3].

Recent evidence suggests that the underlying pathology of preeclampsia, FGR and preterm delivery takes place in the first trimester. Earlier assessment before the establishment of placental dysfunction may have the potential to improve treatment and prognosis for clinical practice. Numerous stutdies have shown that abnormal concentration of first trimester serum markers is related to the onset of preeclampsia, small for gestational age and preterm delivery. With the increased use of first-trimester screening for Down syndrome, there is the opportunity to 'piggy back' screening tests for pre-eclampsia, FGR and preterm delivery onto existing tests.

The purpose of our review was to investigate the accuracy of serum biochemical markers (Pregnancy-Associated Plasma Protein-A (PAPP-A), human Chorionic Gonadotropin (hCG), Placental Growth Factor (PlGF), Placental Protein 13 (PP13) used in first trimester serum

* Correspondence: dylcsu@sina.cn
The Second Xiangya Hospital, Central South University, No.139, Middle Renmin Road, Changsha, Hunan 410011, P.R. China

screening in predicting preelampsia, small for gestational age (SGA) and preterm delivery. We systematically reviewed the available literature and meta-analysed the data.

Methods

Identification of studies

We searched MEDLINE, EMBASE and Cochrane Library from inception to April 2014 for relevant citations. The reference lists of all known primary and review articles were examined to identify cited articles not captured by electronic searches. The search strategy consisted of MeSH (medical subject heading) terms, Emtree terms, and keywords related to the disease (preeclampsia, small for gestational age, preterm birth, preterm delivery, etc.) combined with serum markers(PAPP-A, hCG, PP13, PlGF, etc.). Details of the search strategy are available from the authors. Language restrictions were not applied. A comprehensive database of relevant articles was constructed.

Study selection

The first stage of study selection was the scrutinizing of the database by two reviewers to identify articles from title and/or abstract. In a second stage, a search based on keywords for each of the analytes under review was performed within the Reference Manager database. The results of this search were scrutinized by a second reviewer. In the final stage of study selection the full papers of identified articles were obtained with final inclusion or exclusion decisions made after independent and duplicate examination of the papers. We included studies that reported on singleton pregnancies at low risk in any healthcare setting before the 14th week of gestation. Test accuracy studies allowing generation of 2×2 tables were included.

Data extraction and study quality assessment

Acceptable reference standards for preeclampsia were: persistent systolic blood pressure ≥ 140 mmHg or diastolic blood pressure ≥ 90 mmHg with proteinuria ≥ 0.3 g/24 h or $\geq 1+$ dipstick (= 30 mg/dl in a single urine sample), new after 20 weeks of gestation. Early preeclampsia was defined as preeclampsia resulting in a delivery before 34 weeks of gestation. Late preeclampsia was defined as preeclampsia resulting in a delivery after 34 weeks of gestation. Acceptable reference standards for SGA included birth weight $< 10^{th}$ centile adjusted for gestational age and based on local population values. We also included severe SGA defined as birth weight $< 5^{th}$ centile. Preterm delivery was defined as delivery < 37 weeks. We also included preterm delivery < 34 weeks.

All included manuscripts were assessed by at least one reviewer for study and reporting quality using validated tools. Items considered important for a good quality paper were prospective design with consecutive recruitment,

prospective design, adequate description of selection criteria, patient spectrum,test and use of appropriate reference standard.

Data synthesis and analysis

From the 2×2 tables the following were calculated with their 95 % confidence intervals for individual studies; sensitivity (true positive rate), specificity (true negative rate) and the likelihood ratios (LR). Results were pooled among groups of studies with similar characteristics, the same threshold and same adverse outcomes. Where 2×2 tables contained zero cells, 0.5 was added to each cell to enable calculations. All statistical analyses were performed using Stata 11.0 statistical package.

Results

Literature identification and study quality

Figure 1 summarises the process of literature identification and selection. There were 1575 primary articles that met the selection criteria. The initial electronic search strategy led to screen titles and abstracts of 1406 citations. Fig. 1 shows the screening and selection process that was followed for the identification and inclusion of studies. We retrieved 155 potentially eligible primary studies for detailed evaluation and inclusion in the systematic review, and an additional 14 potentially eligible publications from the reference lists of included studies. Detailed evaluation led to the exclusion of 66 publications that did not meet the selection criteria. Overall, 103 studies were considered relevant and were included in the systematic review. Total number of women in 103 studies is 432,621.

The quality assessment of included studies is summarized in Fig. 2. There was good reporting of prospective design with consecutive recruitment, prospective design, adequate description of selection criteria, patient spectrum, test and use of appropriate reference standard.

Data analysis

For both analysis for preelampsia, SGA and preterm delivery, there was significant heterogeneity in all results. As a consequence of this the random effects model was used throughout the study.

Pregnancy associated plasma protein A (PAPP-A)

The results for PAPPA to predict preeclampsia are summarized in Fig. 3. The total number of women in these studies is 385,643. There were 16 studies for preeclampsia, 10 for early preeclampsia and 3 for late preeclampsia included in the meta-analysis [4–22]. For preeclampsia, thresholds that were most commonly used were $<5^{th}$ centile (5 studies) and $< 10^{th}$ centile (4 studies). The most accurate predictor was PAPPA < 0.4 MoM (multiples of median); LR+ 2.17 (1.48,3.17), LR- 0.91 (0.85,

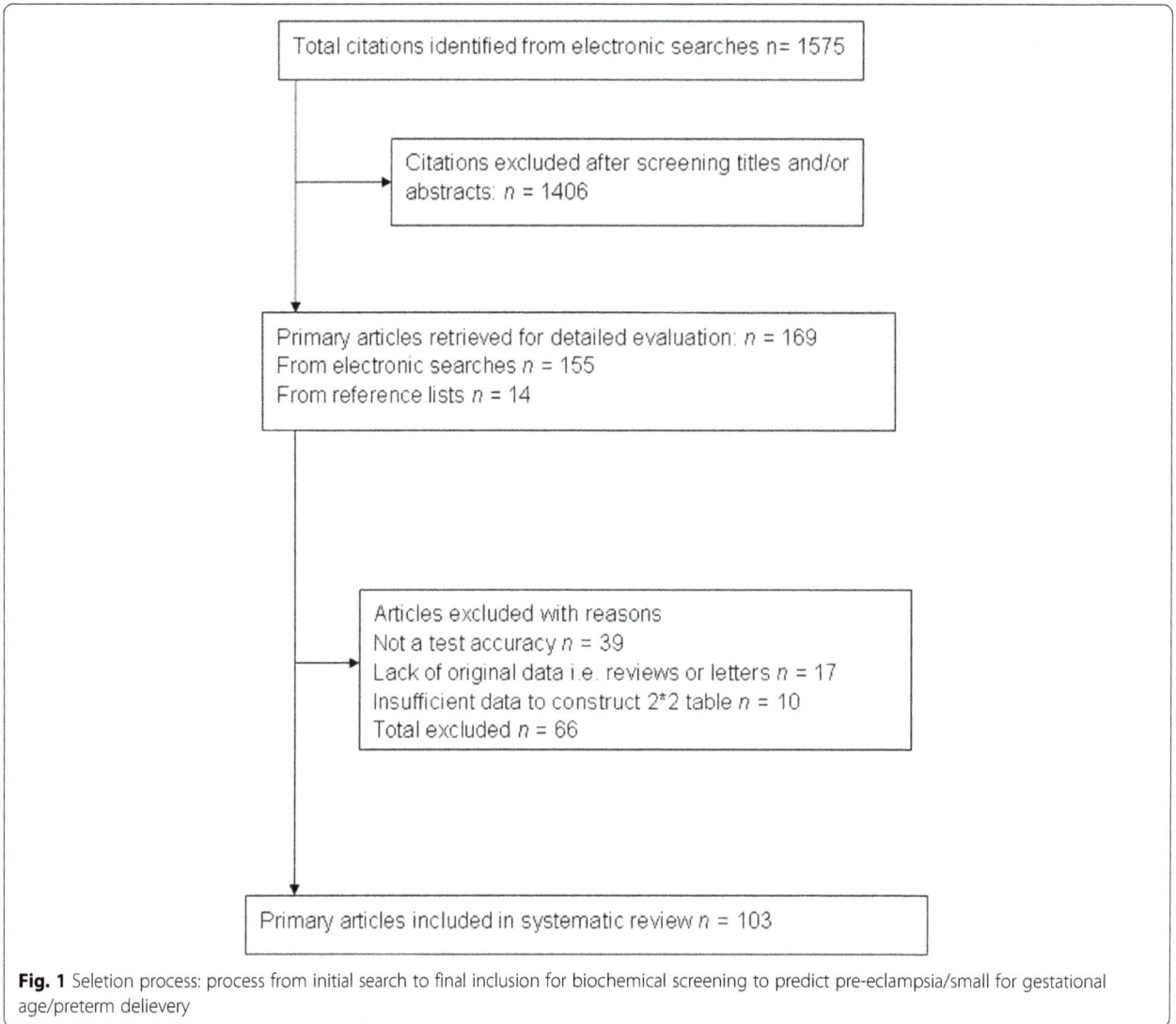

Fig. 1 Seletion process: process from initial search to final inclusion for biochemical screening to predict pre-eclampsia/small for gestational age/preterm delievery

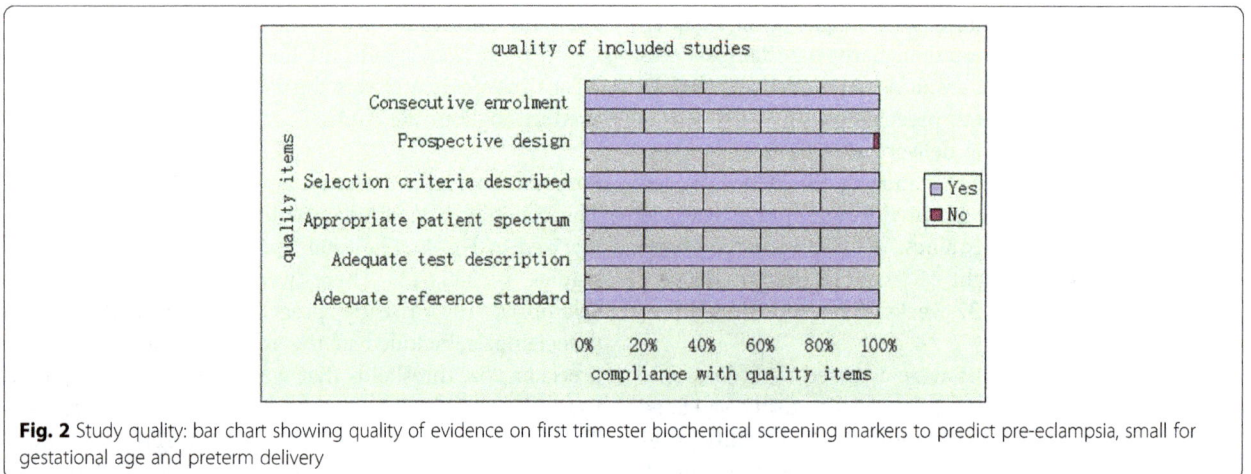

Fig. 2 Study quality: bar chart showing quality of evidence on first trimester biochemical screening markers to predict pre-eclampsia, small for gestational age and preterm delivery

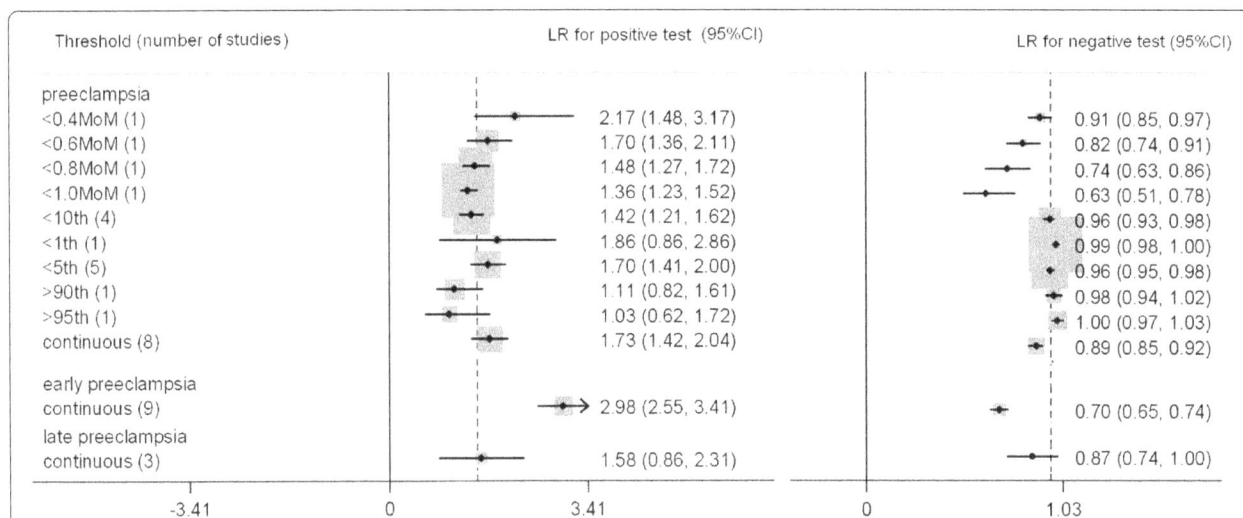

Fig. 3 Forest plot for PAPP-A to predict preeclampsia: forest plot showing likelihood ratio of a positive and negative test result with 95 % confidence intervals (95 % CI) for studies of Pregnancy- Associated Plasma Protein-A (PAPP-A) to predict pre-eclampsia. * continuous: Likelihood ratio calculated from receiver operating curve analysis

0.97), sensitivity 16 % (4 %, 35 %), specificity 93 % (76 %, 99 %), this was a single study. For early preeclampsia, all the predictive value was calculated from receiver operating curve analysis. The predictive value for early preeclampsia (LR+ 2.98 (2.55,3.41), LR-0.70 (0.65, 0.74), sensitivity (39 % (33 %, 47 %)), specificity (87 % (82 %, 90 %)) was generally better than that for preeclampsia and late preeclampsia (LR+ 1.58 (0.86, 2.31), LR-0.87 (0.74, 1.00), sensitivity 29 % (28 %, 30 %), specificity 82 % (81 %, 83 %)).

For SGA there were 19 studies for SGA < 10th centile and 6 studies for SGA < 5th centile included in the meta-analysis [4, 6, 7, 10, 11, 23–36] (Fig. 4). The commonest threshold used to predict SGA < 10th centile were PAPPA < 5th centile (9 studies). The best predictor for SGA <10th centile was PAPPA < 1st centile; LR+ 3.59 (2.77, 4.40), LR- 0.98 (0.97, 0.98), sensitivity 3 % (3 %, 4 %), specificity 99 % (98 %, 99 %). For SGA < 5th centile, PAPPA < 1st centile was also the most accurate predictor,

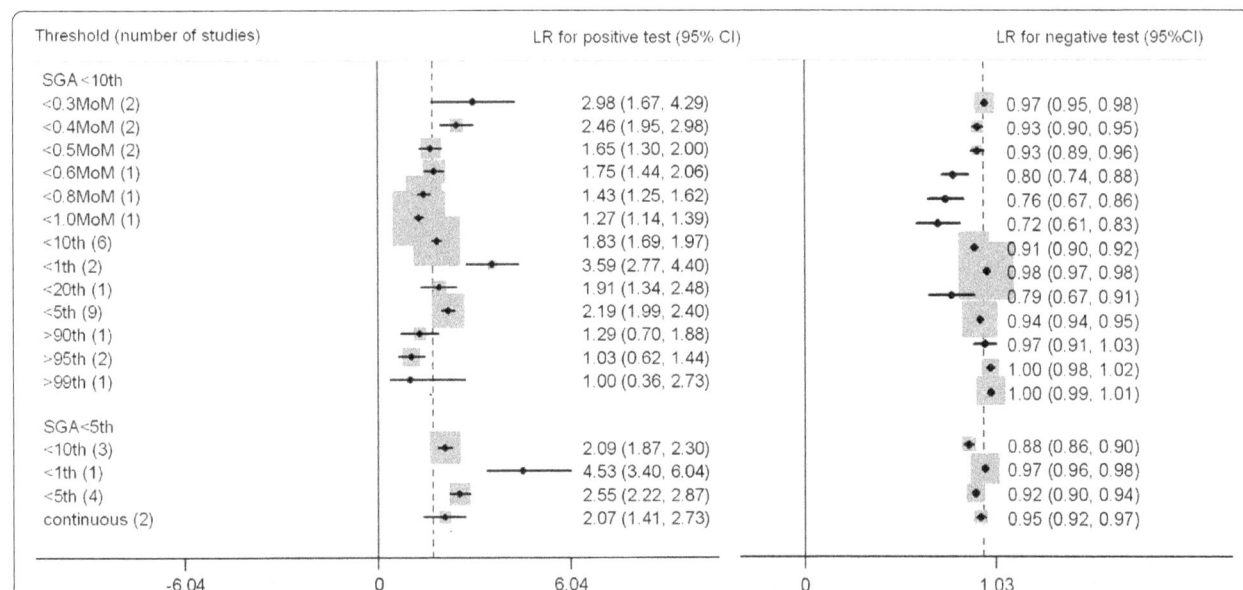

Fig. 4 Forest plot for PAPP-A to predict SGA: forest Plot showing likelihood ratio of a positive and negative test result with 95 % confidence intervals (95 % CI) for studies of Pregnancy- Associated Plasma Protein-A (PAPP-A) to predict small for gestational age (SGA). * continuous: Likelihood ratio calculated from receiver operating curve analysis

LR+ 4.53 (3.40, 6.04), LR-0.97 (0.96, 0.98), sensitivity 4 % (2 %, 5 %), specificity 99 % (98 %, 100 %).

For preterm delivery there were 12 studies for preterm delivery and 6 studies for preterm delivery < 34 weeks included in the meta-analysis [4, 7, 10, 11, 23-25, 33, 35, 37–40] (Fig. 5). The commonest threshold used to predict preterm delivery were <5th centile (6 studies). The best predictor for preterm delivery was calculated from receiver operating curve analysis; LR+ 2.99 (1.95, 4.03), LR- 0.66 (0.60, 0.77), sensitivity 44 % (28 %, 58 %), specificity 85 % (70 %, 93 %). For preterm delivery < 34 weeks, PAPPA < 0.3 MoM was the most accurate predictor, LR+ 3.64 (1.89, 7.02), LR-0.96 (0.93, 1.00), sensitivity 5 % (1 %, 14 %), specifcity 99 % (93 %, 100 %).

Plancenta protein 13 (PP13)

The results for PP13 are summarized in Fig. 6, all the predictive value was calculated from receiver operating curve analysis. The total number of women in these studies is 60,786. For early preeclampsia there were 6 included studies [8, 12, 15, 41-44]. PP13 turns out to be more accurate predictor for early preclampsia; LR+ 4.20 (3.69, 4.71), LR-0.60 (0.53, 0.66), sensitivity 47 % (39 %, 54 %), specificity 89 % (85 %, 91 %). For preeclampsia there were 4 studies[8, 21, 45, 46]; LR+ 2.69 (2.05, 3.32), LR- 0.51 (0.42, 0.59), sensitivity 60 % (50 %, 73 %), specificity 78 % (64 %, 85 %). For SGA <10th there was only one included study[29], LR+ 3.70 (3.39, 4.03), LR- 0.70 (0.67, 0.73), sensitivity 36 % (33 %, 41 %), specificity 90 % (88 %, 92 %). For preterm delivery, there were 2 included studies [39, 45]; LR+ 4.16 (2.72, 5.61), LR- 0.56

(0.45, 0.67), sensitivity 51 % (37 %, 66 %), specificity 88 % (76 %, 93 %).

Placental growth factor (PlGF)

The results for PlGF are summarized in Fig. 7. There were 16 included studies. The total number of women in these studies is 84,424. For preeclampsia there were 2 studies [13, 20]; LR + 4.01(3.74, 4.28), LR-0.67 (0.64, 0.69), sensitivity 40 % (37 %, 43 %), specificity 90 % (88 %, 91 %). PlGF was also shown to be more predictive for early preeclampsia[12-14, 17, 19, 20]; LR + 6.05 (5.55, 6.55), LR- 0.48 (0.43, 0.52), sensitivity 56 % (52 %, 61 %), specificity 91 % (89 %, 92 %). For SGA there were 2 included studies [29, 32]; LR+ 2.65 (2.09, 3.20), LR-0.81 (0.77, 0.85), sensitivity 27 % (20 %, 36 %), specificity 90 % (83 %, 94 %).

Human chorionic gonadotrophin (hCG)

The results for hCG to predict preeclampsia are summarized in Fig. 8. The total number of women in these studies is 112,400. There were 4 included studies in the meta-analysis [7, 10, 11, 18], and there was single study for every threshold. The most accurate predictor was hCG < 0.6MoM; LR+ 1.41 (1.10, 1.82), LR- 0.90 (0.82, 0.99), sensitivity 28 % (2 %, 71 %), specificity 80 % (36 %, 99 %). There were 2 studies and 1 study looking at early preeclampsia [18, 19] and late preeclampsia [19] respectively as the outcome, results showed no improvement in prediction.

For SGA < 10th centile there were 9 included studies in the meta-analysis [7, 11, 23–25, 29, 30, 35, 36] (Fig. 9).

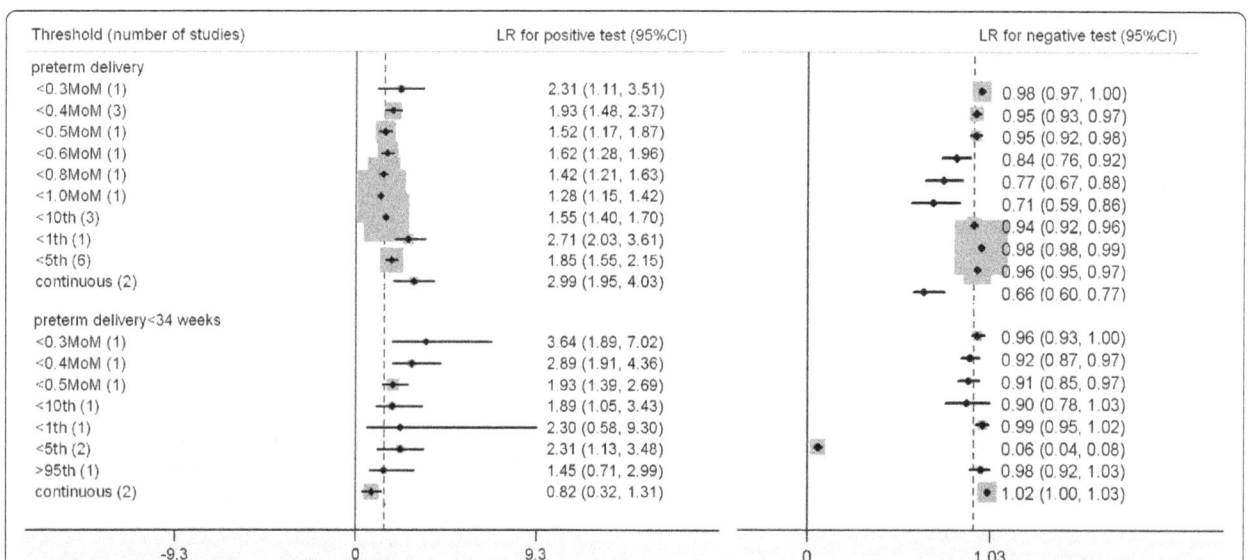

Fig. 5 Forest plot for PAPP-A to predict preterm delivery: forest Plot showing likelihood ratio of a positive and negative test result with 95 % confidence intervals (95 % CI) for studies of Pregnancy- Associated Plasma Protein-A (PAPP-A) to predict preterm delivery. * continuous: Likelihood ratio calculated from receiver operating curve analysis

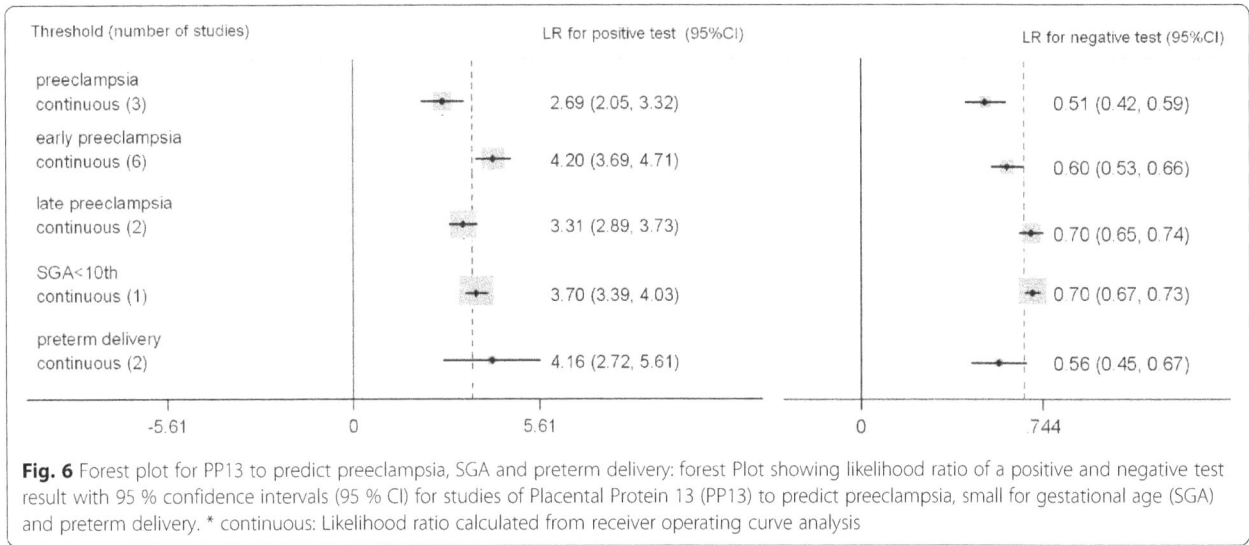

Fig. 6 Forest plot for PP13 to predict preeclampsia, SGA and preterm delivery: forest Plot showing likelihood ratio of a positive and negative test result with 95 % confidence intervals (95 % CI) for studies of Placental Protein 13 (PP13) to predict preeclampsia, small for gestational age (SGA) and preterm delivery. * continuous: Likelihood ratio calculated from receiver operating curve analysis

The commonest thresholds used were hCG < 5th (3 studies) and calculated from receiver operating curve analysis. The most accurate predictor for SGA < 10th centile was calculated from receiver operating curve analysis; LR+ 3.44 (3.26, 3.63), LR-0.73 (0.71, 0.74), sensitivity 34 % (32 %, 37 %), specificity 90 % (89 %, 91 %). For SGA < 5th centile there were only 2 thresholds studied with single study for each[7, 10], hCG < 10th centile was more accurate; LR+ 2.86 (1.97, 4.16), LR-0.90 (0.85, 0.96), sensitivity 15 % (5 %, 26 %), specificity 95 % (87 %, 100 %).

There were 6 studies for preterm delivery [7, 10, 11, 23, 35, 40] and 4 studies for preterm delivery < 34 weeks [7, 23, 25, 40] included in the meta-analysis (Fig. 10). The commonest threshold used to predict preterm delivery were hCG < 5th centile (6 studies). The best predictor for preterm delivery was hCG < 0.5 MoM; LR+ 2.71 (1.88, 3.54), LR- 0.92 (0.89, 0.96), sensitivity 12 % (5 %, 21 %), specificity 96 % (89 %, 98 %). For preterm delivery

< 34 weeks, hCG > 95th was the most accurate predictor, LR+ 1.74 (1.22, 2.47), LR-0.96 (0.93, 0.99), sensitivity 9 % (2 %, 29 %), specificity 95 % (76 %, 99 %).

Discussion

We evaluated the accuracy of five serum screening markers commonly used in first trimester screening for preeclampsia, SGA and preterm delivery. The results showed low predictive accuracy overall. For preeclampsia, the best predictor was PlGF. However, it is important to point out that this threshold was determined from a receiver operating characteristic curve and based only 2 studies. For early and late preeclampsia, the best predictor was also PlGF. Generally, the predictive value of serum markers for early preeclampsia is better than that of late preeclampsia. For SGA the best predictor overall was PP13 while PAPPA < 1st centile was the best predictor of SGA < 5th centile. These results were both based on single studies. For preterm delivery, the best

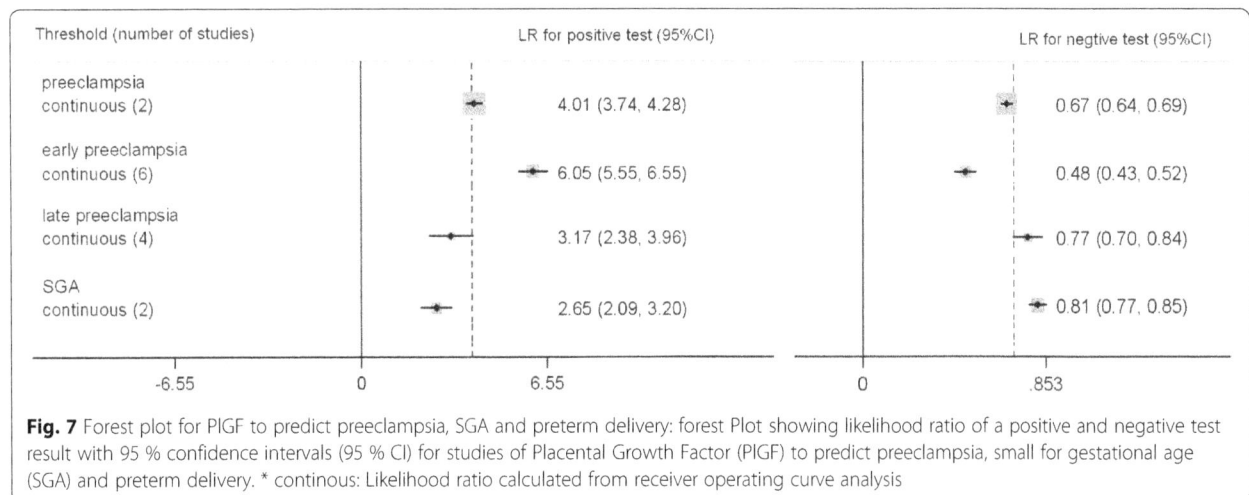

Fig. 7 Forest plot for PlGF to predict preeclampsia, SGA and preterm delivery: forest Plot showing likelihood ratio of a positive and negative test result with 95 % confidence intervals (95 % CI) for studies of Placental Growth Factor (PlGF) to predict preeclampsia, small for gestational age (SGA) and preterm delivery. * continous: Likelihood ratio calculated from receiver operating curve analysis

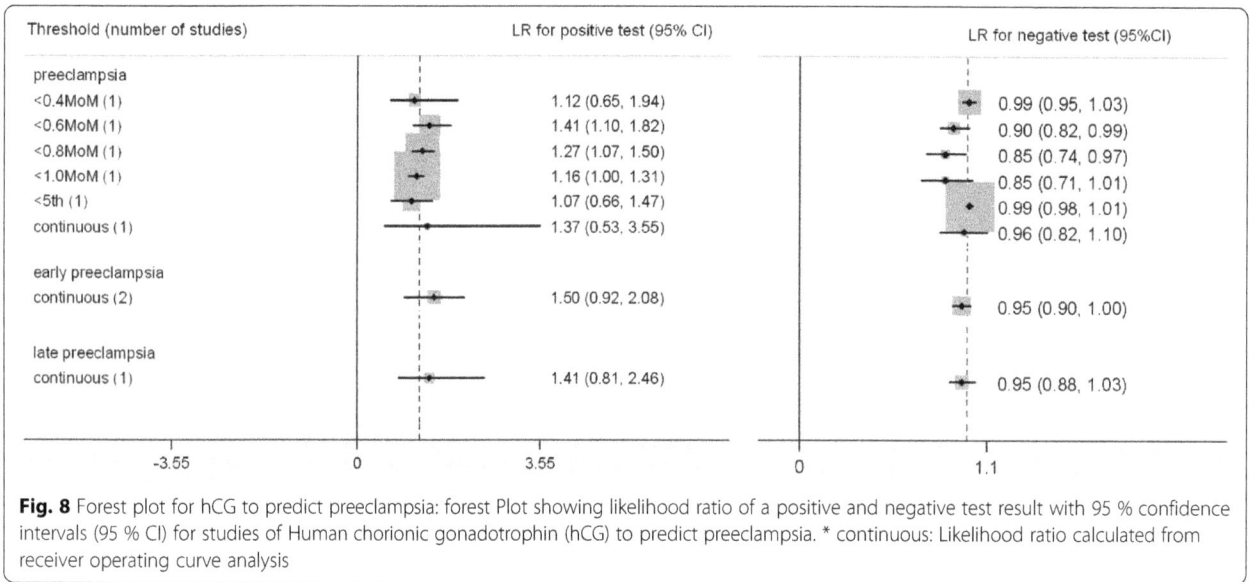

Fig. 8 Forest plot for hCG to predict preeclampsia: forest Plot showing likelihood ratio of a positive and negative test result with 95 % confidence intervals (95 % CI) for studies of Human chorionic gonadotrophin (hCG) to predict preeclampsia. * continuous: Likelihood ratio calculated from receiver operating curve analysis

predictor was PP13 while PAPPA < 0.3 MoM was the best predictor of preterm delivery < 34 weeks.

The predict value of first trimester analytes is not worse compare to that of the second trimester markers. Previous studies show in the second trimester, the most accurate predictor of hCG for preeclampsia was hCG > 2.0 MoM, with LR+ 2.45 (1.57, 3.84), LR- 0.89 (0.83, 0.96); for SGA was hCG > 2.0 MoM, with LR+ 1.74 (1.48, 2.04), LR-0.95 (0.93, 0.96). The most accurate predictor of PAPPA for preeclampsia was PAPP-A < 5th centile, with LR + 2.10 (1.57, 2.81), LR- 0.95 (0.93, 0.98); for SGA was PAPP-A < 1st centile; LR+ 3.50 (2.53, 4.82), LR- 0.98 (0.97, 0.99). On the other hand, our meta-analysis shows the most accurate predictor of hCG for preeclampsia was hCG < 0.6 MoM;

LR+ 1.41 (1.10, 1.82), LR- 0.90 (0.82, 0.99), for SGA was calculated from receiver operating curve analysis; LR+ 3.44 (3.26, 3.63), LR-0.73 (0.71, 0.74). The most accurate predictor of PAPPA for preeclampsia was PAPPA < 0.4 MoM; LR+ 2.17 (1.48, 3.17), LR- 0.91 (0.85, 0.97), for SGA was PAPPA < 1st centile; LR+ 3.59 (2.77, 4.40), LR- 0.98 (0.97, 0.98). A possible explanation for the apparent difference of hCG change between first trimester and second trimester is that the low levels at first trimester are the consequence of impaired placentation and smaller placental mass, whereas the high levels in the second trimester may be the result of 'leakage' or hypoperfusion-related stimulation of production of this hormone [47]. Although the symptoms of preeclampsia and FGR generally

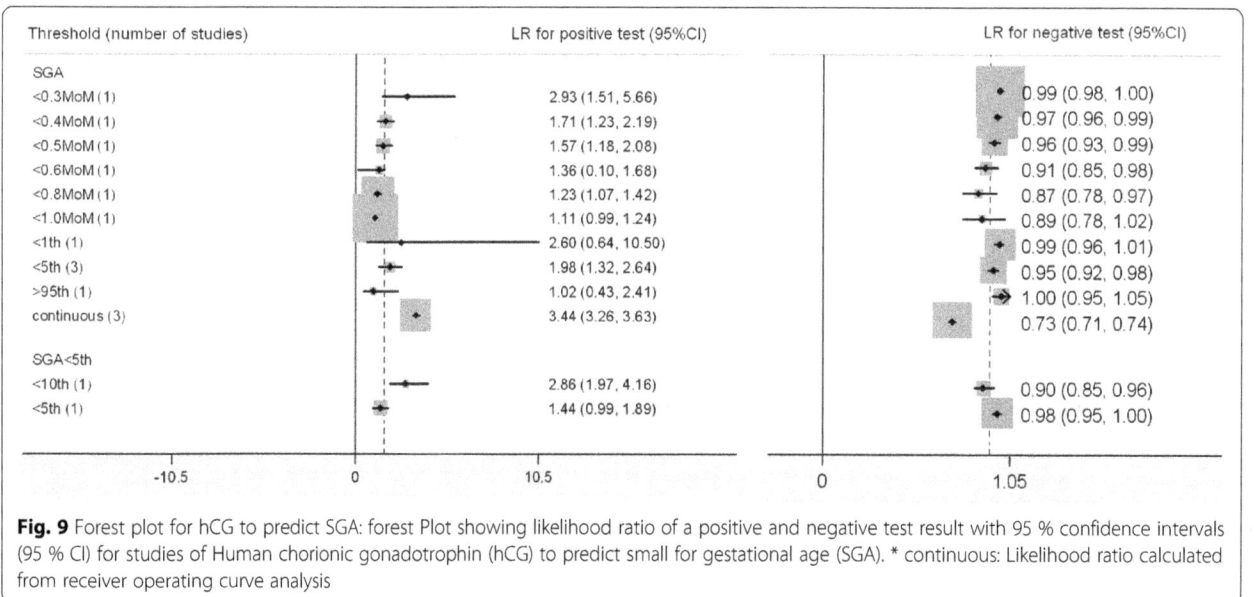

Fig. 9 Forest plot for hCG to predict SGA: forest Plot showing likelihood ratio of a positive and negative test result with 95 % confidence intervals (95 % CI) for studies of Human chorionic gonadotrophin (hCG) to predict small for gestational age (SGA). * continuous: Likelihood ratio calculated from receiver operating curve analysis

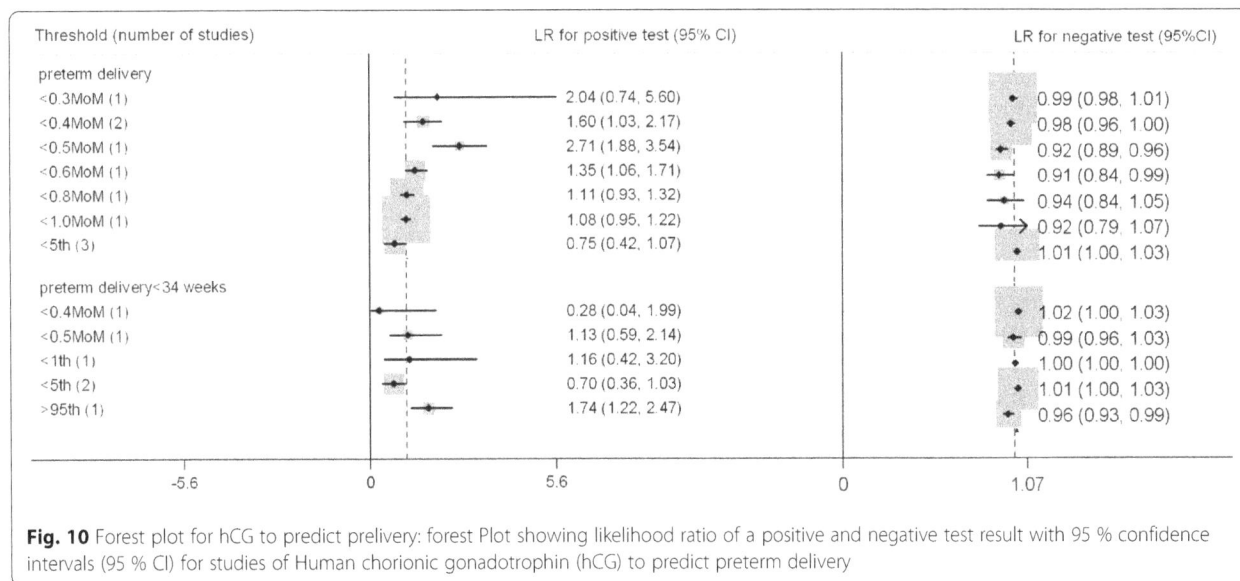

Fig. 10 Forest plot for hCG to predict prelivery: forest Plot showing likelihood ratio of a positive and negative test result with 95 % confidence intervals (95 % CI) for studies of Human chorionic gonadotrophin (hCG) to predict preterm delivery

manifest in the second to third trimester of pregnancy, their underlying pathology takes place in the first trimester. One possible reason why preventive strategies have proven very disappointing at present is that the proposed interventions have commenced in the mid to late second trimester, when the underlying placental dysfunction may already be established. Earlier assessment before the establishment of placental dysfunction may have the potential to improve predictive value for clinical practice. With the increased use of first-trimester screening for Down syndrome, there is the opportunity to 'piggy back' screening tests for preeclampsia, FGR and preterm delivery onto existing tests.

As preeclampsia and SGA are diseases with relatively low prevalence, a clinically useful test would need to have a high positive LR (> 10) and low negative LR (< 0.10) [48]. From the results of this review it is unlikely that any first trimester serum screening marker in isolation will provide this. Future research should thus concentrate in two areas. The first is to improve the knowledge of the biological mechanisms for the abnormal clinical tests by focusing on the exact placental pathology resulting in the changes seen in preeclampsia, FGR and preterm delivery. Preliminary findings suggest that genomic studies can improve our understanding of the early pathophysiology of preeclampsia/FGR/preterm delivery at the molecular level. It is hoped that proteomics, metabolomics, and other techniques will allow us to provide potential targets for the development of biomarkers with high enough predictive and prognostic information to be translated into clinical practice. Secondly, future research should attempt to improve the predictive value by combining Doppler sonography, different maternal serum analytes and clinical characteristics. The use of multiple parameters increases the specificity and sensitivity of the screening possibly because they reflect different pathways to the disease

process, with abnormal Doppler reflecting the inadequate trophoblastic invasion of the maternal spiral arteries and abnormal biomarkers demonstrating the dysregulated secretory activity by the trophoblasts. However, some studies showed no additive effect of combining different markers, likely secondary to correlation between the markers (such as ADAM12 and PAPP-A, sFlt-1 and sEng) [47]. Sequential measurements of markers might also improve the risk assessment as individual changes from the first to second trimesters have been shown to occur in preeclampsia and FGR.

Our result also showed the detection rate of first trimester serum markers for early preeclampsia is better than that for late preeclampsia. This disparity may result from different etiologies between early and late preeclampsia. Early preeclampsia is said to be associated with inadequate and incomplete trophoblast invasion of maternal spiral arteries, and is often complicated with a fetal growth restriction. In contrast, the late onset type of preeclampsia is often related to enlarged placental mass or surface (diabetes, multiple pregnancies, anemia, high altitude). It often shows normal or only slightly altered behavior of the uterine spiral arteries and thus no changes in the blood flow of the umbilical arteries. Fetus with late onset preeclampsia often shows no signs of any growth restriction [49]. Since abnormal concentration of serum markers in the first trimester is caused by intrinsic alteration of the villous trophoblast, it is reasonable that predictive value would be poorer for late onset preeclampsia with normal or only slightly altered trophoblast invasion in the first trimester.

The strength of the study includes generally sufficient quality and a quality assessment of studies based on recognized criteria. However, there are still some limitations. First, there is large discordance in reports of cutoff points, thus, a formal meta-analysis with estimated over-all relative risks was not feasible. Secondly, the number of studies for some cutoffpoints is so small that they lead to some contradictive results. For example, our analysis shows the best predictor for preterm delivery was hCG < 0.5 MoM while the best predictor for preterm delvery < 34 weeks is a hCG > 95th centile. This odd result is probably due to the small numbers of studies since there is only one study for each threshold. Clearly large scale studies are needed for more reliable evaluation. Thirdly, all of the studies we selected are population of low risk so we are unable to perform a sub analysis. We didn't choose the population of high risk since there are few studies on it. More studies are needed to analyse predictive accuracy by the type of population.

Conclusion

First trimester screening analytes have low predictive accuracy for pre-eclampsia, SGA and preterm delivery. However, the predict value of first trimester analytes is not worse compare to that of the second trimester markers. They may be useful in prediction when combined with other tests. Early pathophysiology of preeclampsia/FGR/preterm delivery should be studied to develop biomarkers with high enough predictive and prognostic information to be translated into clinical practice.

Abbreviations
PAPP-A: Pregnancy- associated plasma protein-A; hCG: Human chorionic gonadotropin; PlGF: Placental growth factor; PP13: Placental protein 13; SGA: Small for gestational age; LR: Likelihood ratio.

Competing interests
The authors declare that they have no competing interests.

Authors' contributions
YD and FZ independently selected the articles, and independently extracted data on study characteristics, quality and results. YZ designed the study, performed the statistical analysis, and draft the manuscript. All authors read and approved the final manuscript.

References
1. Ray JG, Vermeulen MJ, Schull MJ, Redelmeier DA. Cardiovascular health after maternal placental syndromes (CHAMPS): population-based retrospective cohort study. Lancet. 2005;366(9499):1797–803.
2. Barker DJ. Adult consequences of fetal growth restriction. Clin Obstet Gynecol. 2006;49(2):270–83.
3. Gluckman PD, Hanson MA, Cooper C, Thornburg KL. Effect of in utero and early-life conditions on adult health and disease. N Engl J Med. 2008;359(1):61–73.
4. Dugoff L, Hobbins JC, Malone FD, Porter TF, Luthy D, Comstock CH, et al. First-trimester maternal serum PAPP-A and free-beta subunit human chorionic gonadotropin concentrations and nuchal translucency are associated with obstetric complications: a population-based screening study (the FASTER Trial). Am J Obstet Gynecol. 2004;191(4):1446–51.
5. Poon LC, Nekrasova E, Anastassopoulos P, Livanos P, Nicolaides KH. First-trimester maternal serum matrix metalloproteinase-9 (MMP-9) and adverse pregnancy outcome. Prenat Diagn. 2009;29(6):553–9.
6. Pilalis A, Souka AP, Antsaklis P, Daskalakis G, Papantoniou N, Mesogitis S, et al. Screening for pre-eclampsia and fetal growth restriction by uterine artery Doppler and PAPP-A at 11–14 weeks' gestation. Ultrasound Obstet Gynecol. 2007;29(2):135–40.
7. LA Ong CT, Spencer K, Munim S, Nicolaides KH. First-trimester maternal serum free beta-human chorionic gonadotropin and pregnancy associated plasma protein-A as predictors of pregnancy complications. Bjog-an International Journal of Obstetrics and Gynaecology. 2000;107:1265–70.
8. Spencer K, Cowans NJ, Chefetz I, Tal J, Meiri H. First-trimester maternal serum PP-13, PAPP-A and second-trimester uterine artery Doppler pulsatility index as markers of pre-eclampsia. Ultrasound Obstet Gynecol. 2007;29(2):128–34.
9. Hedley PL, Placing S, Wojdemann K, Carlsen AL, Shalmi AC, Sundberg K, et al. Free leptin index and PAPP-A: a first trimester maternal serum screening test for pre-eclampsia. Prenat Diagn. 2010;30(2):103–9.
10. Smith GC, Stenhouse EJ, Crossley JA, Aitken DA, Cameron AD, Connor JM. Early pregnancy levels of pregnancy-associated plasma protein a and the risk of intrauterine growth restriction, premature birth, preeclampsia, and stillbirth. J Clin Endocrinol Metab. 2002;87(4):1762–7.
11. Jenni K, Ranta KR. Jarkko Romppanen, Kari Pulkki, Seppo Heinonen Decreased PAPP-A is associated with preeclampsia, premature delivery and small for gestational age infants but not with placental abruption. Eur J Obstet Gynecol Reprod Biol. 2011;157(2011):48–52.
12. Wortelboer EJ, Koster MP, Cuckle HS, Stoutenbeek PH, Schielen PC, Visser GH. First-trimester placental protein 13 and placental growth factor: markers for identification of women destined to develop early-onset pre-eclampsia. BJOG. 2010;117(11):1384–9.
13. Audibert F, Boucoiran I, An N, Aleksandrov N, Delvin E, Bujold E, et al. Screening for preeclampsia using first-trimester serum markers and uterine artery Doppler in nulliparous women. Am J Obstet Gynecol. 2010;203(4):e1–8.
14. Akolekar R, Zaragoza E, Poon LCY, Pepes S, Nicolaides KH. Maternal serum placental growth factor at 11 + 0 to 13 + 6 weeks of gestation in the prediction of pre-eclampsia. Ultrasound Obstet Gynecol. 2008;32(6):732–9.
15. Akolekar R, Syngelaki A, Sarquis R, Zvanca M, Nicolaides KH. Prediction of early, intermediate and late pre-eclampsia from maternal factors, biophysical and biochemical markers at 11–13 weeks. Prenat Diagn. 2011;31(1):66–74.
16. Poon LCY, Maiz N, Valencia C, Plasencia W, Nicolaides KH. First-trimester maternal serum pregnancy-associated plasma protein-A and pre-eclampsia. Ultrasound Obstet Gynecol. 2009;33(1):23–33.
17. Foidart JM, Munaut C, Chantraine F, Akolekar R, Nicolaides KH. Maternal plasma soluble endoglin at 11–13 weeks' gestation in pre-eclampsia. Ultrasound Obstet Gynecol. 2010;35(6):680–7.
18. Keikkala E, Vuorela P, Laivuori H, Romppanen J, Heinonen S, Stenman UH. First trimester hyperglycosylated human chorionic gonadotrophin in serum - a marker of early-onset preeclampsia. Placenta. 2013;34(11):1059–65.
19. Kuc S, Koster MP, Franx A, Schielen PC, Visser GH. Maternal characteristics, mean arterial pressure and serum markers in early prediction of preeclampsia. PLoS One. 2013;8(5), e63546.
20. Akolekar R, Syngelaki A, Poon L, Wright D, Nicolaides KH. Competing risks model in early screening for preeclampsia by biophysical and biochemical markers. Fetal Diagn Ther. 2013;33(1):8–15.
21. Moslemi Zadeh N, Naghshvar F, Peyvandi S, Gheshlaghi P, Ehetshami S. PP13 and PAPP-A in the First and Second Trimesters: Predictive Factors for Preeclampsia? ISRN Obstet Gynecol. 2012;2012:263871.
22. Goetzinger KR, Singla A, Gerkowicz S, Dicke JM, Gray DL, Odibo AO. Predicting the risk of pre-eclampsia between 11 and 13 weeks' gestation by combining maternal characteristics and serum analytes, PAPP-A and free beta-hCG. Prenat Diagn. 2010;30(12–13):1138–42.
23. Kirkegaard I, Henriksen TB, Uldbjerg N. Early fetal growth, PAPP-A and free beta-hCG in relation to risk of delivering a small-for-gestational age infant. Ultrasound Obstet Gynecol. 2011;37(3):341–7.
24. Pihl K, Larsen T, Krebs L, Christiansen M. First trimester maternal serum PAPP-A, beta-hCG and ADAM12 in prediction of small-for-gestational-age fetuses. Prenat Diagn. 2008;28(12):1131–5.
25. Krantz D, Goetzl L, Simpson JL, Thom E, Zachary J, Hallahan TW, et al. Association of extreme first-trimester free human chorionic gonadotropin-beta, pregnancy-associated plasma protein A, and nuchal translucency with intrauterine growth restriction and other adverse pregnancy outcomes. Am J Obstet Gynecol. 2004;191(4):1452–8.
26. Kwik M, Morris J. Association between first trimester maternal serum pregnancy associated plasma protein-A and adverse pregnancy outcome. Aust N Z J Obstet Gynaecol. 2003;43(6):438–42.

27. Leung TY, Sahota DS, Chan LW, Law LW, Fung TY, Leung TN, et al. Prediction of birth weight by fetal crown-rump length and maternal serum levels of pregnancy-associated plasma protein-A in the first trimester. Ultrasound Obstet Gynecol. 2008;31(1):10–4.

28. Goetzinger KR, Singla A, Gerkowicz S, Dicke JM, Gray DL, Odibo AO. The efficiency of first-trimester serum analytes and maternal characteristics in predicting fetal growth disorders. Am J Obstet Gynecol. 2009;201(4):e1–6.

29. Karagiannis G, Akolekar R, Sarquis R, Wright D, Nicolaides KH. Prediction of small-for-gestation neonates from biophysical and biochemical markers at 11–13 weeks. Fetal Diagn Ther. 2011;29(2):148–54.

30. Montanari L, Alfei A, Albonico G, Moratti R, Arossa A, Beneventi F, et al. The impact of first-trimester serum free beta-human chorionic gonadotropin and pregnancy-associated plasma protein A on the diagnosis of fetal growth restriction and small for gestational age infant. Fetal Diagn Ther. 2009;25(1):130–5.

31. Plasencia W, Akolekar R, Dagklis T, Veduta A, Nicolaides KH. Placental volume at 11–13 weeks' gestation in the prediction of birth weight percentile. Fetal Diagn Ther. 2011;30(1):23–8.

32. Poon LC, Zaragoza E, Akolekar R, Anagnostopoulos E, Nicolaides KH. Maternal serum placental growth factor (PlGF) in small for gestational age pregnancy at 11(+0) to 13(+6) weeks of gestation. Prenat Diagn. 2008;28(12):1110–5.

33. Cowans NJ, Spencer K. First-trimester ADAM12 and PAPP-A as markers for intrauterine fetal growth restriction through their roles in the insulin-like growth factor system. Prenat Diagn. 2007;27(3):264–71.

34. Pihl K, Larsen T, Laursen I, Krebs L, Christiansen M. First trimester maternal serum pregnancy-specific beta-1-glycoprotein (SP1) as a marker of adverse pregnancy outcome. Prenat Diagn. 2009;29(13):1256–61.

35. Lain SJ, Algert CS, Tasevski V, Morris JM, Roberts CL. Record linkage to obtain birth outcomes for the evaluation of screening biomarkers in pregnancy: a feasibility study. BMC Med Res Methodol. 2009;9:48.

36. Poon LC, Karagiannis G, Staboulidou I, Shafiei A, Nicolaides KH. Reference range of birth weight with gestation and first-trimester prediction of small-for-gestation neonates. Prenat Diagn. 2011;31(1):58–65.

37. Dane B, Dane C, Kiray M, Cetin A, Koldas M, Erginbas M. Correlation between first-trimester maternal serum markers, second-trimester uterine artery doppler indices and pregnancy outcome. Gynecol Obstet Invest. 2010;70(2):126–31.

38. Goetzinger KR, Cahill AG, Kemna J, Odibo L, Macones GA, Odibo AO. First-trimester prediction of preterm birth using ADAM12, PAPP-A, uterine artery Doppler, and maternal characteristics. Prenat Diagn. 2012;32(10):1002–7.

39. Stout MJ, Goetzinger KR, Tuuli MG, Cahill AG, Macones GA, Odibo AO. First trimester serum analytes, maternal characteristics and ultrasound markers to predict pregnancies at risk for preterm birth. Placenta. 2013;34(1):14–9.

40. Barrett SL, Bower C, Hadlow NC. Use of the combined first-trimester screen result and low PAPP-A to predict risk of adverse fetal outcomes. Prenat Diagn. 2008;28(1):28–35.

41. Nicolaides KH, Bindra R, Turan OM, Chefetz I, Sammar M, Meiri H, et al. A novel approach to first-trimester screening for early pre-eclampsia combining serum PP-13 and Doppler ultrasound. Ultrasound Obstet Gynecol. 2006;27(1):13–7.

42. Romero R, Kusanovic JP, Than NG, Erez O, Gotsch F, Espinoza J, et al. First-trimester maternal serum PP13 in the risk assessment for preeclampsia. Am J Obstet Gynecol. 2008;199(2):e1–e11.

43. Khalil A, Cowans NJ, Spencer K, Goichman S, Meiri H, Harrington K. First trimester maternal serum placental protein 13 for the prediction of pre-eclampsia in women with a priori high risk. Prenat Diagn. 2009;29(8):781–9.

44. Akolekar R, Syngelaki A, Beta J, Kocylowski R, Nicolaides KH. Maternal serum placental protein 13 at 11–13 weeks of gestation in preeclampsia. Prenat Diagn. 2009;23.

45. Chafetz I, Kuhnreich I, Sammar M, Tal Y, Gibor Y, Meiri H, et al. First-trimester placental protein 13 screening for preeclampsia and intrauterine growth restriction. Am J Obstet Gynecol. 2007;197(1):e1–7.

46. Odibo AO, Zhong Y, Goetzinger KR, Odibo L, Bick JL, Bower CR, et al. First-trimester placental protein 13, PAPP-A, uterine artery Doppler and maternal characteristics in the prediction of pre-eclampsia. Placenta. 2011;32(8):598–602.

47. Zhong Y, Tuuli M, Odibo AO. First-trimester assessment of placenta function and the prediction of preeclampsia and intrauterine growth restriction. Prenat Diagn. 2010;30(4):293–308.

48. Deeks JJ, Altman DG. Diagnostic tests 4: likelihood ratios. BMJ. 2004;329(7458):168–9.

49. Huppertz B. Placental origins of preeclampsia: challenging the current hypothesis. Hypertension. 2008;51(4):970–5.

20

How many preterm births in England are due to excision of the cervical transformation zone? Nested case control study

R. Wuntakal[1,2], Alejandra Castanon[3*], R. Landy[3] and P. Sasieni[3]

Abstract

Background: Preterm births (as a proportion of all births) have been increasing in many countries. There is growing evidence of increased risk of preterm birth following excisional treatment of the cervix. We estimate the number of preterm births attributable to excisional treatments with a length of 10 mm or more in England.

Methods: Case–control study nested in a record linkage cohort of women with a histological sample at 13 hospitals in England. We combined observed age at first excisional treatment in our cohort with the weighted distribution of excision length from the case–control study to estimate the length distribution by age at first treatment among the cohort. The number of births after excision for each 5-year age group was estimated using national fertility data; published absolute risks of preterm (<37 gestational weeks) and very preterm birth (<32 weeks) were applied to these to estimate the number of preterm births per 100 women treated. Excess preterm births were estimated assuming all treatments were small. The attributable risk of preterm birth following excisional treatment in England was estimated.

Results: The majority of first excisional treatments at colposcopy were small (47.5 %) or medium (39.1 %), 9.5 % were large and 4.1 % were very large excisions. 4.0 % of women treated before birth had more than one excisional treatment. Thus based on our cohort of 10,711 treated women and the length of treatment observed in the case control study we estimate an excess of 240 preterm births (including 57 very preterm) or 2.2 (including 0.5 very preterm) per 100 women treated. At a population level (for England) we estimate that 39,101 women aged 20–39 would be treated each year and that these treatments will lead to an excess of 840 preterm births (including 196 very preterm) in England each year.

Conclusions: Assuming associations between preterm birth and treatment for cervical disease are causal; we estimate that an excess 840 (2.5 %) preterm birth in England each year are due to excisional treatments of 10 mm or more. Those that go on to become pregnant should be closely monitored during antenatal period to reduce their risk of preterm birth.

Keywords: Preterm birth, Cervical treatment, LLETZ, Attributable risk

Background

A growing body of literature suggests that women who undergo treatment for cervical disease are at increased risk of preterm birth, particularly when the length of the tissue excised is greater than or equal to 10 mm [1–8]. In England, the absolute risk of preterm birth among treated women increased with the length of excision from 7.5 % (with length <10 mm) to 18 % in those with excisions greater than 20 mm [8].

Although the risk of preterm birth following excision is often cited as a reason for not offering cervical screening to young women, we are not aware of any papers formally calculating the risk associated with screening per se. Further whilst preterm births (as a proportion of all births) have been increasing in many countries [9, 10] it is unclear what proportion may be attributable to prior treatment for cervical disease.

In this study, we estimate the number of preterm births among women with cervical excisional treatments,

* Correspondence: a.castanon@qmul.ac.uk
R Wuntakal, A Castanon are joint first authors
[3]Centre for Cancer Prevention, Wolfson Institute of Preventive Medicine, Charterhouse Square, London, England EC1M 6BQ, UK
Full list of author information is available at the end of the article

accounting for age at excision and length of excision, in order to estimate the number and proportion of preterm births in England attributable to cervical tissue excision of 10 mm deep or more.

Methods

Subjects

Women with cervical histology between April 1988 and December 2011 were identified from clinical records in 13 National Health Service (NHS) hospitals (see acknowledgments). The women were linked to hospital obstetric records between April 1998 and March 2011 for the whole of England using their NHS number (a unique identifier) and date of birth by HES (Hospital Episode Statistics), a data warehouse containing details of all admissions to NHS hospitals in England [11]. Minimal details were obtained for this cohort: date of first and last attendance to colposcopy and whether they had a punch biopsy or excisional treatment at these appointments. Excisional treatments were defined as: LLETZ, laser excision, non specified cone excision or knife cone biopsy. Details of women included in this study in comparison to published manuscripts [8, 12] are presented in Fig. 1.

From this cohort we identified women who had at least one singleton live birth with a gestational age of 20–42 weeks. We then selected the first singleton preterm birth (gestational age of 20–36 completed weeks) in each woman and frequency matched these to singleton term births (38–42 completed weeks) in women with no preterm births. Births at 37 weeks gestational age were excluded when performing the matching to allow a clear divide between term and preterm births. Full details on the study design have been published previously [8, 12]. From HES records we obtained detailed obstetric information. Hospitals entered colposcopy details into a study database and additionally submitted anonymised pathology reports to Barts Health NHS Trust. Pathology reports were entered into the study database by two trained individuals (AP and TP) to ensure measurements were entered in a standardised way, facilitating the identification of the length, thickness and circumference of specimens. Participating pathology departments confirmed that usual practice was to record the length of the specimen first on the pathology reports. Individuals searching for and coding colposcopy information were blind to the case–control status of the women.

Women were not eligible for the case–control study if detailed colposcopy information was not available, if colposcopy records were known to be incomplete, if the only pathology sample reported was non-cervical or if the woman was diagnosed with cervical cancer at any time. We also excluded one woman who was recorded as being sterilized whilst pregnant. Details of women excluded from the case–control study have been published previously [8]. Here we further exclude the following women: those attending colposcopy but not receiving excisional treatment, those who had their first treatment aged 40 and over and those with unknown length of their only excisional treatment (see Fig. 1). In our previous publication births as a result of a high risk pregnancy (defined elsewhere [8]) were excluded; however they are included here to determine the age at first excisional treatment, to ensure the sample is representative of the general population.

Ethical approval

This study was approved by the Brompton, Harefield, and NHLI research ethics committee, Charing Cross Hospital, London (study reference number: 09/h0708/65). Since this was a retrospective linkage study using routinely recorded

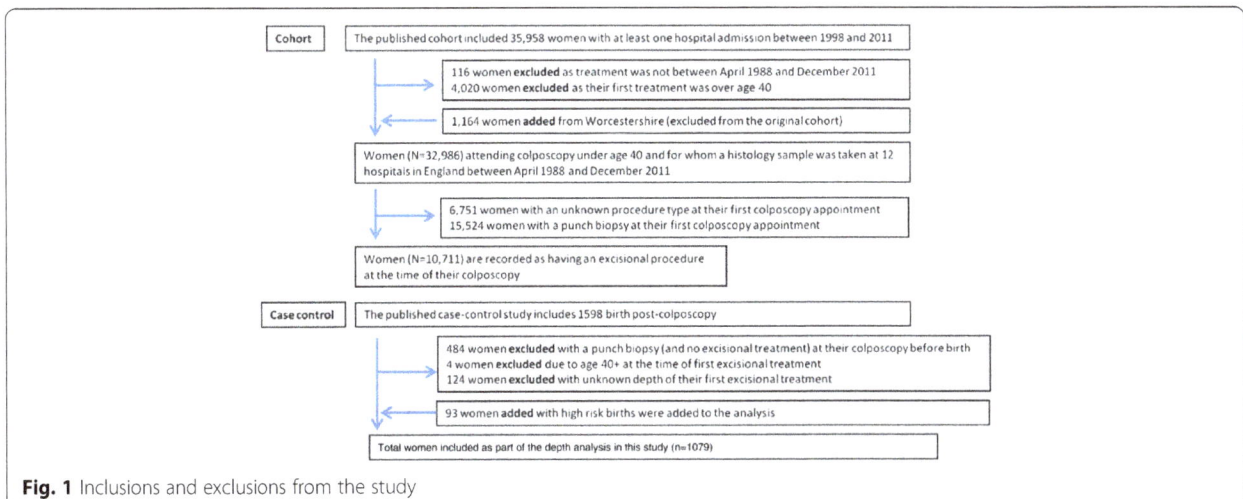

Fig. 1 Inclusions and exclusions from the study

data, informed consent was not required by the research ethics committee. All data received by the researchers were anonymous.

Statistical methods

To assess the concordance between dates at first colposcopy procedure recorded in the cohort and the case–control study we selected all women recorded in the case–control study as having an excisional treatment as their first colposcopic procedure. We used a paired sample t-test to compare the age at first colposcopic appointment in the case–control study and the cohort study.

Length of excision was defined as the distance from the distal or external margin to the proximal or internal margin of the excised specimen, as defined by the IFCPC nomenclature [13]. The length of treatment was coded as per the pre-specified statistical analysis plan: excision with a length of <10 mm (small), 10–14 mm (medium), 15–19 mm (large) and ≥20 mm (very large). When the excision was piecemeal, the largest fragment length was used. For women with more than one excisional treatment ($n = 106$), if the treatments were within a year ($n = 40$), the lengths were summed, as is it is extremely unlikely there would be a birth between the two treatments. Length of treatments that were more than a year apart ($n = 66$) were summed at the time of the later treatment.

The distribution of length of excisional treatment was calculated using all available data for each age group (<20, 20–24, 25–29, 30–34, 35–39) in the case–control study, weighted using the inverse probability of selection into the case–control study to reflect the distribution of cases and eligible controls in the cohort. These data were combined with cohort data on the number of women in each age group who underwent an excisional treatment between April 1988 and December 2011. Using these data we estimate by age group the number of women in the cohort who had an excisional treatment in each length category. We assume that single excisions with unknown length have the same distribution as those with known length in the same age group. Women with an unknown length of first treatment but known length of second treatment within a year were assigned the median length observed among women who had multiple treatments within a year for the unknown length. For women with multiple treatments which were at least a year apart, if either treatment had an unknown length they were proportionally assigned to the length categories of treated women who had multiple treatments within the same age group.

Using age-specific fertility rates for England from 2010, [14] we estimated the expected number of future births per woman in 5-year age groups. We have previously shown that the increased risk of preterm birth remains for all future births, not just the first birth after colposcopy

[15]. Therefore we applied published absolute risks [8] of preterm (20–36 gestational weeks) and very preterm (20–31 gestational weeks) births for each length category to the expected number of future births for women in each age group. The absolute risks of a preterm birth were 7.5 % following small excisions, 9.6 % following medium, 15.3 % following large and 18.0 % following very large excisions (for very preterm they were 2.0 %, 2.3 %, 3.6 % and 6.4 % respectively) [8]. Women with multiple excisional treatments not within a year of each other were assigned the absolute risk appropriate for their first treatment length from the age at their first excisional treatment to their second treatment, and the absolute risk associated with the two treatment lengths summed from the age at the second treatment. The expected number of preterm births was then estimated assuming that all treatments were small, to allow estimation of the excess risk of preterm birth caused by deeper excisions.

To estimate the number of preterm births associated with excisional treatments in England, it was necessary to estimate the number of women per year who have excisional treatments. For this we sourced the number of tests taken and the result of these tests from routinely published screening data for England in the financial year 2013/14 [16]. We then used previously published methodology [17] to estimate (from the published data) the total number of women aged 20–39 who had an excisional treatment in financial year 2013/14. Full details on how this was estimated can be found in Additional file 1, and the results in Additional file 2: Tables S1 and Additional file 3: Table S2.

Analyses were carried out in STATA 12 (StataCorp. College Station, Texas, USA).

Results

Information was available on 32,986 women with a histological sample taken under age 40 at colposcopy between April 1988 and December 2011. From this cohort, around two-fifths ($n = 10,711$) of the women with known treatment at their first colposcopy ($N = 26,235$) were recorded as having an excisional procedure at their first attendance to colposcopy. Most of these women (53.9 %) were aged 25–34 at their first treatment (Table 1). From the case–control study 1079 women treated at colposcopy were eligible for this analysis; of these 894 were treated on their first attendance to colposcopy. This subset of women ($n = 894$) tended to be younger than women in the cohort, with 70.2 % treated age 20–29. This was expected, as women attending colposcopy at a younger age are more likely to go on to have a birth, and therefore be eligible for the case–control study. Comparison of the data from the cohort with that from the case–control study (for these 894 women) showed that the age at first treatment agreed exactly for 49.2 % of women and was within a month for an additional 32.8 %. Only 4.3 % differed by over 6 months. There was no

Table 1 Age among women whose first attendance to colposcopy resulted in excisional treatment. Comparison of cohort and case–control data

Age at treatment	Case–control study Treated at first colposcopy		Treated at first colposcopy in cohort among those included in the case–control study		Cohort study Treated at first colposcopy	
	N	%	N	%	N	%
<20	20	2.2	18	2.0	167	1.6
20–24	286	32.0	286	32.0	2355	22.0
25–29	342	38.3	340	38.0	3417	31.9
30–34	181	20.2	191	21.4	2907	27.1
35–39	65	7.3	59	6.6	1865	17.4
Total	894	100 %	894	100 %	10711	100 %

significant difference in the age distributions (paired t-test p-value = 0.2319).

Estimated (weighted) age at first excisional treatment and proportion in each excisional length category among women in the cohort study is shown in Table 2. Overall the majority of first excisional treatments at colposcopy were small (47.5 %) or medium (39.1 %), 9.5 % were large and 4.1 % were very large excisions. Only 4.0 % of women treated before giving birth are estimated to have had a second excisional treatment more than a year after the first. The estimated number of births following excisional treatment by age group and the estimated excess preterm births due to treatment can be seen in Table 3. Thus based on our cohort of 10,711 treated women and the distribution of treatment lengths observed in the case control study we estimate an excess of 240 preterm births (including 57 very preterm) or 2.2 (including 0.5 very preterm) per 100 women treated.

At a population level (for England) we estimate that 39,101 women aged 20–39 would be treated each year (Table 4, and Additional file 1). We estimate that these treatments will lead to an excess of 840 preterm births (including 196 very preterm) in England each year among women with excisional treatments with a length of ≥10 mm.

Table 2 Estimated (weighted) age at first excisional treatment by length of tissue removed among women in the cohort study

	<10 mm		10–14 mm		15–19 mm		20 + mm		Total
	N	%	N	%	N	%	N	%	
<20	42.1	36.1	64.2	54.9	9.5	8.2	1.0	0.9	116.9
20–24	836.9	52.5	535.7	33.6	154.5	9.7	68.2	4.3	1595.3
25–29	957.8	42.0	974.4	42.8	238.3	10.5	108.4	4.8	2278.8
30–34	510.3	49.8	424.0	41.4	62.7	6.1	27.1	2.6	1024.0
35–39	140.5	58.5	56.7	23.6	32.6	13.6	10.5	4.4	240.3
Total	2487.6	47.3	2054.9	39.1	497.6	9.5	215.2	4.1	5255.3

Discussion

Based on the observed age at first excisional treatment at colposcopy in women under age 40, the observed length of tissue removed, age specific fertility rates and the length specific absolute risks of preterm birth we have estimated that treatment for cervical disease leads to 2.2 preterm (0.5 very preterm) births per 100 women treated under age 40. At a national level this corresponds to 840 preterm births per year in England.

Strengths and limitations

Our results are based on the assumption that the association between preterm birth and treatment for cervical disease is causal. However lifestyle factors (such as smoking) were not adjusted for when estimating the risks used in this study, thus it is possible that residual confounding remains.

The distribution of age at first excisional treatment for women in England is extrapolated from that observed in our study and may not be representative of all women currently being treated in England. For example, women aged 20–24 are no longer invited for cervical screening in England, so we expect the number of preterm births due to excisional treatment among women in this age group to be lower than the number estimated here. Only 2.7 % of all treatments in the study were carried out before age 25, so the impact on the number of preterm birth is likely to be small.

Although the NHS hospital trusts providing data to this study were self selected they did not differ (on the basis of published data) from other colposcopy clinics in England [8]. We therefore think it is justified to assume that the observed distribution of excised tissue length can be extrapolated to all women in England.

Due to the lack of routinely reported data, it was necessary to estimate the number of women treated each year at colposcopy in England. Our estimate ($n = 39,101$) is based on routinely reported cytology and histology data, however

Table 3 Estimated preterm births due to excisional treatment of the cervical transformation zone

Age at first treatment	Women with excisional treatment		Estimated births after first treatment (N)	Preterm births (<37 gestational weeks)			Very preterm births (20–31 gestational weeks)		
	N	%		Estimated births taking into account length distribution*	Estimated births assuming all excisions ≥10 mm were small	Excess births due to treatments	Estimated births taking into account length distribution	Estimated births assuming all excisions ≥10 mm were small	Excess births due to treatments
<20 single excision	167	1.6	323	31	24	7	8	6	1
20–24 single excision	2355	22.0	4043	395	303	91	104	81	23
25–29 single excision	3417	31.9	4332	428	325	103	111	87	24
30–34 single excision	2907	27.1	1929	176	145	31	45	39	7
35–39 single excision	1865	17.4	343	33	26	7	9	7	2
Total	10711	100 %	10970	1063	823	240	276	219	57

it is worth noting that the results are similar to twice the number of CIN3 diagnoses in women under age 40 (*n* = 40,750) [18]. Diagnoses of CIN2 are not routinely recorded or reported, but we think it sensible to assume that the number diagnosed is similar to that of CIN3 and that most of these women would have an excisional treatment as a result. This gives us confidence that our estimate of women treated at colposcopy each year is robust.

We have made assumptions regarding the length of excision among samples where the measurements are unknown, including those with multiple treatments. The risk in those with unknown length was found to be similar to those with medium excisions [8] suggesting that factors other than length (such as piecemeal excisions) are responsible for missing values.

We have applied absolute risks of preterm birth to all future births, not just the first following excisional treatment. We believe this is justified since we have shown that an increased risk of preterm birth remains for all future births, not just the first birth following treatment [15].

We have estimated the excess number of preterm birth attributable to excisional by comparing the observed length distribution in our study to a scenario where all excisions have a length of less than 10 mm (equivalent to the baseline risk in those attending colposcopy). We are not suggesting that clinical practice should change to force all excisions to be small, we are purely estimating the excess risk attributable to excisions with a length greater than 10 mm.

Interpretation

Relative risks of preterm birth following large (17 + mm) treatments compared to small treatments (≤10 mm) have been reported to be between 1.74 [7] and 1.79 [3] in Scandinavian populations and up to 2.4 in an English population [8]. A meta-analysis [5] comparing untreated women to those with excisions deeper than 10 mm found the relative risk of preterm delivery to be 2.61

Table 4 Estimated number of women referred and treated at colposcopy due to cervical intraepithelial neoplasia grade 2 (CIN2+) or worse diagnosis and the resulting excess preterm births each year in England

	N screening tests:	N referred to colposcopy:	N referred with mild	N referred with mod+	N with CIN2+:	Estimated excess number of future preterm births		Estimated excess number of future very preterm births	
						per woman treated	in women treated	per woman treated	in women treated
20–24	46,050	4,668	2,852	1,816	2037	0.04	79	0.01	20
25–29	566,057	46,468	27535	18933	20844	0.03	630	0.01	149
30–34	497,109	24,640	16178	8462	10004	0.01	108	0.00	22
35–39	446,807	16,086	11036	5050	6216	0.00	23	0.00	6
total	1,556,023	91,861	57,600	34,261	39,101		840		196

(95 % CI 1.28–5.34), though a study from Belgium [19] found even higher risks (RR = 4.55, 95 % CI:1.32–15.65). The study in England [8] found that the absolute risk of preterm birth among those who receive a diagnostic biopsy (7.2 %, 95 % CI: 5.9 %–8.5 %) is similar to that of women with small treatments (7.5 %, 95 % CI: 6.0 %–8.9 %). Nevertheless women attending colposcopy following an abnormal cytology result are at a higher risk of preterm birth than the general population in England, where the preterm rate in England is 6.7 % [8]. This is most likely due to the shared risk factors for preterm delivery and cervical disease.

An excess of 2.2 preterm births per 100 women treated may not seem like much, however the average number of births in England between 2000 and 2009 was 510,660 each year and the preterm rate during this period was 6.7 % (or 33,168 births) [12]. Extrapolating the results observed in this study to the whole of England, we would expect 840 preterm births a year (equivalent to 2.5 % of preterm births in England) to be due to excisional treatments of length ≥10 mm.

The risk of preterm birth following treatment for cervical disease can be considered a harm of cervical cancer screening. Nevertheless it needs to be considered against the 20,375 women under age 40 diagnosed and treated for carcinoma in situ of the cervix uteri (CIN3) in 2012 [18], many of whom would have gone on to develop cervical cancer without intervention.

Colposcopists will need to carefully consider whether the benefits of a small excision outweigh the potential risk of leaving diseased tissue on the cervix (i.e. positive margins), risking the need for further treatment. Patients who need a large excision of the cervix should be informed about the risk of preterm birth. Close obstetric monitoring is warranted for women who undergo large excisional treatment and subsequently become pregnant, particularly since recently published evidence suggests that preterm birth in high risk pregnancies can be substantially reduced by measuring fibronectin levels and assessing cervical length [20]. The extra costs of close obstetric monitoring of these women will easily be offset by the saving made in the reduction of preterm births, which cost on average 1.47 % more than term babies up to age 18 [21].

Conclusion

We estimate that 840 or 2.5 % of preterm births in England each year are due to excisional treatments of 10 mm or more. Clinicians (and in particular obstetricians) need to be aware of whether women in their care have undergone treatment of the cervical transformation zone. Those who have must undergo close monitoring and further investigations with the aim of reducing the number of preterm births among these women.

Additional files

Additional file 1: Data and methodology to estimate the number of women receiving excisional treatment for cervical disease each year in England.

Additional file 2: Table S1. Routinely published screening data from England in the financial year 2013/14.

Additional file 3: Table S2. Outcomes of referrals to colposcopy in England in the financial year 2013/14.

Competing interests
The authors declare that they have no competing interests.

Authors' contribution
AC had full access to all of the data in the study and confirms that it is an honest, accurate, and transparent account of the study being reported; that no important aspects of the study have been omitted; and that any discrepancies are disclosed. RL analysed the data and prepared results. AC and RW wrote the first draft of the report. PS and AC participated in the design and establishment of the study. All authors edited the report and approved the final version.

Authors' information
Not applicable.

Acknowledgments

PaCT investigators
Peter Brocklehurst, Heather Evans, Donald Peebles, Naveena Singh, Patrick Walker and Julietta Patnick. Pathology report data entry for the study was done by Anna Parberry and Tim Pyke (Barts Health NHS Trust). Members of PaCT study group (participating hospitals) are responsible for the collection of data included in this study. They include: Hollingworth A and Wuntakal R (Whipps Cross University Hospital London), Singh N and Parberry A (Barts Health NHS Trust), Palmer J (Royal Hallamshire Hospital, Sheffield), Das N, Andrew A and Russ L (Royal Cornwall Hospital), China S, Lenton H and Raghavan R (Worcestershire Acute Hospitals NHS Trust), Wood N and Preston S (Royal Preston Hospital Lancashire), Hannemann M and Fuller D (Royal Devon and Exeter NHS Foundation Trust), Lincoln K, Wheater G and Rolland P (The James Cook University Hospital, South Tees), Ghaem-Maghami S and Soutter P (Hammersmith Hospital, Imperial College), Hutson R (St James University Hospital, Leeds), Senguita P and Dent J (North Durham County and Darlington Trust), Lyons D (St Mary's Hospital, Imperial College), N Gul and A Miles (Wirral University Teaching Hospital). All contributors were paid for their contribution to the data collection in this study.

Funding
This manuscript presents independent research funded by the National Institute for Health Research (NIHR) under its Research for Patient Benefit (RfPB) Programme (Grant Reference Number PB-PG-1208-16187). The views expressed are those of the author(s) and not necessarily those of the NHS, the NIHR or the Department of Health. The funder had no input in the design, conduct, collation, analysis or interpretation of the data or the preparation, review or approval of the manuscript.

Author details
[1]Whipps Cross University Hospital, Barts Health NHS Trust, London, England, UK. [2]Guys and St Thomas' Hospital, London, England, UK. [3]Centre for Cancer Prevention, Wolfson Institute of Preventive Medicine, Charterhouse Square, London, England EC1M 6BQ, UK.

References
1. Albrechtsen S, Rasmussen S, Thoresen S, Irgens LM, Iversen OE. Pregnancy outcome in women before and after cervical conisation: population based cohort study. BMJ. 2008;337:a1343.

2. Sadler L, Saftlas A, Wang W, Exeter M, Whittaker J, McCowan L. Treatment for cervical intraepithelial neoplasia and risk of preterm delivery. JAMA. 2004;291(17):2100–6.

3. Noehr B, Jensen A, Frederiksen K, Tabor A, Kjaer SK. Depth of cervical cone removed by loop electrosurgical excision procedure and subsequent risk of spontaneous preterm delivery. Obstet Gynecol. 2009;114(6):1232–8.

4. Noehr B, Jensen A, Frederiksen K, Tabor A, Kjaer SK. Loop electrosurgical excision of the cervix and subsequent risk for spontaneous preterm delivery: a population-based study of singleton deliveries during a 9-year period. Am J Obstet Gynecol. 2009;201(1):33. e31-36.

5. Kyrgiou M, Koliopoulos G, Martin-Hirsch PL, Arbyn M, Prendiville W, Paraskevaidis E. Obstetric Outcome after conservative treatment for intraepithelial or early invasive cervical lesions: systematic review and meta-analysis. Lancet. 2006;367:489–98.

6. Bruinsma FJ, Quinn MA. The risk of preterm birth following treatment for precancerous changes in the cervix: a systematic review and meta-analysis. BJOG. 2011;118(9):1031–41.

7. Jakobsson M, Gissler M, Paavonen J, Tapper AM. Loop electrosurgical excision procedure and the risk for preterm birth. Obstet Gynecol. 2009;114(3):504–10.

8. Castanon A, Landy R, Brocklehurst P, Evans H, Peebles D, Singh N, et al. Risk of preterm delivery with increasing depth of excision for cervical intraepithelial neoplasia in England: nested case–control study. BMJ. 2014;349:g6223.

9. Zeitlin J, Szamotulska K, Drewniak N, Mohangoo AD, Chalmers J, Sakkeus L, et al. Preterm birth time trends in Europe: a study of 19 countries. BJOG. 2013;120(11):1356–65.

10. Martin JA, Kirmeyer S, Osterman M, Shepherd RA. Born a bit too early: recent trends in late preterm births. NCHS Data Brief. 2009;24:1–8.

11. What is HES? [http://www.hscic.gov.uk/hes]

12. Castanon A, Brocklehurst P, Evans H, Peebles D, Singh N, Walker P, et al. Risk of preterm birth after treatment for cervical intraepithelial neoplasia among women attending colposcopy in England: retrospective-prospective cohort study. BMJ. 2012;345, e5174.

13. Bornstein J, Bentley J, Bosze P, Girardi F, Haefner H, Menton M, et al. 2011 colposcopic terminology of the International Federation for Cervical Pathology and Colposcopy. Obstet Gynecol. 2012;120(1):166–72.

14. Office for National Statistics: Age–specific fertility rates (ASFRs), constituent countries of the UK, 2010. In: Fertility Summary, 2010 http://www.ons.gov.uk/ons/rel/fertility-analysis/fertility-summary/2010/uk-fertility-summary.html. 2010.

15. Castanon A, Landy R, Brocklehurst P, Evans H, Peebles D, Singh N, et al. Is the increased risk of preterm birth following excision for cervical intraepithelial neoplasia restricted to the first birth post treatment?. BJOG 2015;122:1191–1199.

16. Health and Social Care Information Centre: Cervical Screening Programme, England, Statistics for 2013–14. In., 25 November 2014 edn; 2014.

17. Landy R, Birke H, Castanon A, Sasieni P. Benefits and harms of cervical screening from age 20 years compared with screening from age 25 years. Br J Cancer. 2014;110(7):1841–6.

18. Office for National Statistics: Cancer Statistics Registrations, England (Series MB1) No 43, 2012. In., 19 June 2014 edn; 2014.

19. Simoens C, Goffin F, Simon P, Barlow P, Antoine J, Foidart JM, et al. Adverse obstetrical outcomes after treatment of precancerous cervical lesions: a Belgian multicentre study. BJOG. 2012;119(10):1247–55.

20. Foster C, Shennan AH. Fetal fibronectin as a biomarker of preterm labor: a review of the literature and advances in its clinical use. Biomark Med. 2014;8(4):471–84.

21. Mangham LJ, Petrou S, Doyle LW, Draper ES, Marlow N. The cost of preterm birth throughout childhood in England and Wales. Pediatrics. 2009;123(2):e312-327.

21

Maternal history of childhood sexual abuse and preterm birth

Adaeze C. Wosu, Bizu Gelaye[*] and Michelle A. Williams

Abstract

Background: History of childhood sexual abuse (CSA) is highly prevalent with as many as one in four American women being victims. Exposure to CSA or other early life traumatic experiences has been associated with adverse reproductive and pregnancy outcomes. However, the effects of CSA on preterm delivery (PTB), a leading cause of neonatal mortality, remain poorly understood. The objectives of this review are (i) to synthesize the available research investigating the relationship between maternal history of childhood sexual abuse (CSA) and preterm delivery (PTB); (ii) to provide suggestions for improving future research on this topic; and (iii) to highlight implications for clinical practice and public health.

Methods: Relevant articles were identified through searches of four electronic databases (PubMed, CINAHL, Web of Science Core Collection and BIOSIS Online) for studies published before March 2014, as well as through reviewing references of published articles.

Results: A total of six studies published from 1992 to 2010 were included in this review. Overall, findings were inconsistent. Three studies reported statistically significant associations of CSA with PTB (<37 weeks gestation) or shorter mean gestational age at birth. Women with a history of CSA had 2.6 to 4.8-fold increased odds of PTB as compared with women without a history of CSA. Three other studies did not observe statistically significant differences in rates of PTB or mean gestational age at birth in relation to a history of CSA.

Conclusions: Available evidence on this topic is sparse and inconsistent, and limited by a number of methodological challenges. Given the ubiquity of CSA, as well as the clinical and public health significance of PTB, more rigorously designed epidemiologic studies on the association between CSA and PTB are warranted.

Introduction

Definitions, prevalence and correlates of CSA

Childhood sexual abuse (CSA) is a major public health problem with serious immediate and long-term health consequences [1–3]. Although significant variation exists in its definition, CSA is generally recognized as the involvement of a child in sexual activity that is not developmentally appropriate, that he or she does not fully comprehend or is unable to give consent to, by an individual who by age or development is in a relationship of responsibility, trust or power to the child. CSA may involve use of manipulation, coercion, threats or violence to engage a child in sexual activity [4].

Generally, CSA is characterized into three broad categories: (a) *non-contact sexual abuse* (e.g. exhibitionism,

indecent exposure, sexual harassment or voyeurism); (b) *contact sexual abuse without penetration* (e.g. non-genital fondling, kissing, or genital touching); and (c) *contact sexual abuse with penetration* (e.g. anal, oral, or vaginal intercourse) is recognized as the most severe. In addition, CSA may be characterized in terms of frequency, duration, age of onset of abuse, and relationship of the victim to the perpetrator [5].

Recent prevalence estimates of CSA, summarized in meta-analyses and multi-country studies confirm high global prevalence, with markedly higher prevalence among girls as compared with boys; see Table 1 for a summary of CSA estimates from recent studies [5–10]. Briefly, in their study of student and community samples from 22 countries, Pereda *et al.* reported that the average prevalence of CSA was 19.7 % for girls and 7.9 % for boys [10]. These figures were corroborated by other investigators who reported global CSA prevalence estimates of 7.6 % for boys

* Correspondence: bgelaye@hsph.harvard.edu
Department of Epidemiology, Harvard T.H. Chan School of Public Health, 677 Huntington Ave, K505F, Boston, MA 02115, USA

Table 1 Summary of global prevalence of CSA

First author (year)	Definition of CSA	Studies included	Prevalence estimates		
			Overall	Boys	Girls
Andrews (2004) [5]	Contact and non-contact (age varied across studies; upper limit was 18 years)	513 articles or reports	Range 3.8–67.7 %	Range 3.8–35 %	Range 8.4–67.7 %
WHO multi-country study (2005) [9]	Unwanted or forced sexual activity before age 15 years	24,058 individuals in 15 sites in 10 countries around the world	---	---	Range 1–21 %
Pereda (2009a) [6]	Contact and non-contact (age varied across studies; upper limit was 18 years)	38 independent articles representing 21 countries	Range 0–60 %	Range 0–60 %	Range 0–53 %
Pereda (2009b) [10]	Contact and non-contact (age varied across studies; upper limit was 17 years)	65 articles, covering 24 countries	N/A	7.9 % (95 % CI 6.0–10.3 %)	19.7 % (95 % CI 16.7–23.0 %)
Stoltenborgh (2011) [7]	Contact and non-contact (age varied across studies; upper limit was 18 years)	331 independent samples from 217 publications	11.8 % (95 % CI 10.0 – 13.8 %)	7.6 % (95 % CI 6.6–8.8 %)	18 % (95 % CI 16.4–19.7 %)
Barth (2013) [8]	Contact and non-contact (age varied across studies; upper limit was 19 years)	55 studies from 22 countries	Range 3–31 %	Range 3–17 %	Range 8–31 %

Abbreviations: CSA Childhood sexual abuse, *WHO* World Health Organization

and 18 % for girls [7]. It is important to note that CSA rarely occurs as a solitary episode but appears to consist of continued sexual victimization and maltreatment. CSA typically co-occurs with one or more types of childhood maltreatment (i.e., child neglect, physical abuse, and emotional abuse) [5, 11].

The prevalence of CSA in hospital and clinic based studies of pregnant women, primarily from high-income countries, range from 3.2 to 32.2 % [12–22]. As with studies conducted among non-pregnant individuals, much of the heterogeneity in CSA prevalence estimates are attributable to differences in operational definitions of CSA, differences in study setting, study design, sampling methods and sample size. For example, Sørbø *et al.* observed CSA prevalence of 7 % using one question to screen for CSA: "have you been forced to have sexual intercourse (as a child, under 18 years old)?" [13], whilst Yampolsky *et al.* observed a prevalence of 32.2 % using the 14-item Childhood Sexual Assaults Scale [12].

CSA and health outcomes

The relation of CSA with a range of health outcomes has been well documented among men and women. Investigators have reported strong associations of CSA with psychiatric disorders including post-traumatic stress disorder (PTSD) [2], depression [23], suicidal behavior [1, 2], and substance abuse [24, 25]. Investigators have also described dose–response relationships between CSA severity and worsening psychiatric health. For example, the number of suicide attempts was shown to increase with frequency of CSA ($\beta = 0.56$, SE = 0.23, p <0.05) and with use of force during CSA ($\beta = 1.13$, SE = 0.57, $p < 0.05$) among men [26]. Similarly, CSA involving intercourse was found to be more strongly associated with psychiatric and substance use disorders as compared with CSA that did not involve intercourse [24].

CSA is linked to increased odds of a host of adverse reproductive characteristics in women including early age at menarche [27, 28] and adolescent pregnancy [29]. Among pregnant women, history of CSA has been associated with psychiatric disorders [30, 31], physical, sexual, or emotional abuse during pregnancy [30], and lifestyle risk behaviors such as cigarette smoking [30, 32], all of which may endanger the health of both mother and her developing fetus.

Definition, prevalence and correlates of preterm birth

Preterm birth (PTB), defined as birth prior to the completion of 37 weeks gestation [33], is the leading cause of neonatal mortality [34]. Globally, approximately 15 million infants (i.e., 10 % of all births) are delivered preterm and about 1 million of these infants die as a result of their prematurity [34]. Maternal risk factors associated with PTB include cigarette smoking [35], previous preterm birth [36], infection [37], preeclampsia [38], obesity [39], psychiatric disorders [40, 41], psychotropic medication use [42] and exposure to intimate partner violence [43].

Although the majority of preterm births occur in low and middle income countries [34], PTB remains a significant problem in developed countries. In the United States, 1 in 8 infants is born preterm, although PTB rates seem to be on the decline (from 12.8 % in 2006 to 11.6 % of all births in 2012) [33, 44]. Preterm birth is associated with enormous social and economic burdens as outlined in a report from the Institute of Medicine [45]. The report estimated the maternal birth costs, early intervention services, four disabling conditions occurring from preterm birth, and lost household and labor market productivity costs related to PTB to be at least $26.2 billion (or $51,600 per infant born preterm) in 2005 [45]. Compared with term infants, preterm infants are at an increased risk for immediate and long-term health problems

[46, 47]. Notably, an accumulating literature now documents increased risk of later-life cardiovascular-related conditions for mothers of preterm infants [48–50].

Despite its high prevalence, the etiology of PTB is not well understood [45]. However, some investigators suggest that early life stress, such as CSA, may be associated with PTB [51]. Given the importance of CSA and PTB as two public health conditions with major consequences for maternal and child health, our objectives in conducting this review are: (i) to synthesize the limited available research investigating the relationship between maternal history of childhood sexual abuse (CSA) and preterm birth (PTB); (ii) to provide suggestions for improving future research on this topic; and (iii) to highlight implications for clinical practice and public health.

Methods

Search strategy

Relevant studies published before March 2014 were identified from four online databases (PubMed, Cumulative Index of Nursing and Allied Health Literature (CINAHL), Web of Science Core Collection and BIOSIS Online). A full list of search terms used can be found in Additional file 1: Table S1. We also reviewed references of retrieved publications to identify other potentially relevant articles reporting on the association between CSA and PTB.

Selection criteria

The exposure of interest was maternal exposure to CSA, and the outcome of interest was preterm birth or gestational age at birth. To be included, studies had to: (1) define CSA as occurring sometime before age 18 years; (2) report quantitative associations between CSA and PTB or gestational age at birth; (3) be observational studies (cross-sectional, prospective cohort, retrospective cohort, and case–control studies); and (4) be full-length papers (conference abstracts, case studies, gray literature, editorials were excluded).

Results

The electronic database search identified 2,207 titles, of which 1955 were duplicates or rejected upon title review. The abstracts of the remaining unique 252 articles were read. Of these, 34 were selected for full-text screening (Fig. 1 summarizes the selection and screening process). Six full-length papers met the inclusion criteria and were included in this review (Table 2—papers in table are arranged by year of publication). The studies were published from 1992 to 2010 and in English. Four of the studies were from the United States while the other two were from Norway and Germany, respectively. Three studies used a prospective cohort design, two were retrospective cohort studies, and one was a case–control study. Findings were inconsistent, with only three studies reporting statistically significant positive associations of CSA with PTB or shorter mean gestational age at birth. In the sections below, we describe each study.

Steven-Simons and colleagues analyzed data for 127 women who were <19 years old at the time of conception of pregnancy. History of current or prior physical or sexual abuse was obtained through interviews and was defined as answering "yes" to the question "Have you ever been physically or sexually abused?" or other related

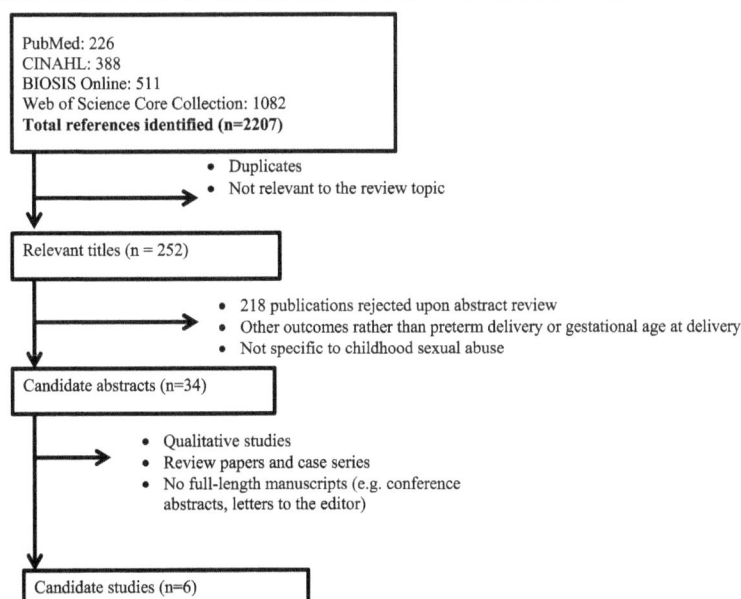

Fig. 1 Flowchart showing selection of articles reporting on the relationship between CSA and preterm birth

Table 2 Summary of original studies examining the association of maternal history of CSA with preterm birth or gestational age at birth

First author (year)	Country	Study design	Sample size	Recruitment	CSA definition	PTB definition	CSA and PTB findings
Jacobs (1992) [56]	United States	Retrospective	15 CSA-exposed, 13 controls	CSA-exposed women recruited from survivors' group, mental health center and through therapists; controls recruited from evening psychology class taught in the community	CSA definition not specified	Mean gestational age at birth	No significant correlation between being a victim of CSA and gestational age at birth in the entire sample ($r = 0.12$, $p > 0.05$). However, the authors reported a positive correlation between gestational age at birth and maternal history of being sexually touched as a child ($r = 0.34$, $p < 0.05$).
Stevens-Simon (1994) [52]	United States	Prospective cohort	127 women	Participants in the Rochester Study of Adolescent Pregnancy	Physical or sexual abuse (<19 years)	<37 weeks gestation	CSA-exposed women had shorter mean gestational lengths (38.0 ± 3.4 weeks) compared with non-exposed (39.1 ± 1.7 weeks, $p \leq 0.05$). PTB more common among exposed women (19.1 % vs. 4.7 %, $p \leq 0.05$; OR = 4.76, 95 % CI: 1.34, 16.89)
Benedict (1999) [55]	United States	Prospective cohort	357 women	Prenatal clinics in a large university-based hospital; women interviewed at 28–32 weeks gestation	≥1 non-consensual and non-experimental contact or non-contact sexual episode (<18 years) by a perpetrator who was ≥5 years older than victim	<37 weeks gestation	No statistically significant association between CSA and gestational age at birth
Grimstad (1999) [32]	Norway	Case–control	82 women with low birth weight infants, 91 women with normal birth weight infants	Department of Obstetrics, the University Hospital of Trondheim	Adverse sexual experiences (<18 years)	Not defined	PTB prevalence similar for abused and non-abused women (36 % vs. 32 %, $p = 0.68$)
Noll (2007) [53]	United States	Prospective cohort	40 CSA-exposed, 31 controls	CSA-exposed girls were referred by CPS; unexposed girls were recruited through community advertisements	Substantiated contact sexual abuse perpetuated by a family member (between 6 and 16 years)	<37 weeks gestation	PTB risk increased among women with CSA vs. non-abused women (21 % vs. 11 %; OR = 2.80, $p < 0.05$)
Leeners (2010) [54]	Germany	Retrospective cohort	85 CSA-exposed, 170 controls	CSA-exposed women recruited through sexual abuse survivor centers in large cities; unexposed women were recruited through local kindergartens	Contact and non-contact sexual abuse (<18 years)	<37 weeks gestation	PTB risk increased among women with CSA history vs non-abused women (18.8 % vs. 8.2 %, $p = 0.02$; OR = 2.58, 95 % CI: 1.19 – 5.59)

Abbreviations: CPS Child protective services, *CSA* Childhood sexual abuse, *PTB* Preterm birth

questions. Overall, 42 women (33 %) reported exposure to childhood physical or sexual abuse. The authors noted that abused women delivered approximately 1 week earlier, on average, as compared with non-abused women (mean gestational age at birth: 38.0 ± 3.4 vs. 39.1 ± 1.7 weeks, $p \leq 0.05$). Also, the frequency of PTB was higher among abused women as compared with non-abused women (19.1 % vs. 4.7 %, $p < 0.05$; unadjusted OR = 4.76, 95 % CI: 1.34, 16.89). However, the authors reported that when controlling for maternal stress, depression, social support, and substance abuse, the association between abuse and gestational age at birth was not statistically significant (quantitative summary not reported) [52]. It is possible that some of these factors may be indirect effects of CSA. A major strength of this study is the use of various methods to substantiate infant gestational age at birth. However, inference from this study is limited by the lack of differentiation between childhood sexual and physical abuse, and lack of adjustment for age. Since the sample ranged from 12 to 18 years old, youngest members of the sample may have been at particularly high risk for preterm birth.

In a prospective cohort study of 40 women with CSA history and 31 without a history of CSA, Noll and colleagues reported that the odds of PTB was elevated among women with a history of CSA as compared with those who had no such history of abuse (21 % vs. 11 %; adjusted OR = 2.80, $p < 0.05$, adjusted for minority status and sibling number). Prenatal alcohol use, but not maternal cortisol concentrations, mediated this relationship [53]. Important strengths of this study included the prospective study design, and clear definition of CSA (i.e., contact sexual abuse by a family member that occurred while participants were between the ages of 6–16 years, and was reported to Child Protection Services), and major improvements in statistical analyses over preceding studies.

Recently, Leeners *et al.* conducted a retrospective cohort study of 85 women with CSA history who were attending sexual abuse support centers and 170 women without a history of CSA. CSA was defined as contact or non-contact sexual abuse prior to age 18 years and delivery information was ascertained from medical records. The investigators found that abused women were more likely to deliver preterm as compared with non-abused women (18.8 % vs. 8.2 %, $p = 0.02$; unadjusted OR = 2.58, 95 % CI: 1.19, 5.59) [54].

In contrast to the studies described above, three other studies did not observe significant associations of CSA with PTB or mean gestational age at birth. In a case–control study conducted in Norway, Grimstad and colleagues analyzed data for 82 women who delivered low birth weight (<2500 g) infants, and 91 women with normal birth weight (≥2500 g) infants. A positive history

of CSA was determined on the basis of participants' response to a single question as to whether they had negative sexual experiences prior to age 18 years. The authors did not observe a significant difference in the prevalence of preterm birth (definition not specified) among women with CSA history (36 %) and women with no CSA history (32 %, $p = 0.68$) [32].

Benedict and colleagues conducted a prospective cohort study to examine the association of CSA with depressive symptomatology, negative life events, and selected pregnancy outcomes, including gestational age at birth among 357 women aged ≥18 years. CSA was defined as ≥ 1 episode of non-consensual and non-experimental contact or non-contact sexual abuse prior to 18 years by a perpetrator ≥ 5 years older than the victim. However, if force was used, women were considered as CSA-exposed regardless of age difference with perpetrator. Thirty-seven percent of participants reported exposure to CSA and prevalence of PTB in the entire sample was 13 %. The authors reported no significant association of CSA with mean number of gestational weeks at birth or PTB observed (no quantitative summary was shown) [55]. Finally, in a small ($N = 28$) retrospective cohort study, Jacobs reported no statistically significant association between being a victim of CSA and PTB or gestational age at birth. However, the authors reported a positive correlation between gestational age at birth and maternal history of being sexually touched as a child (r = 0.34, $p < 0.05$). Due to a number of methodological challenges, one being an extremely small sample size, findings from this study, particularly those on the CSA sub-category of being sexually touched as a child, should be interpreted with caution [56].

Limitations of available evidence

These studies on the association of CSA with PTB or gestational age at birth had some common limitations. First, the majority of studies were based on convenience samples with relatively small sizes (range from 28 to 357 women), which limited statistical power and hindered inferences that could be made from the studies. Second, there was significant heterogeneity across studies with regard to the definition of CSA, i.e., level of contact considered, mode of ascertainment of CSA history, and the maximum cutoff age for CSA (range from 16 to 19 years of age). These differences in the operational definition of CSA may have contributed to variations in CSA prevalence and observed associations of CSA with PTB and gestational age at birth. Third, the mode of ascertainment of PTB or gestational age at birth varied, from maternal self-report [56], to extraction from medical records [53–55], to ultrasound dating [32, 52]. Fourth, most of the studies were not specifically designed to determine the extent to which, if at all, maternal history of exposure to CSA is associated with PTB risk, rather they were secondary analyses of data collected for other purposes. Thus, most analyses of the CSA-PTB relationship were preliminary and did not adequately account for important confounding factors, mediators and modifiers such as maternal preconception and antepartum exposures to cigarette smoking, mood and anxiety symptomatology, and stressors such as intimate partner violence and sexual abuse in adulthood. Fifth, CSA histories were assessed retrospectively for the majority of studies, and so may have been subject to reporting errors. Lastly, all studies were from high-income countries (US, Norway and Germany). Thus, results may not be generalizable to women in low and middle-income countries.

Hypothesized biological mechanisms

Pathophysiological mechanisms that may account for observed associations of CSA exposure histories with PTB are not well known. However, investigators have suggested that CSA, an early life stressor, contributes to psychological stress and promotes dysregulation of the hypothalamic-pituitary-adrenal (HPA) axis, one of two major neuroendocrine pathways activated in stress response [51]. HPA axis activation begins with discharge of corticotrophin-releasing hormone (CRH) from the hypothalamus, which then triggers the secretion of adrenocorticotropic hormone (ACTH) by the pituitary and the subsequent release of cortisol by the adrenal cortex [57]. CRH is also found in other sites including the placenta, ovaries, and adrenal glands [57, 58]. During pregnancy, maternal CRH concentrations rise due to increased CRH synthesis in the fetus, placenta and uterine lining, resulting in increases in maternal ACTH and cortisol concentrations [58].

In their review paper, Horan and colleagues propose that the trauma, stress and fear associated with CSA may stimulate enhanced CRH gene expression and chronic overproduction of CRH in the brain, making a woman susceptible to elevated placental CRH gene expression during pregnancy and consequently, increased risk of PTB [51]. This thesis is supported by animal studies that showed that infusion of CRH initiated early labor [59] and a Type I CRH receptor antagonist delayed parturition [60]. In humans, elevated third trimester placental CRH concentrations have been associated with increased risks of spontaneous PTB and/or fetal growth restriction [61–63]. These studies support CRH's role in labor initiation, particularly its function as a placental clock that may regulate the length of human gestation [64]. CSA may also increase risk for PTB through mediators such as psychiatric disorders [40], obesity [25], and lifestyle factors such as alcohol use [53], and cigarette smoking [65], which have been shown to be associated with CSA [24, 30] and with increased risk for PTB [45]. As observed by Noll and colleagues (in one of the studies

included in this review) maternal prenatal alcohol use was a mediator of the CSA-PTB relationship [53].

Discussion

CSA is a highly prevalent early life stressor with wide-ranging immediate and long-term biological and psychological sequelae [5]. Among pregnant women, some investigators have documented associations of CSA history with cigarette smoking [30, 32], psychiatric disorders [31], and abuse during pregnancy [30], known risk factors for preterm birth. Preterm birth occurs in 10 % of all births globally, and has tremendous medical, economic, and health implications for mother, infant, and society at-large [45]. Available evidence suggest that maternal history of early life adversity may play a role in PTB [51]. However, only a limited number of studies have empirically examined associations of CSA, a common stressor in the lives of young girls and women, with PTB.

As reported in this review of the six published studies on the topic to date, only three studies observed statistically significant associations of CSA with PTB or shorter mean gestational age at birth [52–54]. Three other studies did not observe substantial or statistically significant associations [32, 55, 56], although one study reported higher prevalence of PTB for women with a history of CSA (36 %) compared to women with no such history (32 %) [32] and another study observed an increased gestational age at birth with one sub-category of women with a history of CSA [56]. Inferences from the majority of available studies on the CSA-PTB relationship are hindered by small sample sizes, and incomplete control of confounding factors. Of note, these studies did not adequately distinguish the effects of CSA from the effects of other forms of childhood maltreatment or trauma, or later-life abuse. CSA and PTB are common and have significant clinical and developmental consequences for mothers and children. There is need for longitudinal and rigorously designed studies to improve understanding of the CSA-PTB relationship. Here, we offer some considerations for improving future studies on this topic:

1. The use of detailed CSA questionnaires (e.g., The Childhood Trauma Questionnaire and The Sexual and Physical Abuse Questionnaire) in future CSA-PTB studies would allow for more uniform exposure collection efforts and capture of a wide range of CSA severities to enable nuanced analyses and interpretation of findings.
2. Studies should distinguish between sub-categories of preterm birth (i.e., extremely preterm, very preterm, and moderate to late preterm) to add greater specificity to the existing literature and further inform the development of clinical risk stratification and risk management protocols.

3. Longitudinal studies incorporating the use of biological samples may facilitate understanding of biological mechanisms and identify important mediators and modifiers of the CSA-PTB relationship.

4. Study design and analytical approaches to account for confounders and potential mediators (e.g., other forms of child maltreatment and trauma, adult traumatic experiences, socioeconomic status, prenatal cigarette smoking, illicit drug or alcohol use) will improve validity and precision of measured CSA-PTB associations.

5. Efforts should be made to quantify the contribution of CSA to PTB incidence in middle and low-income countries, particularly those countries with high prevalence of CSA. Such efforts would expand current knowledge and may be informative for PTB prevention in these settings.

6. Prevention of both CSA and PTB requires a multi-sectorial response. Prevention and risk management efforts should engage individuals from health services, educational, advocacy, institutions, with better recognition of the social, cultural and environmental milieu within which CSA and PTB occur.

Conclusions
Clinical and public health implications

In spite of the great strides that have been made towards elucidating the medical, environmental, psychosocial and genetic risk factors of PTB [45], this review underscores that much remains to be done to fully understand the contribution of CSA to PTB. Given (1) the high prevalence of history of CSA among women, (2) the relationships between CSA and adverse reproductive characteristics and risk behaviors during pregnancy, (3) the accumulating evidence linking PTB to adverse long-term maternal and child health outcomes, and (4) the observed associations of maternal history of CSA with PTB, identifying women with a history of CSA, and providing them with increased attention and care during pregnancy may be one important strategy for PTB prevention. Finally, women with a history of CSA may also benefit from additional education and intervention (e.g., psychosocial support) targeted at modifying health risk behaviors for better maternal and infant health outcomes.

Abbreviations
ACTH: Adrenocorticotropic hormone; CI: Confidence interval; CINAHL: Cumulative index to nursing and allied health literature; CRH: Corticotrophin-releasing hormone; CSA: Childhood sexual abuse; HPA: Hypothalamic-pituitary-adrenal; OR: Odds ratio; PTB: Preterm birth; US: United States; WHO: World Health Organization.

Competing interests
The authors declare that they have no competing interests.

Authors' contributions
ACW performed the literature search and screening of articles. ACW, BG, and MAW participated in the evaluation of relevant articles, and writing of the manuscript. All authors have read and approved the final manuscript.

Acknowledgments
This research was supported by awards from the National Institutes of Health, the Eunice Kennedy Shriver Institute of Child Health and Human Development (5R01-HD-059827 and 1R01-HD-059835), and National Institute of Minority Health and Health Disparities (T37-MD-001449). The National Institutes of Health had no further role in the study design, in the collection, analysis and interpretation of data, in the writing of the report, or in the decision to submit the paper for publication.

References
1. Molnar B, Berkman L, Buka S. Psychopathology, childhood sexual abuse and other childhood adversities: relative links to subsequent suicidal behaviour in the US. Psychol Med. 2001;31(6):965–77.
2. Molnar B, Buka S, Kessler R. Child sexual abuse and subsequent psychopathology: results from the National Comorbidity Survey. Am J Public Health. 2001;91(5):753–60.
3. Lindert J, von Ehrenstein OS, Grashow R, Gal G, Braehler E, Weisskopf MG. Sexual and physical abuse in childhood is associated with depression and anxiety over the life course: systematic review and meta-analysis. Int J Public Health. 2014;59(2):359–72.
4. World Health Organization. Guidelines for Medico-Legal Care for Victims of Sexual Violence. Geneva: World Health Organization; 2003.
5. Andrews G, Corry J, Slade T, Issakidis C, Swanston H. Child Sexual Abuse. In: Ezzati M, Lopez A, Rodgers A, Murray C, editors. Comparative Quantification of Health Risks : Global and Regional Burden of Disease Attributable to Selected Major Risk Factors. Volume 2, edn. Geneva: World Health Organization; 2004. p. 1851–940.
6. Pereda N, Guilera G, Forns M, Gomez-Benito J. The international epidemiology of child sexual abuse: a continuation of Finkelhor (1994). Child Abuse Negl. 2009;33(6):331–42.
7. Stoltenborgh M, van Ijzendoorn M, Euser E, Bakermans-Kranenburg M. A global perspective on child sexual abuse: meta-analysis of prevalence around the world. Child Maltreatment. 2011;16(2):79–101.
8. Barth J, Bermetz L, Heim E, Trelle S, Tonia T. The current prevalence of child sexual abuse worldwide: a systematic review and meta-analysis. Int J Public Health. 2013;58(3):469–83.
9. WHO multi-country study on women's health and domestic violence against women: summary report of initial results on prevalence health outcomes and women's responses. Geneva: World Health Organization 2005. available at: http://www.who.int/gender/violence/who_multicountry_study/summary_report/summary_report_English2.pdf. Accessed on 08/11/2015.
10. Pereda N, Guilera G, Forns M, Gomez-Benito J. The prevalence of child sexual abuse in community and student samples: a meta-analysis. Clin Psychol Rev. 2009;29(4):328–38.
11. Ehlert U. Enduring psychobiological effects of childhood adversity. Psychoneuroendocrinology. 2013;38(9):1850–7.
12. Yampolsky L, Lev-Wiesel R, Ben-Zion I. Child sexual abuse: is it a risk factor for pregnancy? J Adv Nurs. 2010;66(9):2025–37.
13. Sorbo MF, Grimstad H, Bjorngaard JH, Schei B, Lukasse M. Prevalence of sexual, physical and emotional abuse in the Norwegian mother and child cohort study. BMC Public Health. 2013;13. doi:10.1186/1471-2458-1113-1186.
14. Robertson-Blackmore E, Putnam F, Rubinow D, Matthieu M, Hunn J, Putnam K, et al. Antecedent trauma exposure and risk of depression in the perinatal period. J Clin Psychiatry. 2013;74(10):942–8.

15. Lukasse M, Vangen S, Øian P, Kumle M, Ryding E, Schei B. Childhood abuse and fear of childbirth - a population-based study. Birth. 2010;37(4):267–74.

16. Cammack A, Buss C, Entringer S, Hogue C, Hobel C, Wadhwa P. The association between early life adversity and bacterial vaginosis during pregnancy. Am J Obstet Gynecol. 2011;204(5):431.e431–8.

17. Eide J, Hovengen R, Nordhagen R. Childhood abuse and later worries about the baby's health in pregnancy. Acta Obstet Gynecol Scand. 2010;89(12):1523–31.

18. Nelson D, Lepore S. The role of stress, depression, and violence on unintended pregnancy among young urban women. J Womens Health. 2013;22(8):673–80.

19. Schei B, Lukasse M, Ryding E, Campbell J, Karro H, Kristjansdottir H, et al. A history of abuse and operative delivery - results from a European multi-country cohort study. PLoS One. 2014;9(1):e87579.

20. Dunkle KL, Jewkes RK, Brown HC, Yoshihama M, Gray GE, McIntyre JA, et al. Prevalence and patterns of gender-based violence and revictimization among women attending antenatal clinics in Soweto, South Africa. Am J Epidemiol. 2004;160(3):230–9.

21. Hutchinson GA, Jameson EM. Prevalence and risk factors for HIV infection in pregnant women in north Trinidad. West Indian Med J. 2006;55(5):346–50.

22. Audi CA, Segall-Correa AM, Santiago SM, Andrade Mda G, Perez-Escamila R. Violence against pregnant women: prevalence and associated factors. Rev Saude Publica. 2008;42(5):877–85.

23. Dinwiddie S, Heath A, Dunne M, Bucholz K, Madden P, Slutske W, et al. Early sexual abuse and lifetime psychopathology: a co-twin-control study. Psychol Med. 2000;30(1):41–52.

24. Kendler K, Bulik C, Silberg J, Hettema J, Myers J, Prescott C. Childhood sexual abuse and adult psychiatric and substance use disorders in women: an epidemiological and cotwin control analysis. Arch Gen Psychiat. 2000;57(10):953–9.

25. Chartier M, Walker J, Naimark B. Health risk behaviors and mental health problems as mediators of the relationship between childhood abuse and adult health. Am J Public Health. 2009;99(5):847–54.

26. Easton SD, Renner LM, O'Leary P. Suicide attempts among men with histories of child sexual abuse: examining abuse severity, mental health, and masculine norms. Child Abuse Negl. 2013;37(6):380–7.

27. Henrichs KL, McCauley HL, Miller E, Styne DM, Saito N, Breslau J. Early menarche and childhood adversities in a nationally representative sample. Int J Pediatr Endocrinol. 2014, 2014;(1). doi:10.1186/1687-9856-2014-1114.

28. Boynton-Jarrett R, Wright RJ, Putnam FW, Lividoti Hibert E, Michels KB, Forman MR, et al. Childhood abuse and age at menarche. J Adolesc Health. 2013;52(2):241–7.

29. Noll JG, Shenk CE, Putnam KT. Childhood sexual abuse and adolescent pregnancy: a meta-analytic update. J Pediatr Psychol. 2009;34(4):366–78.

30. Leeners B, Rath W, Block E, Gorres G, Tschudin S. Risk factors for unfavorable pregnancy outcome in women with adverse childhood experiences. J Perinat Med. 2014;42(2):171–8.

31. Seng JS, Sperlich M, Low LK. Mental health, demographic, and risk behavior profiles of pregnant survivors of childhood and adult abuse. J Midwifery Womens Health. 2008;53(6):511–21.

32. Grimstad H, Schei B. Pregnancy and delivery for women with a history of child sexual abuse. Child Abuse Negl. 1999;23(1):81–90.

33. McCormick M, Litt J, Smith V, Zupancic J. Prematurity: an overview and public health implications. Annu Rev Public Health. 2011;32(1):367–79.

34. March of Dimes, PMNCH, Save the Children, WHO. Born too soon : the global action report on preterm birth. In: Howson CP, Kinney MV, Lawn JE, editors. Geneva: 2012:1–126. available at: http://www.who.int/pmnch/media/news/2012/introduction.pdf, accessed on 08/11/2015.

35. Baba S, Wikstrom AK, Stephansson O, Cnattingius S. Influence of smoking and snuff cessation on risk of preterm birth. Eur J Epidemiol. 2012;27(4):297–304.

36. Schaaf JM, Hof MH, Mol BW, Abu-Hanna A, Ravelli AC. Recurrence risk of preterm birth in subsequent twin pregnancy after preterm singleton delivery. BJOG. 2012;119(13):1624–9.

37. Noble A, Ning Y, Woelk GB, Mahomed K, Williams MA. Preterm delivery risk in relation to maternal HIV infection, history of malaria and other infections among urban Zimbabwean women. Cent Afr J Med. 2005;51(5–6):53–8.

38. Bilano VL, Ota E, Ganchimeg T, Mori R, Souza JP. Risk factors of pre-eclampsia/eclampsia and its adverse outcomes in low- and middle-income countries: a WHO secondary analysis. PLoS One. 2014;9(3):e91198.

39. Cnattingius S, Villamor E, Johansson S, Edstedt Bonamy AK, Persson M, Wikstrom AK, et al. Maternal obesity and risk of preterm delivery. JAMA. 2013;309(22):2362–70.

40. Yonkers K, Smith MV, Forray A, Epperson CN, Costello D, Lin H, et al. Pregnant women with posttraumatic stress disorder and risk of preterm birth. JAMA Psychiatry. 2014;71(8):897–904.

41. Sanchez SE, Puente GC, Atencio G, Qiu C, Yanez D, Gelaye B, et al. Risk of spontaneous preterm birth in relation to maternal depressive, anxiety, and stress symptoms. J Reprod Med. 2013;58(1–2):25–33.

42. Calderon-Margalit R, Qiu C, Ornoy A, Siscovick DS, Williams MA. Risk of preterm delivery and other adverse perinatal outcomes in relation to maternal use of psychotropic medications during pregnancy. Am J Obstet Gynecol. 2009;201(6):579 e571–578.

43. Sanchez SE, Alva AV, Diez Chang G, Qiu C, Yanez D, Gelaye B, et al. Risk of spontaneous preterm birth in relation to maternal exposure to intimate partner violence during pregnancy in Peru. Matern Child Health J. 2013;17(3):485–92.

44. Martin J, Hamilton B, Osterman M, Curtin S, Mathews T. Births: Final Data for 2012. Vol. 62. Hyattsville: Department of Health and Human Services, Centers for Disease Control and Prevention, National Center for Health Statistics, National Vital Statistics System; 2013. p. 1–87.

45. Institute of Medicine (IOM). Preterm Birth: Causes, Consequences, and Prevention. In: National Research Council (NRC), editor. National Academies Press: Washington DC; 2007.

46. Fawke J, Lum S, Kirkby J, Hennessy E, Marlow N, Rowell V, et al. Lung function and respiratory symptoms at 11 years in children born extremely preterm: the EPICure study. Am J Respir Crit Care Med. 2010;182(2):237–45.

47. Kajantie E, Osmond C, Barker DJ, Eriksson JG. Preterm birth—a risk factor for type 2 diabetes? The Helsinki birth cohort study. Diabetes Care. 2010;33(12):2623–5.

48. Smith GD, Sterne J, Tynelius P, Lawlor DA, Rasmussen F. Birth weight of offspring and subsequent cardiovascular mortality of the parents. Epidemiology (Cambridge, Mass). 2005;16(4):563–9.

49. Robbins CL, Hutchings Y, Dietz PM, Kuklina EV, Callaghan WM. History of preterm birth and subsequent cardiovascular disease: a systematic review. Am J Obstet Gynecol. 2013;210(4):285–97.

50. Catov JM, Wu CS, Olsen J, Sutton-Tyrrell K, Li J, Nohr EA. Early or recurrent preterm birth and maternal cardiovascular disease risk. Ann Epidemiol. 2010;20(8):604–9.

51. Horan D, Hill L, Schulkin J. Childhood sexual abuse and preterm labor in adulthood: an endocrinological hypothesis. Womens Health Issues. 2000;10(1):27–33.

52. Stevens-Simon C, McAnarney E. Childhood victimization: relationship to adolescent pregnancy outcome. Child Abuse Negl. 1994;18(7):569–75.

53. Noll J, Schulkin J, Penelope T, Susman E, Breech L, Putnam F. Differential pathways to preterm delivery for sexually abused and comparison women. J Pediatr Psychol. 2007;32(10):1238–48.

54. Leeners B, Stiller R, Block E, Görres G, Rath W. Pregnancy complications in women with childhood sexual abuse experiences. J Psychosom Res. 2010;69(5):503–10.

55. Benedict M, Paine L, Paine L, Brandt D, Stallings R. The association of childhood sexual abuse with depressive symptoms during pregnancy, and selected pregnancy outcomes. Child Abuse Negl. 1999;23(7):659–70.

56. Jacobs J. Child sexual abuse victimization and later sequelae during pregnancy and childbirth. J Child Sex Abuse. 1992;1(1):111–21.

57. O'Connor T, O'Halloran D, Shanahan F. The stress response and the hypothalamic-pituitary-adrenal axis: from molecule to melancholia. QJM. 2000;93(6):323–33.

58. Mastorakos G, Ilias I. Maternal and fetal hypothalamic-pituitary-adrenal axes during pregnancy and postpartum. Ann N Y Acad Sci. 2003;997:136–49.

59. Wintour E, Bell R, Carson R, MacIsaac R, Tregear G, Vale W, et al. Effect of long-term infusion of ovine corticotrophin-releasing factor in the immature ovine fetus. J Endocrinol. 1986;111(3):469–75.

60. Chan E, Falconer J, Madsen G, Rice K, Webster E, Chrousos G, et al. A corticotropin-releasing hormone type I receptor antagonist delays parturition in sheep. Endocrinology. 1998;139(7):3357–60.

61. Korebrits C, Ramirez M, Watson L, Brinkman E, Bocking A, Challis J.

Maternal corticotropin-releasing hormone is increased with impending preterm birth. J Clin Endocrinol Metab. 1998;83(5):1585–91.

62. Stamatelou F, Deligeoroglou E, Farmakides G, Creatsas G. Abnormal progesterone and corticotropin releasing hormone levels are associated with preterm labour. Ann Acad Med Singapore. 2009;38(11):1011–6.

63. Wadhwa P, Garite T, Porto M, Glynn L, Chicz-DeMet A, Dunkel-Schetter C, et al. Placental corticotropin-releasing hormone (CRH), spontaneous preterm birth, and fetal growth restriction: a prospective investigation. Am J Obstet Gynecol. 2004;191(4):1063–9.

64. McLean M, Smith R. Corticotropin-releasing hormone in human pregnancy and parturition. Trends Endocrin Met. 1999;10(5):174–8.

65. Grimstad H, Backe B, Jacobsen G, Schei B. Abuse history and health risk behaviors in pregnancy. Acta Obstet Gynecol Scand. 1998;77(9):893–7.

Permissions

All chapters in this book were first published in P&C, by BioMed Central; hereby published with permission under the Creative Commons Attribution License or equivalent. Every chapter published in this book has been scrutinized by our experts. Their significance has been extensively debated. The topics covered herein carry significant findings which will fuel the growth of the discipline. They may even be implemented as practical applications or may be referred to as a beginning point for another development.

The contributors of this book come from diverse backgrounds, making this book a truly international effort. This book will bring forth new frontiers with its revolutionizing research information and detailed analysis of the nascent developments around the world.

We would like to thank all the contributing authors for lending their expertise to make the book truly unique. They have played a crucial role in the development of this book. Without their invaluable contributions this book wouldn't have been possible. They have made vital efforts to compile up to date information on the varied aspects of this subject to make this book a valuable addition to the collection of many professionals and students.

This book was conceptualized with the vision of imparting up-to-date information and advanced data in this field. To ensure the same, a matchless editorial board was set up. Every individual on the board went through rigorous rounds of assessment to prove their worth. After which they invested a large part of their time researching and compiling the most relevant data for our readers.

The editorial board has been involved in producing this book since its inception. They have spent rigorous hours researching and exploring the diverse topics which have resulted in the successful publishing of this book. They have passed on their knowledge of decades through this book. To expedite this challenging task, the publisher supported the team at every step. A small team of assistant editors was also appointed to further simplify the editing procedure and attain best results for the readers.

Apart from the editorial board, the designing team has also invested a significant amount of their time in understanding the subject and creating the most relevant covers. They scrutinized every image to scout for the most suitable representation of the subject and create an appropriate cover for the book.

The publishing team has been an ardent support to the editorial, designing and production team. Their endless efforts to recruit the best for this project, has resulted in the accomplishment of this book. They are a veteran in the field of academics and their pool of knowledge is as vast as their experience in printing. Their expertise and guidance has proved useful at every step. Their uncompromising quality standards have made this book an exceptional effort. Their encouragement from time to time has been an inspiration for everyone.

The publisher and the editorial board hope that this book will prove to be a valuable piece of knowledge for researchers, students, practitioners and scholars across the globe.

List of Contributors

Grace Liu
Antenatal Corticosteroids Working Group of the UN Commodities Commission, Cambridge, MA, USA

Joel Segrè
Antenatal Corticosteroids Working Group of the UN Commodities Commission, Oakland, CA, USA

A Metin Gülmezoglu
UNDP/UNFPA/UNICEF/WHO/World Bank Special Programme of Research, Development and Research Training in Human Reproduction (HRP), Department of Reproductive Health and Research, World Health Organization, 20 Avenue Appia, 1211 Geneva 27, Switzerland

Matthews Mathai
Department of Maternal, Newborn, Child & Adolescent Health, World Health Organization, 20 Avenue Appia, 1211 Geneva 27, Switzerland

Jeffrey M Smith
Jhpiego, 1615 Thames St., Baltimore, MD, 21231, USA

Jorge Hermida
University Research Co., LLC, 7200 Wisconsin Avenue, Suite 600, Bethesda, MD 20814, USA

Aline Simen-Kapeu and Kim E Dickson
Health Section, Programme Division, UNICEF Headquarters, 3 United Nations Plaza, New York, NY 10017, USA

Pierre Barker
Institute for Healthcare Improvement, 20 University Road, Cambridge, MA 02138, USA
Gillings School of Global Public Health, University of North Carolina at Chapel Hill, 135 Dauer Drive, Chapel Hill, NC 27599, USA

Mercy Jere and Edward Moses
MaiKhanda Trust, House number 14/56 Off Presidential Drive - Area 14, 265 Lilongwe, Malawi

Sarah G Moxon and Joy E Lawn
Maternal, Adolescent, Reproductive and Child Health (MARCH) Centre, London School of Hygiene and Tropical Medicine, London, WC1E 7HT, UK
Saving Newborn Lives, Save the Children, 2000 L Street NW, Suite 500, Washington, DC 20036, USA
Department of Infectious Disease Epidemiology, London School of Hygiene and Tropical Medicine, London, WC1E 7HT, UK

Fernando Althabe
Institute for Clinical Effectiveness and Health Policy (IECS), Dr. Emilio Ravignani 2024, Buenos Aires, C1414CPV, Argentina

Haiqing Xu, Qiong Dai, Yusong Xu, Zhengtao Gong, Guohong Dai and Zubin Hu
Department of Child Health Care, Hubei Maternal and Child Health Hospital, Wuhan, China

Ming Ding and Frank B. Hu
Department of Nutrition, Harvard School of Public Health, 655 Huntington Ave, Boston, MA 02115, USA

Christopher Duggan
Department of Nutrition, Harvard School of Public Health, 655 Huntington Ave, Boston, MA 02115, USA
Boston Children's Hospita, Boston, Massachusetts, USA

Laura Aoife Linehan, Jennifer Walsh, Aoife Morris, Keelin O'Donoghue and Noirin Russell
The Department of Obstetrics and Gynaecology, University College Cork and Cork University Hospital, Cork, Ireland

Louise Kenny
The Department of Obstetrics and Gynaecology, University College Cork and Cork University Hospital, Cork, Ireland
The Irish Centre for Fetal and Neonatal Translational Research, Cork, Ireland

Eugene Dempsey
The Department of Paediatrics and Child Health, University College Cork, Cork, Ireland

Honorati Masanja
Ifakara Health Institute, Kiko Avenue, Mikocheni, Dar es Salaam, Tanzania

Salum Mshamu and Mohamed Bakari
Africa Academy for Public Health, CM Plaza Building, Mwai Kibaki Road, Mikocheni, Dar es Salaam, Tanzania

Alfa Muhihi
Ifakara Health Institute, Kiko Avenue, Mikocheni, Dar es Salaam, Tanzania
Africa Academy for Public Health, CM Plaza Building, Mwai Kibaki Road, Mikocheni, Dar es Salaam, Tanzania

Christopher R. Sudfeld and Emily R. Smith
Department of Global Health and Population, Harvard T. H. Chan School of Public Health, Boston, USA

Ramadhani A. Noor
Africa Academy for Public Health, CM Plaza Building, Mwai Kibaki Road, Mikocheni, Dar es Salaam, Tanzania
Department of Global Health and Population, Harvard T. H. Chan School of Public Health, Boston, USA

Christina Briegleb
Department of Nutrition, Harvard T. H. Chan School of Public Health, Boston, USA

Wafaie Fawzi
Department of Global Health and Population, Harvard T. H. Chan School of Public Health, Boston, USA
Department of Nutrition, Harvard T. H. Chan School of Public Health, Boston, USA
Department of Epidemiology, Harvard T. H. Chan School of Public Health, Boston, USA

Grace Jean-Yee Chan
Department of Global Health and Population, Harvard T. H. Chan School of Public Health, Boston, USA
Department of Medicine, Boston Children's Hospital, Boston, USA

Margarete Erika Vollrath
Domain of Mental and Physical Health, Norwegian Institute of Public Health, Oslo, Norway
Psychological Institute, University of Oslo, Oslo, Norway

Verena Sengpiel
Department of Obstetrics and Gynecology, Sahlgrenska University Hospital, Gothenburg, Sweden

Markus A. Landolt
University Children's Hospital Zurich, Zurich, Switzerland
Department of Child and Adolescent Health Psychology, Institute of Psychology, University of Zurich, Zurich, Switzerland

Bo Jacobsson
Department of Obstetrics and Gynaecology, Sahlgrenska Academy, Gothenburg University, Gothenburg, Sweden
Department of Genes and Environment, Norwegian Institute of Public Health, Oslo, Norway

Beatrice Latal
Child Development Center, University Children's Hospital Zurich, Zurich, Switzerland

Anne Lise Brantsæter, Margareta Haugen, Helle Katrine Knutsen and Helle Margrete Meltzer
Department of Environmental Exposure and Epidemiology, Domain of Infection Control and Environmental Health, Norwegian Institute of Public Health, Nydalen, NO-0403 Oslo, Norway

Linda Englund-Ögge and Verena Sengpiel
Department of Obstetrics and Gynecology, Sahlgrenska University Hospital, Gothenburg, Sweden

Bryndis Eva Birgisdottir
Unit for Nutrition Research, Landspitali University Hospital and University of Iceland, Reykjavik, Iceland

Ronny Myhre
Department of Genetics and Bioinformatics, Domain of Health Data and Digitalisation, Norwegian Institute of Public Health, Oslo, Norway

Jan Alexander
Office of the Director-General, Norwegian Institute of Public Health, Oslo, Norway

Roy M. Nilsen
Department of Health and Social Sciences, Bergen University College, Bergen, Norway

Bo Jacobsson
Department of Genetics and Bioinformatics, Domain of Health Data and Digitalisation, Norwegian Institute of Public Health, Oslo, Norway
Department of Obstetrics and Gynecology, Sahlgrenska Academy, Gothenburg University, Gothenburg, Sweden

Reem Malouf and Maggie Redshaw
Policy Research Unit in Maternal Health and Care, National Perinatal Epidemiology Unit, Nuffield Department of Population Health, University of Oxford, Old Road Campus, Headington, Oxford OX3 7LF, UK

Alex Y Wang and Elizabeth A. Sullivan
Faculty of Health, University of Technology Sydney, Broadway, NSW 2007, Australia

Abrar A. Chughtai
School of Public Health and Community Medicine, University of New South Wales, Sydney, NSW 2031, Australia

Kei Lui
School of Women's and Children's Health, University of New South Wales, Sydney, NSW 2031, Australia

Veronica Samedi and Essa Al Awad
Department of Pediatrics, Section of Neonatology, Cumming School of Medicine, University of Calgary, Calgary, AB, Canada

Stephen K. Field
Department of Medicine, Section of Respiratory Medicine, Cumming School of Medicine, University of Calgary, Calgary, AB, Canada

Gregory Ratcliffe
Department of Radiology, Section of Neuroradiology, Cumming School of Medicine, University of Calgary, Calgary, AB, Canada

Kamran Yusuf
Department of Pediatrics, Section of Neonatology, Cumming School of Medicine, University of Calgary, Calgary, AB, Canada
Department of Radiology, Section of Neuroradiology, Cumming School of Medicine, University of Calgary, Calgary, AB, Canada
Rm 273, Heritage Medical Research Building 3330 Hospital Drive NW, Calgary, AB T2N 4N1, Canada

Shi Chen, Huijuan Zhu, Hongbo Yang, Fengying Gong, Linjie Wang and Hui Pan
Department of Endocrinology, Key Laboratory of Endocrinology of Ministry of Health, Chinese Academy of Medical Sciences & Peking Union Medical College, Peking Union Medical College Hospital, No.1, Shuaifuyuan Road, Beijing, Dongcheng district 100730, China

Rong Zhu
Intern of medicine, PUMCH, Beijing 100730, China
Department of Gynaecology and Obsterics, Peking University First Hospital, Beijing 100034, China

Yu Jiang
School of public health, PUMC, Beijing 100730, China

Bill Q. Lian
University of Massachusetts Medical Center, 55 Lake Ave., North Worcester, MA 01655, USA

Chengsheng Yan
Hebei Center for women and children's health, Shijiazhuang 050031, China

Jianqiang Li
School of Software Engineering, Beijing University of Technology, Beijing 100124, China

Qing Wang
Tsinghua National Laboratory for Info. Science and Technology, Tsinghua University, Beijing 100084, China

Shi-kun Zhang
Research association for women and children's health, Beijing 100081, China

Laura Fernandes Martin, Natália Prearo Moço, Hélio Amante Miot, Camila Renata Corrêa and Márcia Guimarães da Silva
Department of Pathology, Botucatu Medical School, São Paulo State University (UNESP), Distrito de Rubião Júnior, Botucatu, São Paulo CEP 18618-686, Brazil

Moisés Diôgo de Lima
Department of Gynecology and Obstetrics, Federal University of Paraíba, UFPB, João Pessoa, Brazil

Jossimara Polettini
The University of Western São Paulo, UNOESTE, Presidente Prudente, Brazil

Ramkumar Menon
Department of Obstetrics & Gynecology, The University of Texas Medical Branch at Galveston, Galveston, TX, USA

Catherine Dagenais
Department of Obstetrics & Gynecology, McMaster University, 1280 Main St W, HSC 3N52B, Hamilton, ON L8S 4K1, Canada

Anne-Mary Lewis-Mikhael and Marinela Grabovac
Department of Health Research Methods, Evidence, and Impact, McMaster University, 1280 Main St W, Hamilton, ON L8S 4K1, Canada

Amit Mukerji
Department of Pediatrics, McMaster University, 1280 Main St W, Hamilton, ON L8S 4K1, Canada

Sarah D. McDonald
Department of Obstetrics & Gynecology, McMaster University, 1280 Main St W, HSC 3N52B, Hamilton, ON L8S 4K1, Canada
Department of Health Research Methods, Evidence, and Impact, McMaster University, 1280 Main St W, Hamilton, ON L8S 4K1, Canada

Paola Algeri, Francesca Pelizzoni, Francesca Russo, Maddalena Incerti, Sabrina Cozzolino, Salvatore Andrea Mastrolia and Patrizia Vergani
Department of Obstetrics and Gynecology, University of Milano-Bicocca, S. Gerardo Hospital, MBBM Foundation, Via Pergolesi 33, Monza, 20900 Monza, Monza e Brianza, Italy

Davide Paolo Bernasconi
Department of Health Sciences, Center of Biostatistic for Clinical Epidemiology, University of Milan-Bicocca, Via Pergolesi 33, Monza, 20900 Monza, Monza e Brianza, Italy

Peter Wagura, Aggrey Wasunna, Ahmed Laving and Dalton Wamalwa
Department of Paediatrics and Child Health, College of Health Sciences, University of Nairobi, Nairobi, Kenya

Paul Ng'ang'a
Division of Neglected Tropical Diseases, Ministry of Health, Nairobi, Kenya

Geum Joon Cho, Yung-Taek Ouh, Ki Hoon Ahn, Soon-Cheol Hong, Min-Jeong Oh and Hai-Joong Kim
Department of Obstetrics and Gynecology, Korea University College of Medicine, Seoul, Republic of Korea

Log Young Kim and Tae-Seon Lee
The Health Insurance Review and Assessment Service of Korea, Seoul, South Korea

Geun U. Park
Department of applied statistics, Chung-Ang University, Seoul, South Korea

Naomi Mitsuda, Masamitsu Eitoku, Kahoko Yasumitsu-Lovell and Narufumi Suganuma
Department of Environmental Medicine, Kochi Medical School, Kochi University, Kohasu, Oko-cho, Nankoku, Kochi 783-8505, Japan

Keiko Yamasaki
Integrated Center for Advanced Medical Technologies, Kochi Medical School, Kochi University, Kochi, Japan

Masahiko Sakaguchi
Integrated Center for Advanced Medical Technologies, Kochi Medical School, Kochi University, Kochi, Japan
Cancer Prevention and Control Division, Kanagawa Cancer Center Research Institute, Kanagawa, Japan

Nagamasa Maeda
Department of Obstetrics and Gynecology, Kochi Medical School, Kochi University, Kochi, Japan

Mikiya Fujieda
Department of Pediatrics, Kochi Medical School, Kochi University, Kochi, Japan

Zuoqi Peng, Ya Zhang, Ying Yang, Yuan He and Jihong Xu
National Research Institute for Family Planning, No. 12, Dahuisi Road, Haidian District, Beijing 100081, China

Yuanyuan Wang, Zongfu Cao, Xiaona Xin and Xu Ma
National Research Institute for Family Planning, No. 12, Dahuisi Road, Haidian District, Beijing 100081, China
Graduate School of Peking Union Medical College, No. 9, Dongdansantiao, Dongcheng District, Beijing 100730, China

Xiaoli Sun, Xiping Luo and Chunmei Zhao
Gynecology Department, Guangdong Women and Children Hospital, No. 521, Xingnan Road, Panyu District, Guangzhou 511442, China

Rachel Wai Chung Ng
Sydney South West Clinical School, Faculty of Medicine, University of New South Wales, Sydney, Australia

Chi Eung Danforn Lim
Sydney South West Clinical School, Faculty of Medicine, University of New South Wales, Sydney, Australia
Faculty of Science, University of Technology Sydney, Ultimo, Australia

Bo Zhang
Department of Preventive Medicine, School of Public Health, Sun Yat-sen University, Guangzhou 510080, China

Tao Liu
Guangdong Provincial Institute of Public Health, Guangdong Provincial Center for Disease Control and Prevention, No. 160, Qunxian Road, Panyu District, Guangzhou 511430, China
Environment and Health, Guangdong Provincial Key Medical Discipline of Twelfth Five-Year Plan, Guangzhou 511430, China

Yan Zhong, Fufan Zhu and Yiling Ding
The Second Xiangya Hospital, Central South University, No.139, Middle Renmin Road, Changsha, Hunan 410011, P.R. China

R. Wuntakal
Whipps Cross University Hospital, Barts Health NHS Trust, London, England, UK
Guys and St Thomas' Hospital, London, England, UK

Alejandra Castanon, R. Landy and P. Sasieni
Centre for Cancer Prevention, Wolfson Institute of Preventive Medicine, Charterhouse Square, London, England EC1M 6BQ, UK

Adaeze C. Wosu, Bizu Gelaye and Michelle A. Williams
Department of Epidemiology, Harvard T.H. Chan School of Public Health, 677 Huntington Ave, K505F, Boston, MA 02115, USA

Index

A

Abortion, 50, 81, 145, 147-148, 150, 153, 158

Adverse Pregnancy Outcome, 102, 111, 160, 171, 180-181

Antenatal Corticosteroids, 1-7, 9, 11-16, 28, 118

Antepartum Hemorrhage, 132-133, 138

Antioxidant Capacity, 105-110

Artificial Insemination, 83-84, 91

Assisted Reproductive Technology, 17-19, 21-25, 83-84, 91-92, 94, 126

B

Birthweight, 25, 34-35, 43, 63-65, 82, 84, 89, 91-92, 94, 104, 118, 123-124, 129, 133, 138-139, 159, 171

Breech Presentation, 113

C

Caesarean Section, 2, 4, 113-123, 134, 137-138

Cephalic/non-cephalic Twin Pairs, 113-114, 117, 119-120, 122

Cerclage, 67, 75, 78-79, 82, 140-143

Cervical Conization, 140-143

Cervical Incompetence, 140, 142

Cervical Transformation Zone, 182, 186-187

Cervical Treatment, 182

Chorionic Gonadotrophin, 145, 150, 176, 178-180

Congenital Tuberculosis, 93, 96

Curettage, 140

E

Early Pregnancy, 18, 50, 64, 102, 150, 158-159, 167, 180

Embryo, 84, 89-92, 102-104, 150, 152, 157

Enzymatic Antioxidants, 105

Extremely Low Birth Weight, 113, 121

Extremely Preterm, 15, 31, 78, 93, 113, 117-123, 145-149, 194, 196

F

Finnstrom Score, 132-134, 136

First Trimester, 14, 28, 37, 39, 126, 145-146, 151, 153-157, 165, 167-168, 171-172, 174, 177-181

Folic Acid Supplement, 99, 151, 155-156

Folic Acid Supplementation, 40, 97, 102, 104, 151, 158-159

Food Frequency Questionnaire, 51, 63-64

G

Gestational Age, 1-2, 8-10, 14, 24, 27, 29-30, 33, 37-38, 41, 43, 47, 67, 69, 76, 82-88, 92, 94, 98, 101, 104, 108, 114, 116-124, 126, 134, 136, 138-139, 142, 146, 152, 158, 175, 178, 180, 191, 194

H

Head Circumference, 28, 64, 123

High Risk Pregnancy, 66, 68, 75, 82, 183

Histologic Chorioamnionitis, 105-106, 108-110, 112

Hyper-ovulation, 83-84

I

In Vitro Fertilization (IVF), 91-92, 94

Infant Mortality, 17-18, 21, 24, 43, 91, 114, 124, 140, 143

Intrauterine Fetal Growth Restriction (IUGR), 34

L

Large for Gestational Age, 104, 126, 130

Last Menstrual Period, 14, 18, 34, 40, 54, 99, 103, 106, 126, 146, 153

M

Maternal Body Mass Index, 64, 151, 159

Maternal Diet, 62

Maternal Pm2.5 Exposure, 160-161, 163, 165, 170

Maternal Preconception, 99, 151, 153, 194

Maternal Trait Anxiety, 45, 49

Maternal Weight Gain, 125-126, 128, 130

Mental Health, 45, 50, 79-80, 196

Midtrimester Pprom, 26-29

N

Nausea and Vomiting During Pregnancy, 145, 149-150

Neonatal Intensive Care Units (NICU), 84

Neonatal Morbidity, 15, 31, 45, 51, 90, 123-124

Neonatal Mortality, 2, 4-5, 11-12, 14-15, 18, 25-26, 34, 79, 82-83, 92, 101, 123-124, 132, 158, 189-190

Non-enzymatic Antioxidants, 105

O

Oral Contraceptive, 97, 99, 101-102

Oxidative Stress, 105-106, 108, 110-112, 165

P

Perinatal Morbidity, 66-67, 92, 123

Placenta, 26, 28, 30, 68, 81, 93-96, 102, 106, 110-112, 115, 149, 167, 180-181, 194

Preconception, 83, 90, 98-99, 103-104, 151-158, 194

Premature Birth, 17-18, 24, 138, 161, 171, 180

Prematurity, 2, 17-18, 21-22, 24, 31, 67-68, 78, 82, 84, 89, 92, 96, 102, 114, 116, 123-124, 127, 129-130, 134, 158, 161, 190, 196

Preterm Birth, 1-2, 4-28, 33-34, 43-44, 49-50, 62, 64-69, 75-76, 78-86, 89-92, 97, 102, 104-106, 109-111, 123, 129, 132-150, 152, 156-163, 165, 167-171, 173, 181-191, 193-197

Preterm Delivery, 21, 25, 45-46, 49-55, 57-64, 78, 82, 97, 104-105, 125-126, 128-130, 132-135, 137-138, 140-143, 151-152, 155-156, 158-159, 161, 170-174, 176-180, 186-189, 196

Preterm Labor, 16, 23, 82, 93, 108-109, 111-112, 125, 133, 138, 140, 152, 158, 188, 196

Preterm Neonate, 93

Preterm Premature Rupture of Membranes (PPROM), 26-27, 105-106

Preterm-aga, 33-40

Preterm-sga, 33-40

Protein Oxidative Damage, 105, 108, 110

Provider-initiated Deliveries, 45-49

R

Random-effects Model, 160, 163, 170

Risk Factors, 17-18, 20, 25, 33-35, 37, 39-40, 43-45, 79, 97-101, 104-105, 108, 123, 133-134, 139, 142-143, 149, 153, 155-156, 158-159, 170, 187, 190, 194-196

Risks of Preterm, 20, 39, 101, 158, 182, 185-186

S

Seafood Consumption, 51-53, 62-65

Sepsis, 26-31, 118, 127, 129-130

Serum Screening, 172, 177, 179-180

Severe Brain Injury, 113, 115, 117-120, 122

Singleton Pregnancies, 67, 125-126, 158, 173

Small for Gestational Age, 33, 35, 37-38, 41, 43, 83-84, 87, 91, 97-98, 103-104, 126, 129-130, 172-175, 177-178, 180-181

T

Term-sga, 33-40

Tuberculosis, 93-96

Twin Pregnancy, 123, 125-126, 130, 134, 196

V

Vaginal Delivery, 94, 113-116, 118-119, 121-123, 128, 141

Very Preterm Birth, 68, 78, 83, 90, 145, 147-149, 182

Very Preterm Singletons, 83-90

W

Weight Gain, 40, 44, 50, 125-131, 139, 158

www.ingramcontent.com/pod-product-compliance
Lightning Source LLC
Chambersburg PA
CBHW082026190326
41458CB00010B/3291